WESLEY O. YOUNG, D.M.D., M.P.H.

Professor and Chairman of the Department of Community Dentistry, College of Dentistry, University of Kentucky, Lexington.

DAVID F. STRIFFLER, D.D.S., M.P.H.

Professor of Public Health Dentistry, School of Public Health, and Professor of Dentistry (Community Dentistry), School of Dentistry, The University of Michigan, Ann Arbor.

In Collaboration With
A. L. RUSSELL, D.D.S., M.P.H.

Professor of Dental Public Health, School of Public Health, and Professor of Dentistry (Community Dentistry), School of Dentistry, The University of Michigan, Ann Arbor. (Formerly Chief, Epidemiology and Biometry Branch, National Institute of Dental Research, National Institutes of Health, Public Health Service, Bethesda, Maryland).

This text is the successor to, and contains material from, the second edition of *Dentistry in Public Health*, edited by Walter J. Pelton and Jacob M. Wisan.

THE DENTIST, HIS PRACTICE, AND HIS COMMUNITY

SECOND EDITION

W. B. SAUNDERS COMPANY
Philadelphia   London   Toronto

W. B. Saunders Company: West Washington Square
Philadelphia, Pa. 19105

12 Dyott Street
London, WC1A 1DB

833 Oxford Street
Toronto 18, Ontario

THE DENTIST, HIS PRACTICE, AND HIS COMMUNITY   ISBN 0-7216-9051-1

© 1969 by W. B. Saunders Company. Copyright 1964 by W. B. Saunders Company. Copyright under the International Copyright Union. All rights reserved. This book is protected by copyright. No part of it may be duplicated or reproduced in any manner without written permission from the publisher. Made in the United States of America. Press of W. B. Saunders Company. Library of Congress catalog card number 69-17807.

Print No.:   9   8   7   6

With respect and admiration this book is dedicated to Kenneth A. Easlick, an inspiring teacher and critic, and Walter J. Pelton, a dynamic and imaginative administrator.

Great economic and social forces flow like a tide over half-conscious people. The wise are those who foresee the coming event and seek to shape their institutions and mold the thinking of the people in accordance with the most constructive change. The unwise are those who add nothing constructive to the process, either because of ignorance on the one hand or ignorant opposition on the other.

Attributed to JOHN STUART MILL

FOREWORD TO THE FIRST EDITION

In the foreword to the second edition (1955) of the predecessor to this book, itself "completely revised and rewritten," I had the prophetic good judgment to say that "the story of dentistry in public health has many chapters as yet unwritten. If the progress in this important field of health continues, one can look with assurance in the next few years to another edition 'completely revised and rewritten.'" Progress has continued. The predicted chapters have been written. The result is the third edition of *Dentistry in Public Health* so substantially revised and enlarged in scope and so changed in orientation that it deserves, and has received, a new name, *The Dentist, His Practice, and His Community*.

The book provides the links, too long unforged, between dental public health and the practitioners and prospective practitioners of dentistry and dental hygiene; between the dentist, his practice, and his community. There is no comparable book and, because there is not, this book should claim a total audience of all of those thousands who participate in providing dental health services.

Some of the material from the first two editions, from the pens of Pelton, Wisan, Fulton, Knutson, and Russell, has been retained although in substantially revised form. The two new principal authors, Young and Striffler, have provided new material and new orientation which give currency and excitement to the role of the dentist in his community. They have given social, technical, and professional perspectives to all who treat either the patient or the community in the interests of better dental health.

The enlarged scope of the revised volume may be more fully appreciated by scanning some of the new topics which have been included: fluoridation, mass dental inspections, mouth protectors, group-purchase programs, "socialization" (appropriately placed in quotation marks), specialists, manpower, auxiliary personnel, health education, and aids to young practitioners. In addition, of course, the reader will find the bone-essential chapters on the assessment of the problems of dental diseases, the epidemiology, prevention, and control of dental diseases, dental needs, and demand.

The authors speak forthrightly on topics that currently hold forum in public and professional discussions and, not in the least part, the value of the book lies in this frank, although scholarly and scientific, approach to questions that are moot for some or many.

For example, the authors refuse to equate the word "socialized" with every minute change or proposal that appears to outrage comfort or the *status quo*; they point, instead, to constructive programs which can minimize the increasingly sturdy challenge of what they properly term "state medicine." The problems of manpower and of manpower distribution are confronted unemotionally, as they should be, and there are reasoned and reasonable sections on the increasing productivity of the dentist and on the effective utilization of auxiliary personnel. They treat fairly the problems of dental service corporations and the resulting questions of fees for services. They evaluate mass dental inspections and bring themselves to less than an unqualified approval of this traditional procedure.

The revised edition, therefore, is not a technical treatise on dental public health, as it was intended that it should not be. It is, instead, a perceptive exposition of the role of the practicing dentist in serving his patient and his community by understanding and using the full resources of his profession and of dental public health procedures. It should create new horizons for many and illumine them for others. It should prove, if proof be needed, that the totality of related knowledge must be brought to bear intelligently on improving dental health which, in turn, contributes to the totality of personal and community health, which is the dental profession's reason for working and being.

It is hoped that this edition will have such impact and stimulate such further progress that, in less time than weary authors care to contemplate, it will be high time for the fourth and "completely revised and rewritten" edition.

HAROLD HILLENBRAND, D.D.S.
Secretary, American Dental Association
Chicago, Illinois

PREFACE

The Dental Health Section of the American Public Health Association initiated the effort to produce a textbook describing the place of dentistry in public health, resulting in the publication, in 1949, of the first edition of *Dentistry in Public Health*, edited by Walter J. Pelton and the late Jacob M. Wisan. Rapid developments in dental public health practice made it necessary to revise and rewrite the second edition, published in 1955.

Advances in scientific knowledge and technical procedures in the fields of dentistry and dental public health continued. In addition, concepts of dental public health instruction most appropriate for dental and dental hygiene students underwent a transformation. The concept of a department of social (or community) dentistry to be responsible for "subjects of social import," as advocated by Philip Blackerby, Jr., and others, gained increasing acceptance. Reports of the Joint Committee on Professional Education of the Dental Health Section of the American Public Health Association and the American Association of Public Health Dentists pointed out that the dental student need not be expected to develop skills which parallel those of the dentist in public health. Instead, undergraduate instruction should emphasize those skills and concepts relevant to public health which will be of value to the dentist and dental hygienist in private practice. The 1964 edition was written to reflect this changing philosophy of instruction, a change which may be said to have shifted the emphasis, in each edition, from "dentistry in public health" to "public health aspects of dental practice and the role of the practitioner in his community." Because of this change, it seemed reasonable to adopt the current title.

The content and organization of the material covered were modified considerably in the 1964 edition. Dental survey procedures and statistical methods, treated separately previously, were included in a section on epidemiology. Information on the prevention and control of dental diseases was brought up to date and a new section on the application of preventive procedures in the dental office and in the community added. The classic chapter by Knutson, "What Is Public Health?", was reprinted from the 1955 edition of *Dentistry in Public Health* without substantive change. Selected excerpts from the 1955 edition also were used throughout the book as well as portions of those sections of *The Survey of Dentistry; The Final Report* which were prepared by the writers.

The present edition is both similar and different from its immediate predecessor. The concept of creating departments of social (or community) dentistry has gained wide acceptance, and the 1964 edition has appeared to meet the needs of these departments. Therefore, the general organization and the approach to the subject matter has stayed essentially the same. On the other hand, all of the chapters have been updated and revised. Particularly substantial changes have been made in discussing dental epidemiology, preventive dentistry, and group health care programs. Major changes are taking place, of course, in the provision of dental care in public programs — changes so rapid that they represent the "current events" of the profession rather than appropriate material for detailed treatment in a text. Chapter 12 attempts to give the historical background of public care programs and outline the basic principles involved to prepare the student to understand day-to-day events.

This text naturally reflects the background and experience of those who collaborated in its preparation. Before entering the field of dental public health, all three engaged in the private practice of dentistry. They also have served as directors of dental programs in state health departments. In addition, Striffler has directed the health program of a large urban school system; Young has headed a medical rehabilitation program in a state health department; and Russell has had extensive experience in epidemiological research.

No attempt has been made to avoid controversial issues when these issues seemed relevant to the practice of dentistry and the role of the dentist and the dental hygienist in the life of their communities. When discussing issues about which debate might be expected, the writers have attempted to be as objective as possible. It is believed that the viewpoints expressed in the book generally reflect the current consensus of the dental profession as stated by official actions of the House of Delegates of the American Dental Association.

Many individuals have assisted with this edition. Particular thanks are due Dr. Viron Diefenbach (Chief of the Division of Dental Health, Public Health Service) and members of his staff, including Miss Ruth Bothwell and Drs. Harry Bruce and Edward Campbell. The revision probably could not have been accomplished without the substantial professional assistance of Misses Joan Keevil, Ann Miller, Mr. Samuel Lam, and Mrs. Ruth Striffler at Michigan and Mrs. Jean Shannon at Kentucky.

In the Foreword to the 1964 edition Dr. Harold Hillenbrand predicted "... that, in less time than weary authors care to contemplate, it will be high time for the [next] and 'completely revised and rewritten' edition." Five years later the "weary authors" recognize that Dr. Hillenbrand was more prophetic than had been realized. This half-decade has been one of the most significant periods in the history of our profession—a period in which the rate of change will probably be exceeded only during the coming five to 10 years. The fatigue of the authors is the satisfying one that results from the rigors and excitement of analyzing developing trends as well as participating in them and teaching about them.

Lexington, Kentucky
Ann Arbor, Michigan

WESLEY O. YOUNG
DAVID F. STRIFFLER

CONTENTS

Section One Dentistry and Public Health

Chapter 1
PATIENTS, THE PUBLIC, AND DENTAL PRACTICE 3

Chapter 2
WHAT IS PUBLIC HEALTH? 8

Chapter 3
THE DENTIST AND DENTAL HYGIENIST IN PUBLIC HEALTH 17

Section Two Assessment of the Problem of Dental Disease

Chapter 4
EPIDEMIOLOGY AND THE RATIONAL BASES OF DENTAL PUBLIC HEALTH AND DENTAL PRACTICE 35
    By A. L. Russell

Chapter 5
THE INTERPRETATION OF DATA AND THE EVALUATION OF SCIENTIFIC LITERATURE 63
    By A. L. Russell

Chapter 6
THE EPIDEMIOLOGY OF DENTAL CARIES AND PERIODONTAL DISEASES 73
    By A. L. Russell

Section Three Prevention and Control of Dental Diseases

Chapter 7

MEASURES AVAILABLE FOR THE PREVENTION AND CONTROL OF DENTAL CARIES 89
   By A. L. Russell

Chapter 8

MEASURES AVAILABLE FOR THE PREVENTION AND CONTROL OF PERIODONTAL AND OTHER ORAL DISEASES 126
   By A. L. Russell

Chapter 9

THE APPLICATION OF PREVENTIVE AND CONTROL MEASURES ... 143

Section Four Meeting the Demand for Dental Care

Chapter 10

DENTAL TREATMENT NEEDS AND THE DEMAND FOR CARE 183

Chapter 11

THE PURCHASE OF DENTAL CARE 208

Chapter 12

PUBLIC DENTAL CARE PROGRAMS 236

Chapter 13

DENTAL MANPOWER RESOURCES 266

Section Five Dental Health Education

Chapter 14

DENTAL HEALTH EDUCATION 295

Section Six The Dentist, His Practice, and His Community

Chapter 15

THE ROLE OF THE DENTIST AND DENTAL HYGIENIST IN MAINTAINING THE HEALTH OF THE COMMUNITY 325

INDEX 343

Section One

DENTISTRY AND PUBLIC HEALTH

CHAPTER 1
Patients, the Public, and Dental Practice

CHAPTER 2
What Is Public Health?

CHAPTER 3
The Dentist and Dental Hygienist in Public Health

When Jim Smith, D.D.S., heard his home phone ring, he offered a silent prayer that it did not mean a dental emergency. "Jim, it's Jack (the president of the local dental society). The town council has advanced the hearing date on fluoridation, and we want you to join a group of us who will be testifying. Can we pick you up in half an hour?" In the second that it took Jim to say "yes," he had made a decision to be a truly professional person who recognizes not only his obligations to his patients but also his obligations to his community. When the president of the P.T.A. and the president of the Jaycees said "thanks" at the end of the council hearings, Jim had the feeling that he had accomplished something—something for his town—and he felt good about it.

And that is what this book is all about. The health of the public, the first concern of a health profession, can be improved through the application of the unique combination of the knowledge and skills of dental public health, community dentistry, and clinical dentistry. In applying their knowledge and skills in behalf of the community, the dentist and dental hygienist fulfill the obligation emphasized by the Principles of Ethics of the American Dental Association.*

> The dentist has the obligation of providing freely of his skills, knowledge and experience to society in those fields in which his qualifications entitle him to speak with professional competence. The dentist should be a leader in his community, especially in all efforts leading to the improvement of the dental health of the public.

---

*Principles of ethics with official advisory opinions as revised June, 1967. Am. Dent. A. J., 76:678-84, Sept. 1967.

CHAPTER 1

PATIENTS, THE PUBLIC, AND DENTAL PRACTICE

A primary purpose of a book on dental public health or community dentistry is to give dental and dental hygiene students a better understanding of the patients for whom they will assume professional responsibility. Instead of emphasizing the patient and his oral disabilities as a specific "case" requiring treatment, this text will attempt to consider the patient as a part of the community in which he lives.* Such an approach makes it possible to measure oral health status in terms of how the patient's problems are similar to those of other individuals like him, and how they differ. The available knowledge about attitudes toward dental care and the factors which influence people to follow desirable oral health practices should give some insight into patients' motivations and provide guidance in building a practice, in planning treatment for individual patients, and in assuming the responsibilities of a professional man in the community.

The practice of dentistry involves a personal relation between the dentist, the dental hygienist, the dental assistant, and the patients who elect to seek professional service from them. Within the walls of his office the dentist creates a professional world of his own. In this

---

*The word "community" has a variety of meanings. As used in this book, the term will ordinarily refer to the setting in which the dentist lives and practices his profession.

Webster's New International Dictionary, Second Edition, gives as one meaning: "A body of people having common organizations, or living in the same place under the same laws and regulations."[5] This definition would encompass not only a city, but also would apply to a state, a region, or the entire nation. For the purposes of clarity, the writers will usually restrict the use of the term to the village, county, or city (or, in a large metropolitan area, the local neighborhood) in which the dentist practices.

"Community" may sometimes be used in the broader sense of "society at large" or "people in general," as "in the interests of the community."

world, the conscientious dentist continually is confronted by the problem of dental diseases. He struggles with the young child suffering from rampant caries and seeks to secure the parental cooperation necessary to bring the caries attack under control. He faces the discouraging prospect of attempting to restore normal function for the young adult in whom loss of teeth has destroyed the integrity of the dental arches. All too frequently he must try to save teeth that have lost a major portion of their supporting structures because of long neglect of periodontal diseases.

Within the limits of his own ability and available current knowledge, the practitioner attempts to conduct a practice based on regular maintenance care and the utilization of all practical preventive procedures. He and his auxiliary personnel try to emphasize health education, to correct misconceptions about proper oral health practices, and to attack apathy about dental health.

The world that the successful practitioner creates within his office should be a creative and satisfying environment. He faces the challenge, and enjoys the satisfaction, of building a practice composed largely of congenial patients who trust his ability and judgment, who accept his professional supervision, and who can pay fees adequate to provide him with a comfortable income.

The environment in a dental office is somewhat artificial, because the patients who present themselves for treatment are not necessarily representative of the entire population. They will reflect the dentist's own age since the younger dentists tend to serve the younger segment of the population while the older men see older patients.[2, 4] In general, the patients will be better educated and have better incomes than the population at large. There will be more women than men seeking routine care. In the older age groups, more of the patients will be those with low caries attack rates, or those who consistently have received regular dental care, for the others probably will be edentulous and will seek professional service infrequently.

Consequently, the dentist's own personal experience probably will not give an accurate indication of the occurrence of dental diseases or the full extent of the unmet dental needs in the community. Because children who experience dental caries may be the children most likely to be brought to the dentist, a dentist in a fluoride area may not see, in his own office, the full benefits of fluoridation in the community. Similarly, experience in a private practice may provide only a casual glimpse of the dental problems of the indigent families in the community. Patients with special problems, such as mentally retarded or cerebral-palsied children, may never appear in the dental office.

Since the patients in his practice probably will come from the segment of the population with higher income and educational attainment, the dentist is likely to underestimate the extent of general public ignorance about dental health. It is easy to assume that his own interest and concern for proper oral health, or at least that of his best patients, is shared generally. The possibility of making this error is increased since many patients may be reluctant to discuss their attitudes toward dental care frankly with a professional person such as a dentist, who may represent "a figure of authority."

An analysis of the dental needs and the attitudes toward dental care of the entire community, therefore, provides valuable insights ordinarily not gained in private practice.

Another important objective of a book on dental public health or community dentistry is to help dental and dental hygiene students understand the forces in the American culture which determine the manner in which dentistry is practiced. An awareness of the way in which social factors influence methods of providing health care is necessary if the professional person is to exercise informed leadership in his community.

Because of their special education and competence, the members of the health professions alone have been accorded by the public the privilege of providing certain health services. In order to ensure the availability of quality dental service, the public has established and maintained dental schools and has set up legal restrictions to forbid the practice of dentistry by those who are not members of the dental profession. To a large extent, the public has permitted the organized profession to regulate itself and to govern the practice of dentistry. Because of the unique privileges granted to them, the members of the dental profession have the responsibility of providing a high type of service to their patients and of exercising leadership in the community in which they reside. As professional individuals, dentists and dental hygienists should assume these responsibilities freely and voluntarily. In addition to the moral implications, it must be recognized that the dental profession has a selfish interest in maintaining its leadership role. The provision of dental care in American society involves a two-way relation between the dentist as a provider of service and the public as the purchaser of service. The relation must continue to be satisfactory, not only to the dental profession, but also to the majority of the public, if dentistry is to continue in its privileged position.

The relation of a profession to the society it serves must be an ever changing one; as the society evolves, the profession must change and develop if it is to continue to be effective. Tremendous social changes have taken place in this country, and in the world, during the past half century. The luxuries of pioneer days have become the necessities of today. The public expectation of a minimum standard of living compatible with decency has risen constantly. Attitudes toward medical care, in particular, appear to have changed quite rapidly within the last quarter century. In recent years, there has been a growing assertion that health is a basic human right.[7] The Committee on Public Policy and the Executive Board of the American Public Health Association have proposed a policy statement which is introduced with the following sentence: "The APHA supports the principle that a good and healthful life is a basic human right that must be available to all persons and that a sufficient share of the nation's resources should be devoted to the assurance of this right."[1]

For one thing, the cost, as well as the effectiveness, of medical care has increased rapidly and, as a result, the total cost of medical care has become a public issue. Although not immediately in the forefront of controversies about the provision of physicians' services and hospital care, dentistry cannot remain aloof from any general changes that take place in methods of providing health care. Patterns established in relation to medical and hospital care may be expected to influence the future development of dental services. Such changes may revolutionize the practice of dentistry as it is known today.

If the dental profession is to maintain its integrity and continue to provide a high standard of oral health care, it is important that it be prepared to provide professional leadership during this period of rapid social change. The professional individual entering practice must, therefore, be aware of the changing social scene, recognize some of the factors that are motivating changes in public attitudes, and be knowledgeable about the approaches that can be used to bring dental care to a larger proportion of the public. General ignorance of these factors on the part of the profession well could be suicidal.

The third major objective of a book on dental public health or community dentistry is to provide the dentist and the dental hygienist with specialized skills and knowledge which will enhance the practice of dentistry. Some acquaintance with epidemiology and biostatistics, for example, is necessary if the practitioner is to interpret research findings and make a rational selection of procedures to be used in the office. Similarly, information about the factors which influence individual attitudes toward health and about the principles of health education is useful in dealing with individual patients as well as in providing professional guidance for community efforts.

The public health approach to dental problems emphasizes the problems of dental diseases as they occur in the total population. Such an emphasis underscores the deficiencies of current efforts to maintain oral health. The fact that only about 40 percent of all Americans even see a dentist once a year,[6] despite annual personal expenditures for dental care which are approaching three billion dollars with approximately 10 percent of the medical care dollar spent on dental services,[8] emphasizes the necessity for greater effort to solve the dental health problem. Members of the dental and dental hygiene professions play the most important part in improving the oral health of the public. Their most basic contribution to this end is the conduct of dental practices of the highest caliber—practices which provide modern comprehensive operative and surgical dental care, which include the use of recognized preventive procedures, and which assume a responsibility for health education.

Even if all dentists and dental hygienists maintained this type of practice, only part of the goal of complete oral health care for the entire population could be attained. First, only 15 to 20 percent of the public seeks regular dental care and is in a position, therefore, to receive full benefit from dental services.[3] Second, there are procedures which cannot be secured as easily by individuals as by organized group action. The benefits of water fluoridation, for example, will reach a majority of children only as successful group effort results in a community fluoridation program.

The purpose of a book on dental public health or community dentistry is, therefore, to prepare the practicing dentist and dental hygienist to fulfill their complete role as professional people, both in the office and in the community in which they reside. This book should help dentists and dental hygienists recognize community dental health problems and suggest sound approaches to be taken for their correction; it should help them to serve their community as sources of current and reliable information on concepts, resources, and methods related to the maintenance and improvement of oral health; it should assist them to participate effectively in the planning and promotion of dental health activities, and, when necessary, in the implementation and evaluation of such activities. As a result, the professional outlook of the practitioner should advance beyond a concern with the technical aspects of restoring teeth to a concern for the total dental health of the population and the effect of dental health on its general health and well being. Extending the sights and objectives of dental practice should make it a more satisfying and rewarding career.

BIBLIOGRAPHY

1. American Public Health Association, Committee on Public Policy and Executive Board. Health and poverty—a proposed policy statement of APHA. this is the news, n.v.: 1-3, Mar. 1968.
2. Haddon, William, Jr., Carlos, J. P., and Ast, D. B. Frequency of dental x-ray examination in a New York county. Pub. Health Rep., 77:525-32, June 1962.
3. Kegeles, S. S. Why people seek dental care: a review of present knowledge. Am. J. Pub. Health, 51:1306-11, Sept. 1961.
4. Mitchell, G. E., and Young, W. O. The 1957 survey of dental practice in Idaho, characteristics of patients and types of services. Boise, Idaho Department Health, 1959. 9 p. mimeog.
5. Neilson, W. A., ed. Webster's new international dictionary of the English language; unabridged. 2nd ed. Springfield, Mass., Merriam, c1957. CXXXVI + 3194 p. (p. 542)
6. Public Health Service, National Center for Health Statistics. Dental visits; time interval since last visit; United States—July 1963–June 1964. Washington, Government Printing Office, 1966. 54 p. (p. 1)
7. The real issue: our right to be healthy. Edit. Look, 31:54, Mar. 21, 1967.
8. U.S. Department of Commerce, Office of Business Economics. Personal consumption expenditures by type of product. Surv. Current Business, 46:20, July 1966.

CHAPTER 2

WHAT IS PUBLIC HEALTH?*

Among the many definitions of public health which have been formulated, that of Winslow is most widely accepted and quoted by public health workers. Winslow defines public health as "the science and art of preventing disease, prolonging life, and promoting physical health and efficiency through organized community efforts. . . ."[2] This definition is comprehensive and encompasses aims which are noble indeed. Undoubtedly these characteristics of the definition have had much to do with its widespread acceptance among the public health profession. It is doubtful, however, that it gives the private dental practitioner or the student of dentistry or of dental hygiene a working knowledge of public health. A clear understanding, not just a general nor vague concept, is essential if the private practitioner is to fulfill with competence his direct and indirect roles in shaping his community's public health programs.

The Private Practitioner's Role in Public Health

Perhaps the dental student's most common aim is to become a successful private practitioner, either as a "generalist" or as a specialist. Because of the personal nature of the services he will render, success ordinarily will be directly related to the number of people in the community who place confidence in his abilities. That confidence will not be limited to his technical dental services but will extend over a broad scope of day-to-day community affairs. The community affairs may include proposals to build a new schoolhouse, fluoridate the drinking water supply, expand the recreational facilities for

---

*Written for the second edition of *Dentistry in Public Health* by John W. Knutson, D.D.S., Dr. P.H., Professor of Preventive Dentistry, School of Dentistry, and Professor of Public Health, School of Public Health, University of California at Los Angeles.

children, build a community health center, construct a new water treatment plant, increase the salaries of school teachers, and a wide diversity of projects. Whatever the proposal at issue, many persons will want the advice and guidance of their family dentist. Furthermore, they will expect good advice because their dentist is a good dentist. In particular, they will expect expert advice on community proposals for health improvement. Moreover, they will not understand nor be satisfied with a disclaimer of competency to advise because a particular proposal is of a nondental nature. The patient seeking the advice is a layman. He may be chairman of the school health committee, which has been charged with the responsibility of considering the proposal and of making specific recommendations for its approval or rejection.

A prominent characteristic of successful public health administrators is the ability to stimulate broad discussion of community health problems by local civic, social, and professional groups and organizations and to encourage wide participation in designing plans and providing continuing financial support for an organized community program. An evasive reply arising from the dentist's lack of knowledge in these matters will be interpreted by the patient as indifference. It may inadvertently influence the patient to assume a similar attitude. On the other hand, response based on inaccurate information is likely to be poor advice. In either event, the dentist has materially, although indirectly, shaped the pattern of his community's action on a public health problem. Therefore, the responsiblity of being an adviser or counselor on community affairs resides in the practicing dentist whether he wills it or not.

The dentist's opportunities to exercise his responsibilities directly are also very great. The chances are excellent that he will be appointed to community health committees of civic, social, or voluntary organizations or to school, industrial, city, or county health councils. How well and how long he serves will depend on the quality of the knowledge, advice, and guidance which he brings to such councils. Furthermore, his own professional organizations, such as local or state dental societies, will have their own councils on dental health. Here, too, effective participation requires a clear concept of public health and the procedures employed in solving public health problems. Thus, the opportunities of a dentist to serve his community and his profession well will inevitably arise. Whether or not his professional life is enriched by active participation in community affairs will be determined by the manner in which these opportunities are accepted and handled.

Public Health Is People's Health

Since "public" means "of or pertaining to the people of a community, state, or nation," the simplest yet most comprehensive definition of public health might be the literal one—public health is people's health. It is concerned with the aggregate health of a group, a community, a state, or a nation. Public health, in accordance with this broad definition, is not limited to the health of poor folks, or by methods of rendering health services, or by the nature of health problems. Nor is it defined by the method of payment for health services, nor by the type of agency responsible for supplying those services. It is simply concern for and activity directed toward the improvement and protection of the health of a population group in the aggregate.

Leavell and Clark attempted to clarify the meaning of public health by pointing to the essential differences between the public health director and the private practitioner in the exercise of their professions.[1] The opposite approach will be adopted here, emphasizing the marked similarity in methods and procedures employed by the private dental practitioner and by the public health officer. The dental student receives long and intensive training to equip him to care for his patients effectively and efficiently. He is encouraged to develop a pattern of thinking and a method of approach which, when followed, are most likely to lead to desirable results. If it is recognized, then, that the same pattern of thinking and the same methods of procedure are employed in public health, the task of comprehending the meaning of public health should be greatly simplified. In the one case the individual patient is the object of concern. In the other, it is the people of a community. Although the tools employed in handling each may vary somewhat, the basic procedural pattern is virtually identical.

PERSONAL VERSUS COMMUNITY HEALTH

Examination—Survey

When a patient comes to the dental office or clinic, the first thing the dentist does is to perform a careful examination. The examination ordinarily starts with a case history, which may be obtained in many ways. The usual way is to ask the patient what his difficulty is or what problem brought him to the office for service. If the patient has a chief complaint, the time of onset, the mode of development, and the symptomatology are determined. The history also will include identifying data such as name, age, sex, address, occupation, and previous health experience. The dental examination may be simple or complex, but it usually includes examination of lips, oral mucosa, tongue, pharynx, and teeth. The examining dentist will observe the occlusion and signs of abnormal functional stresses; lost, carious, and devitalized teeth; condition of restorations; and arch relations. He may want a series of dental radiographs, a blood analysis, a urinalysis, or biopsy studies. He may examine the regional lymph nodes, and may seek information of a general medical nature which has a bearing on the patient's dental health or on his ability to undergo successful treatment. The dentist will use judgment in availing himself of the modern chemical and laboratory aids which can assist him in arriving at a correct diagnosis.

The first step in modern public health procedure is identical to that used by the dental clinician, only here it is the community which must be examined. It is called a survey instead of an examination; nevertheless, it is an examination, and the technics and purposes of the survey are the same. Furthermore, the survey or examination of the community may be initiated by a chief complaint. One of the school teachers may complain that there are no facilities for caring for the toothaches of children of indigent parents. The school health committee, after studying reports of experiences with a new preventive measure applied in a neighboring community, may raise the question, "Why aren't we doing something about it in our community?" Whatever the specific health problem, the initial approach to its solution should involve an examination to determine its dimensions and its particular characteristics. If, for example, the health problem is tuberculosis, one might obtain information first on the size of the population involved, its age and sex distribution, its occupational composition, its tuberculosis mortality rates, the number of cases diagnosed, and the frequency of hospitalization. One may augment this information by conducting a community chest radiographic examination program for screening selected groups of the population. Such a survey is designed to determine the amount of active tuberculosis in a community, and to screen out or identify cases which have not been diagnosed or recognized. The survey would include an examination of the community's resources for doing something about the problem, the hospital facilities, the physicians, the nursing care, the facilities for modern therapeutic treatment, the economic status of the community, and the nature of the distribution of the community's wealth.

The problem may be the widespread occurrence of mottled enamel, and the survey might be limited to a diagnosis of the condition and determination of the degree of mottling. The survey would include a chemical analysis of the local water supply to determine its precise fluoride content. But the purpose of the survey in either case would be to determine the nature and extent of the problem, just as was done when a patient came to his dentist with a complaint.

Diagnosis — Analysis

The examination or the survey is not an end in itself. It is an important beginning — an essential first step — which, when taken carefully, increases the likelihood that subsequent action will be correct and effective. The second step is diagnosis. An accurate diagnosis is essential if a proper course of treatment is to be prescribed. A need for additional information or supplementation in order to make a differential diagnosis may not become apparent until the data initially collected have been analyzed. This analysis also may indicate a need for the services of expert consultants or specialists.

The same methodology is used in public health. However, in public health, the diagnosis, or second step, is referred to frequently as analysis of the survey data. Information collected in the survey is analyzed in order to define the characteristics of specific community health problems. Here one is dealing with groups of people instead of with the individual and it becomes necessary in most instances to organize the data in such a way as to obtain meaningful figures. Such figures can then be used for comparisons and to help simplify the description of the situation at hand. For this purpose statistical tools may be used in order to derive such common descriptive constants as the mean, the median, the range, and the standard deviation. Rates may be calculated to determine the number of times an event occurs among the number of persons exposed to the risk of its occurrence during a given interval of time. Examples would be birth, death, and sickness rates. Ratios, or relative figures in fractional form, are used to indicate the relations of two factors to each other. These are some of the means of converting raw data, or absolute numbers collected in an examination or survey, into meaningful figures or statistics. They are the material that the public health worker uses to obtain a description of the problem and its characteristics. They are the material he uses to arrive at a correct diagnosis or analysis, just as the dental clinician uses his examination data to guide him to an accurate diagnosis.

Treatment Planning—Program Planning

Once the diagnosis has been made, one can proceed to make plans for effective treatment. The job of treatment planning may be simple or extremely complex, more frequently the latter than the former. To most persons in need of dental treatment the cost of treatment is an important factor, and in many instances alternative methods of treatment at varying costs must be considered. In fact, the problem may be resolved in a variety of ways, ranging from the patient's refusal to undergo treatment at all because of a lack of appreciation of its importance, to acceptance of the ideal solution recommended by the dentist who made the examination and diagnosis and designed the treatment plan. For example, the ideal treatment plan may call for balancing of occlusion, construction of one or more dental bridges, restoration of several carious teeth, treatment of gingivitis, changes in diet, and institution of a specific home care regimen. Baked porcelain inlays may have been prescribed as the ideal restorative material for cavities in the anterior teeth. However, the reaction of the individual patient can vary widely. As previously suggested, he may decide to do nothing. He may decide to have the carious anterior teeth restored and let the rest go till later. He may choose a temporary appliance instead of a fixed bridge. He may accept the advice on dietary changes, but the length of time he adheres to the change may vary widely. Similarly, the instructions given for home care may be followed explicitly; they may be carried out indifferently; or they may be ignored completely.

The broad range of factors which influence the reaction of the patient to treatment plans has been emphasized to point up the need for considering alternative methods of treating a patient's problem. The patient becomes an active party in making the decision. His financial resources, the value he places on health services, his health habits, and his whole background of correct and incorrect health information will affect the decision. The same factors influence the third step of the public health worker, namely, program planning, in a similar fashion. Both dental clinicians and public health workers desire to have the optimum treatment or program plan accepted without question. However, the community's reaction to such a plan, like that of the patient, may be to do nothing, to carry out only part of the plan, or to adopt an alternative, less comprehensive, and probably less costly program. It is the community which makes the decision either directly or indirectly through its administrative officials. The decision will reflect the relative value which the community places on solving the particular health problem in comparison with the many other community problems which are in need of attention. Therefore, if the community's decision is to be a realistic one, it must be based on community-wide knowledge of the survey findings, on an understanding of the analysis of these findings, and on a familiarity with proposals for a control program. Each of these areas of need for information can be filled through appropriate health education technics. However, the most certain and effective way of ensuring not only that the community will be informed but also that the facts will be understood correctly is through broad community participation in the conduct of the survey, in the analysis, and in the program planning.

Treatment — Program Operation

When the plan has been accepted by the patient, the dental clinician arranges a specific schedule for carrying out the indicated treatments. If the treatment plan is rather complex, it may involve referring the patient to an oral surgeon for needed extractions, to a prosthodontist for partial dentures, or to a periodontist for treatment of the supporting tissues of the teeth. A variety of specialists within the field of dentistry may be called upon to carry out the treatment plan. However, responsibility for coordination of these efforts will rest with the patient's primary dentist. He will be held responsible for successful administration of the plan. Similarly, when a specific community public health program has been adopted, a variety of disciplines may be called upon for execution of the program. If, for example, the program is water fluoridation, local dentists may be asked to collect base-line data on the prevalence of dental caries, engineers will determine the type of equipment needed to carry out the fluoridation procedure, chemists will make water analyses, and the waterworks operators will be given the job of adding the proper amounts of fluorides to the water supply. Since fluoridation is a continuing program, there will be the overall problem of administration, or responsibility for seeing that the work of the different specialists is coordinated and carried out effectively and efficiently.

Payment—Financing

Mutually agreeable methods of paying for dental services usually are arranged between the patient and his dentist before the treatment plan is undertaken. The arrangement may vary, but a common pattern provides for a cash down payment and for subsequent payments to be made at the time of each clinic session in the course of the treatment. This arrangement assures the dentist payment for services rendered and ensures against nonpayment in case dental service is terminated prior to completion of the treatment plan. For many reasons it is not uncommon for the patient to decide to discontinue treatment before it has been completed. Unforeseen or emergency demands on his financial resources may be one cause for discontinuance. Dissatisfaction with the treatment may be another. A lower value on dental service may have been engendered by competing desires for such items as a new car or a new television set. However, in many cases, the successfully competing value may realistically require a higher priority of attention than the dental treatment. Usually, community public health programs are financed by funds appropriated by the governing body of the community. Occasionally, local funds are supplemented by state or federal funds. Frequently, the program plan may be approved, but funds are not appropriated for carrying out the activity and the program may die aborning. Since appropriations are made usually on an annual or biennial basis, the program may get under way only to be terminated through lack of subsequent appropriations. If this occurs, it should be clear that competing needs have been given a higher priority. However, funds for supporting a community health program also may be derived from contributions by local civic, social, or voluntary organizations. But whether the program is dependent for support on official or voluntary agencies of the community, continuance of that support will, in each case, be determined by community awareness of a real need.

Evaluation—Program Appraisal

Evaluation of the effectiveness of treatment rendered may begin during the course of treatment or be made at subsequent intervals of time, depending on the conditions under treatment. For example, the simple restoration of a carious tooth may have stopped sensitivity to cold or sweet food and may have restored function. These are immediate gains, but subsequent observations will determine whether or not the cavity was prepared properly so that the carious process was interrupted; whether or not the preparation was extended sufficiently to deter recurrence of caries; whether or not the occluding and contact portions of the tooth were restored properly so that the tooth does not suffer from traumatic occlusal forces. These observations can be evaluated from time to time as the patient returns for periodic examination and service. The evaluation can be an objective one only if careful examination records of initial conditions were made and are available for study and comparison. Similarly, data collected in the initial survey by the public health worker for community program planning purposes must serve as the base line against which appraisals can be made to assess the effectiveness of the program. The public health worker is accountable to the community for a periodic appraisal of his performances, just as the dental clinician is accountable to his patient for the effectiveness of the course of treatment which he has rendered. In each case, the evaluation by the dentist or the appraisal by the public health worker should be performed in a spirit of self-discipline and for one's own guidance in developing competence. But it is the value assigned by the patient or the community which will determine ultimately the confidence placed in the private dentist or the public health worker.

Procedural Pattern

The foregoing analogy between the procedures employed by the dental clinician and the public health worker may be summarized as follows:

Patient	Community
1. Examination	1. Survey
2. Diagnosis	2. Analysis
3. Treatment planning	3. Program planning
4. Treatment	4. Program operation
5. Payment for services	5. Finance
6. Evaluation	6. Appraisal

[Education of the patient (or public) is an important part of each of the steps listed in this analogy. Successful practice of clinical dentistry or dental public health requires continuing emphasis on education before and during the six procedures outlined (D.F.S., W.O.Y.).]

Although the terms used to describe the public health worker's approach to community health problems differ from those used to describe the dentist's approach to his patient's dental problem, their meanings are similar. Fundamentally, the procedures are identical. Thus, the training in procedural skills received by the dental student provides him with a basic pattern of approach to problems which should be helpful in enabling him to fill with competence and distinction the role of adviser and counselor on community health programs.

Bibliography

1. Leavell, H. R., and Clark, E. G. Preventive medicine for the doctor in his community; an epidemiologic approach. 3rd ed. New York, McGraw-Hill, 1965. XVI + 684 p. (p. 19-38)
2. Winslow, C. E. A. The untilled fields of public health. Mod. Med., 2:183-91, Mar. 1920.

Additional Readings

Confrey, E. A., ed. Administration of community health services. Chicago, International City Manager's Association, 1961. XV + 560 p.
Dunning, J. M. Principles of dental public health. Cambridge, Mass., Harvard University Press, 1962. XI + 543 p.
Easlick, K. A., ed. The administration of local dental programs; proceedings of the fifth workshop on public health dentistry. Ann Arbor, University Michigan School Public Health Continued Education Service, 1963. VIII + 278 p.
―――. The practice of dental public health; proceedings of the fourth workshop on dental public health. "Objectives and evaluation of a state's dental program." Rev. ed. Ann Arbor, University Michigan School Public Health Continued Education Service, 1960. IV + 198 p.
Freeman, Ruth B., and Holmes, E. M., Jr. Administration of public health services. Philadelphia, Saunders, c1960. XIII + 507 p.
Hanlon, J. J. Principles of public health administration. 5th ed. St. Louis, Mosby, 1969. XVII + 658 p.
Pelton, W. J., and Wisan, J. M., eds. Dentistry in public health. 2nd ed. Philadelphia, Saunders, 1955. X + 282 p.
Podshadley, D. W., Weiss, R. L., and Pipe, Peter. Introduction to dental public health; a self-instruction course. Washington, Government Printing Office, 1964. VII + 183 p.

CHAPTER 3

THE DENTIST AND DENTAL HYGIENIST IN PUBLIC HEALTH

Dentists have been taught to provide dental care for children, and most do so as part of their practices. Some dentists have had special education or experience and elect to limit their practices to dentistry for children. Still others undertake graduate education to qualify for examination by the American Board of Pedodontics and certification as specialists in this field. The same variation in the degree of interest and skill exists in other specialized areas of dental practice, including dental public health. Almost all dentists engage in some type of public health activity during their professional careers. Some, in effect, have limited their practices to dental public health by accepting positions with a health department, dental society, or dental service corporation—positions that require dental public health skills. The specialist in this field has completed a graduate curriculum in public health and has met the requirements for certification as a diplomate of the American Board of Dental Public Health.

Because dental hygienists do not engage in independent practice, and because of the highly specialized nature of their clinical responsibilities, the analogy between the character of general practice, limited practice, and specialization is not as clear as in the practice of dentistry. Nevertheless, there are marked differences in the functions of the hygienist in clinical practice and in public health. Although the unique characteristics of a public health dental hygienist are not identified by specialty board certification, the knowledge and skills she must possess and the nature of the responsibilities she is expected to assume indicate that she functions as a specialist.

DENTAL PUBLIC HEALTH AS A SPECIALTY OF DENTISTRY

Background

Dental public health was not recognized formally as a specialty area until relatively recently, although dentists were active in the field of public health during most of the first half of the twentieth century. Initially, the only identifying characteristic of a "public health dentist" was an interest in improving the oral health conditions of the public. As various types of dental health programs were developed, and as dentists gained experience in their organization and operation, a unique body of knowledge was accumulated, and the special skills of public health dentistry became identified.

The foundation for dentistry in public health was developed in the first decade of this century. The National Dental Association (forerunner of the American Dental Association) appointed its first Committee on Oral Hygiene in 1900, and many state and local dental societies were active in efforts to improve the dental health of the public in that era.[9] Since studies of the oral health of school children indicated appalling neglect, the first programs were directed toward the promotion of dental treatment for all children and the organization of clinics to provide care for children from indigent families. Because of the early emphasis on dental care for children, public health dentistry and pedodontics were identified closely during their early development. For example, Easlick, the first teacher of dental public health, is a pedodontist, and Pelton holds the distinction of being a founding member of the specialty boards in both pedodontics and dental public health. The American Society of Dentistry for Children, founded in 1927 to promote better oral health care for children, has counted many public health dentists among its leaders.[14]

The first clearly identifiable dental public health program was created by the North Carolina State Board of Health in 1918.[8] This program, reflecting the times, emphasized the provision of corrective dental service for rural school children, supplemented by a statewide educational program. Despite the emphasis on treatment, dental programs in this developmental period did attempt to provide both educational and preventive services, although these efforts were largely empirical and lacked a sound scientific basis for action. Toothbrushing was emphasized, frequently on the basis of the now discredited slogan, "a clean tooth never decays." The emphasis on oral hygiene had led Fones to establish a training program to prepare young women to provide oral prophylaxes and to teach toothbrushing to the school children in Bridgeport, Connecticut.[10] Although the efforts of dental hygienists, as they were named, did not fulfill the expectation that dental caries attack would be reduced, this adjunctive profession to dentistry has played an important role in the development of both preventive dental practice and dental public health programs.

After 1930, dental public health made rapid progress.[11, 15] Following Congressional approval of the Social Security Act in 1935, which made grants-in-aid available to the states for extending public health services, dental divisions in state health departments grew from 13 in 1935, to 23 in 1940, to 45 in 1951, and to 48 in 1968. During the 1930's the Public Health Service, which commissioned dentists as early as 1919 to render dental care,[17] assigned officers to research and dental public health projects. The first graduate curriculum in public health dentistry was instituted at The University of Michigan in the latter part of the decade. A growing number of experienced public health dentists, many of whom had completed graduate courses, were available to staff the expanded dental health programs. These men were able to develop a scientific basis for their activities with relatively precise investigative methods and specific preventive procedures.

Early concepts of oral disease were based on dentists' study of individual patients. McKay, in an attempt to determine the cause of a condition of unknown etiology observed in dental practice, moved outside the dental office to study the occurrence of endemic fluorosis in entire communities. By 1931, the discovery of the role of fluorides in the production of endemic fluorosis had demonstrated the value of observing the occurrence of dental diseases in various populations in contrast to clinical observations of individual patients. On this basis, Dean performed "... investigations on mottled enamel or dental fluorosis in the Western United States [which] justifiably rank among epidemiologic classics...."[12] Dean and McKay later became the first dentists to be awarded the coveted Lasker Award of the American Public Health Association for their pioneering work in dental epidemiology.

The epidemiological study of the relation between fluorides and oral health was made possible by the development of a method for classifying mottled enamel and by the DMF index for the quantitative measurement of dental caries experience in permanent teeth (technics which will be outlined in Chapter Four). The DMF index, which soon became a basic tool in dental public health research, was used in Dean's classic study of 21 cities to establish the fluoride-dental caries relation, the Hagerstown studies of the occurrence of dental caries among children, and many subsequent epidemiological investigations. In later years, public health dentists developed epidemiological measurements of dental caries experience in primary teeth, periodontal diseases, oral hygiene, and malocclusion.

In the 1940's the epidemiological studies of dental caries resulted in the development of specific preventive procedures for this disease. Public health dentists were pioneers in the application of community water fluoridation and in topical applications of fluorides.

The contribution of public health dentists to the profession and the unique nature of their practice were recognized officially in 1951 when the American Dental Association approved the American Board of Dental Public Health to certify specialists in this field.[2] Since that time, dentists in public health have continued to explore new horizons in dentistry. Dental care study programs in Richmond, Indiana, and Woonsocket, Rhode Island, demonstrated that dental care provided to school children, on an annual basis, eliminated the backlog of neglect and cut treatment time by as much as one third.[18] These projects further demonstrated that the proper use of auxiliary dental personnel at the chair could increase a dentist's output, reduce operating fatigue, and provide better service to patients at lower costs. Dentistry made an important contribution to the multidisciplined team approach to the rehabilitation of patients with clefts of the lip and palate.

Surveys of dental practice, dental manpower, and dental education have provided a factual background for the analysis of problems facing the dental profession and the basis for planning for the future. When the profession found itself faced for the first time with a demand by organized groups for the group purchase of dental care, the studies that had been conducted by public health dentists on dental needs and treatment requirements made possible the orderly development of prepayment programs. More recently, dental public health has pioneered in applying the skills and knowledge of psychologists, sociologists, anthropologists, and other specialists in the field of social science to the problems of dentistry.

Education and Certification

The dentist in public health should possess two types of specialized skills. First, he must have the same basic public health background as other professional individuals who work in public health — such as physicians, nurses, and engineers. The Committee on Professional Education of the American Public Health Association requires that the graduate course of study for the degree of Master of Public Health include the following fields of instruction:[4]

 1. The nature of man, his physical and social environment, and his personal and social interaction — as they affect his health.
 2. The basic technics of investigation, measurement, and evaluation, including biostatistics and epidemiology.
 3. The basic technics of administration (organization and management), particularly as applicable to comprehensive health care programs.
 4. The economic and political setting relevant to health services.
 5. The application of these knowledges in the promotion of community health.

These fundamental areas of knowledge should prepare the dentist to assume an effective role as a member of the team of specialists that promotes the health of the public.

Second, the dentist must learn specialized skills needed for the practice of dental public health. For this purpose, instruction in graduate dentistry and the special administrative problems of dental programs is recommended. Since the diagnostic, preventive, and restorative technics of dentistry change rapidly, it is important that dentists preparing for a career in public health review the most recent advances in the basic sciences, in clinical dentistry, and in preventive procedures. Furthermore, the graduate student must develop a habit of continuing study and skill in evaluating dental literature critically so that he is prepared to keep pace with future developments in his profession.

Instruction in the administrative phases of dental public health programs (which should be taught by a public health dentist) includes: (1) the social and economic pressures on the dental profession and on dental practice; (2) the blocks to the development of dental public health programs; (3) the critical appraisal of technical information to be used in educational media; (4) the planning and conducting of comprehensive surveys to determine the nature and extent of dental problems and the resources and facilities available to meet those problems; (5) the planning, financing, budgeting, operation, and evaluation of dental public health programs; (6) the use of indices and other methods of measurement in epidemiological studies; and (7) the basic principles of research as applied to dental public health.

The American Board of Dental Public Health requires that diplomates be engaged in administration, teaching, or research limited to dental public health or preventive dentistry as a full-time specialty. Among the chief requirements that must be met by candidates for examination are: (1) graduation from an accredited dental school; (2) membership in the American (or National) Dental Association, the American Public Health Association, and the American Association of Public Health Dentists; (3) licensure to practice dentistry in at least one state; and (4) professional experience and special training in public health which shall include (a) at least two calendar years of clinical or other professional experience following graduation from a dental school, (b) successful completion of at least one academic year of graduate study leading to the degree of Master of Public Health or an equivalent degree or diploma from an institution accredited for this purpose by the American Public Health Association or the American Dental Association, (c) successful completion, under competent direction, of one calendar year of field training or residency acceptable to the Board, and (d) at least four years' experience in the practice of dental public health or preventive dentistry which may include administration, teaching, or research related to dental public health or preventive dentistry.[1]

Functions

The basic procedures of clinical dentistry can be summarized quite simply, as was done in the previous chapter. Similarly, the steps in an individual phase of treatment can be expressed easily. Prosthetic full-denture service, for example, can be said to consist of examination, diagnosis, and development of a treatment plan; full-mouth extractions and surgical preparation of the ridges; securing of impressions and registration of jaw relations; setting up of artificial teeth; processing and finishing of dentures; and insertion and adjustment of the finished prosthetic appliances. This description, although accurate, provides little insight into the many detailed procedures involved or the variety of technical and professional skills required.

The same problem arises in attempting to describe the functions of public health dentists; easy to outline, they are difficult to describe in detail. This difficulty is created partly by the fact that the problems faced by the public health dentist cannot be attacked as directly as can those seen by the dentist in clinical practice. The construction of even a complicated fixed prosthesis can be accomplished in a relatively short period of time by the dentist and those working under his supervision. In contrast, the public health dentist who attempts to reduce tooth loss in the population from periodontal diseases faces a much more complex task. Since there is no specific public health preventive procedure available, improvement in the oral health status of the public will necessitate motivating a larger number of individuals to seek regular professional care—a demanding and long-range task. To be successful, such a project requires a sufficient supply of professional personnel, adequately trained in the most advanced treatment procedures. The sponsorship of postgraduate courses, strengthening of emphasis on periodontal therapy in scientific meetings, and promotion of the utilization of dental hygienists—each a formidable project in itself—are among the first efforts that may have to be made in order to attempt to reduce the loss of teeth from periodontal diseases.

Some indication of the variety of activities that may be included in dental public health programs is provided by a questionnaire used by the Council on Dental Health of the American Dental Association in 1958 to survey state dental health programs.[3] Although designed to reflect activities at the state level, this listing also indicates the nature of dental public health practice in local and federal programs, since the functions at each level differ primarily in emphasis and in the setting in which they are performed. Among the approximately 100 possible activities and functions included were:

1. Program administration
    a. Cooperation in dental health matters with other units within the health agency, and with official and voluntary agencies outside the health department.

    b. Determining and publicizing private practice opportunities in areas with a shortage of dentists.
    c. Recruiting dental and dental hygiene students.
    d. Compiling adequate dental statistics for records, legislative purposes, program planning, and program evaluation.

2. Preventive, diagnostic, and corrective services
    a. Provision of topical fluoride applications for school children or the promotion of local dental programs for this purpose.
    b. Promotion of water fluoridation, or of defluoridation in areas with excessive natural fluorides.
    c. Provision of laboratory services such as lactobacillus counts, cancer biopsy, fluoride analysis of water.
    d. Provision of dental inspections and parent consultation for pre-school and school children or the promotion of dental referral programs to assure that children are seen by dentists in practice.
    e. Provision of dental treatment for the indigent, for those in isolated areas without dental service, and for residents in institutions.
    f. Provision of treatment and rehabilitation of the handicapped, including children with cleft lip and palate or other dentofacial deformities, and for other physically handicapped persons.

3. Program promotion and consultative services
    a. Provision of adequate consultation to local dental programs conducted by local health departments, welfare departments, boards of education, or voluntary organizations.
    b. Provision of funds or personnel to aid local dental programs.
    c. Making dental health consultation available to other state agencies such as departments of education or welfare.

4. Public health training and teaching
    a. Provision of in-service training for state and local health department staffs.
    b. Sponsorship or participation in lectures, conferences, or workshops in public health or allied subjects for practitioners in dentistry, dental hygiene, medicine, or nursing.
    c. Sponsorship of postgraduate refresher courses in areas such as dentistry for children, periodontal therapy, or oral cancer detection.
    d. Teaching dental health in teacher training courses, schools of nursing, medicine, dental hygiene, or public health.
    e. Promoting the utilization of auxiliary personnel by dental practitioners.

5. Dental health education and information
    a. Utilization of newspaper, radio, and television to increase understanding about dental health.
    b. Use of films, filmstrips, and exhibits to promote interest in dental health.
    c. Preparation and distribution of dental health education materials to schools, health personnel, and the public.
    d. Training of teachers through workshops, seminars, personal contact, and participation in classroom instruction.

6. Research and study projects
    a. Conducting surveys to establish the nature and extent of dental disease.
    b. Conducting surveys to determine the dental needs of

special groups such as pre-school children, the handicapped, or the institutionalized.

c. Utilization of special studies for program evaluation to determine the effectiveness of fluoridation, training, treatment, or referral programs.

d. Organizing studies of dental practice to determine dental manpower resources, need for training facilities, usage of auxiliary personnel, or the economic or social barriers to dental care.

Local Programs. To reach the public most effectively any organized program of prevention, education, or treatment should operate in the local community. Dental public health activities are strongest when they are organized and operated in the local setting but, unfortunately, only a few communities maintain comprehensive dental health programs.

Local dental programs staffed by qualified full-time personnel usually are limited to the larger cities or populous counties which include a good-sized city. Some school systems have extensive dental programs emphasizing dental health education and, in some instances, treatment of children from indigent families. Even in the major population centers, however, the scope of local programs varies widely. In smaller cities and counties good dental programs are the exception, not the rule. Some make a partial effort by employing a part-time dentist or hygienist or by operating a voluntary community clinic; the majority are completely dependent on state dental programs for service.[19] A census of local dental health programs, for example, indicated that only 178 of the nation's some 1,600 local health departments have dental health programs staffed by at least one full-time dentist or dental hygienist.[16]

State Programs. State public health dentists have been employed in dental health programs in all states but Alaska. State programs traditionally have been the backbone of dental public health. As might be expected, the scope of activities differs widely, partly because of regional differences of philosophy. In some areas of the country treatment of the indigent is emphasized and large care programs are operated. In other areas, health departments do not offer treatment directly, although they promote the organization of dental care programs for certain segments of the population to be operated by other agencies. The variation in programs also reflects differences in the size of the states and the adequacy of their financial support. Staffs of state dental units range from a single public health dentist and a secretary to large programs with a variety of professional personnel. In a few states, the majority of the functions listed in the questionnaire developed by the Council on Dental Health are performed; in others, staffs are sufficient only to work on three or four of the items of highest priority.

Federal Programs. Most public health dentists employed by the federal government are commissioned officers of the Public

Health Service, a uniformed federal service similar in many respects to the Army, Navy, and Air Force. The Public Health Service is a branch of the Department of Health, Education, and Welfare. The major emphasis in dental public health practice at the federal level is on attacking oral health problems of national significance and, when requested, providing consultation and assistance to state and local health departments.

Public Health Service officers have pioneered the attack on many oral health problems, such as in the study of fluorides, predictions of manpower supply, analysis of plans for the group purchase of dental care, and development of topical applications of fluoride. Consultation to the dental health staffs of state and local health agencies is provided both by dentists on the Washington staff and by consultants located in nine regional offices throughout the country. Dentists at the federal level also develop special demonstration projects, operated either directly or through financial arrangements with states, to test new methods of solving dental health problems, to develop basic information on costs and effectiveness, and to demonstrate the value of new approaches to health problems. A considerable number of Public Health Service officers perform only clinical dentistry, providing care for wards and beneficiaries of the federal government. A few public health dentists serve in these divisions in an administrative capacity.

In recent years, the federal armed forces have been placing great emphasis on preventive dentistry, and there are a number of public health dentists employed as commissioned officers with the Army, Air Force, and Navy.[6]

THE PUBLIC HEALTH DENTAL HYGIENIST

Background

Although dental hygienists were prepared first to work only with children in schools, and although most dental hygienists now are employed in private dental offices, the dental hygienist does have an important role to play in the area of public health. Even in the early years, a small number of dental hygienists were employed in public service by health departments and school systems, fulfilling the initial concept of the hygienist. The number of hygienists engaged in dental public health has increased in recent years as a result of several factors. The first has been a modest but continuing expansion of dental health programs. Whereas, in some instances, small dental public health programs have tended to rely only upon the services of a public health dentist, other small programs, particularly at the local level, have utilized only the services of the public health dental hygienist. In the larger programs, expanding and improving as more funds become available, additional positions for dental hygienists usually are created. A second factor probably has been an increasing recognition of the value of dental hygienists by public health dentists. A third factor, not unrelated to the second, has been the utilization of topical applications of fluoride in community dental programs, which added a new clinical function for hygienists working in public programs. In these types of programs, dental hygienists have demonstrated their worth to the public health dentists who have employed them, and they also have seen the need for further education in public health for themselves. The development of educational programs for public health dental hygienists and the availability of federal traineeship support for students have helped to increase the supply of personnel, but not sufficiently to meet the increasing demand.

Although no accurate data are available, a reasonable guess would be that about 10 to 25 percent of the dental hygienists in the country who are presently employed are working for an official or voluntary agency.[7, 13] Quite likely a considerable number of these hygienists are engaged only in the practice of clinical dental hygiene, and the majority of them are working in dental health programs in city, county, and state health departments or in school health programs. Recently there has been a trend toward the employment of public health dental hygienists by departments of community dentistry in schools of dentistry and in the dental public health units of schools of public health.

Education

There are three levels of educational qualifications of dental hygienists in public health and, in general, the types of responsibilities assumed are related to the educational background.[5] All schools now offer at least the minimum two-year collegiate course which meets the requirements for certification in dental hygiene. The certificate in dental hygiene and successful completion of the state board examination qualifies an individual to practice clinical dental hygiene. A number of schools also offer a four-year degree program. In some cases, this program consists of the standard two-year certificate program preceded by two years of study in the arts and sciences. In other schools the sequence of courses is optional or the certificate course is taken in the first two years. In the latter instances, the additional two years of instruction can be designed specifically to develop skills of particular value in public dental programs. Dental hygienists who have received a bachelor's degree, and who qualify for entrance to the graduate programs in schools of public health, may complete a course of study leading to the master's degree in public health.

The dental hygienist who has completed only the standard two-year certificate course fulfills a valuable function in public health programs, but, because of the limited preparation, her primary responsibilities are in clinical dental hygiene. Provision of oral prophylaxes, patient education at the chair, the application of topical medications to the teeth, and, to some extent, serving as a resource person to teachers and other community leaders comprise the primary functions of the certificate hygienist. The public health dental hygienist, on the other hand, should have completed at least a bachelor's degree in dental hygiene. Completion of the master's program in public health provides a depth of education which, for all practical purposes, approaches that of the public health dentist. Only a relatively few dental hygienists have completed this program, but the number may be expected to increase.

The education and experience of the public health dental hygienist should provide skills which will permit her to carry out specialized functions in a professional field in which she has gained basic skills through the certificate program. Basically, these skills are much the same as those required by the public health dentist. The hygienist should have a general understanding of the field of public health including public health administration, epidemiology, statistics, and the organization of related public health programs. She also should possess knowledge of school health programs including the role of schools in health maintenance and special problems in the administration of school health programs. In the field of dental public health she must understand dental survey methods and special problems of administering dental public health programs, and she must have a detailed knowledge of the application of preventive and control procedures, particularly on a community basis. Because health education is a fundamental part of a dental hygienist's role, she must have background in the principles of education, including basic knowledge about the educational process and specific technics for teaching both individuals and groups.

Hygienists who have been graduated with the degree of Master of Public Health have been or are presently employed as dental health consultants or supervising dental hygienists in state departments of health, the Public Health Service, and the World Health Organization, or as faculty members in schools of dentistry and public health, and several of them now are directing programs of dental hygiene education in universities and community colleges.

Functions

The functions of the dentist and hygienist in clinical practice are very different because of the varying degrees of technical and professional instruction they have received and because of the legal limitations of state dental practice acts. This distinction does not hold true in public dental programs. The dental hygienist has a knowledge of dental theory sufficient to permit her to function effectively in most aspects of dental public health. In accordance with the administrative policy of the program, and under the supervision of a licensed dentist, the dental hygienist in a dental public health program:[5]

1. Provides dental prophylaxis and other oral hygiene measures, including instruction in home care of the mouth.
2. Applies caries preventive measures, such as topical application of fluorides.
3. Demonstrates new dental preventive methods and procedures to other dental hygienists and allied health workers.
4. Participates as a dental health adviser in community health activities, such as well child conferences, expectant parent classes, prenatal conferences, and readiness for school programs.
5. Assists in community dental surveys, including the inspection, recording, analysis, and interpretation of the data to the community.
6. Assists a community in planning, organizing, and conducting a dental health program suitable to the needs and resources of the area.
7. Assists in planning and conducting preservice and inservice training programs in dental health for: (a) other public health personnel, (b) school personnel, and (c) civic groups interested in dental health.
8. Assists in planning and conducting dental public health activities and field experiences for student dental hygienists and student nurses.
9. Assists in planning and conducting school dental health programs by: (a) serving as a resource person in dental health to teachers, administrators, and other school personnel, (b) performing dental inspections of school children, establishing referral and follow-through systems for dental care, (c) maintaining records on the dental status of school children, (d) providing dental prophylaxis and topical fluoride treatments for school children on either demonstration or service basis, (e) evaluating, developing, and making available effective dental health educational material to interested persons.
10. Assists voluntary health agencies, civic groups, and dental, or allied professional groups in carrying out special dental health activities.

SPECIAL KNOWLEDGE AND SKILL REQUIRED

Dental Practice

The public health dentist and dental hygienist need first to be skilled in the field of dental practice. Although they cannot develop specialized skills in every area, they should be knowledgeable about current developments in all phases of dental and dental hygiene practice. For example, since the public health dentist frequently supervises dental care programs or is asked to offer consultation to programs operated by other agencies, he must be able to evaluate the latest developments in dental equipment, in the utilization of auxiliary personnel, and in technical operative procedures. A knowledge of child growth and development and of modern concepts of rehabilitation is necessary if he works with cleft palate rehabilitation teams and other rehabilitation agencies. One of the important functions of the public health dentist is to provide advice and consultation to dentists in private practice, to nondental programs in his own agency, to schools, to welfare agencies, and to custodial institutions. Similarly, the dental hygienist must be prepared to offer consultation to hygienists in clinical practice, other health workers, and teachers.

In all of these functions, a comprehensive knowledge of dental practice is a prerequisite to successful practice in dental public health. To maintain current knowledge, it is necessary to scan many dental journals, evaluate selected articles carefully, consult with other dental specialists (and nondental experts in their areas of competence), and attend refresher courses and dental meetings regularly.

Research and Evaluation

Epidemiology, traditionally conceived as a science that studies only acute infections in populations, has been extended to aid in the investigation of chronic conditions such as dental caries and periodontal diseases. Dentists have the chief responsibility for applying epidemiology to dental problems, since a sound understanding of clinical behavior is the foundation for the study of any disease. Because public health dentists are the specialists in the profession concerned primarily with the occurrence of disease in population groups, they should assume the responsibility for pioneering in this field. It is important that they know the principles and methods of general epidemiology and the closely interwoven science of biostatistics. In addition to a general knowledge of vital statistics, the public health dentist must have a working understanding of sampling procedures, methods of data processing and tabulation, analysis and use of tests of significance, and the presentation and interpretation of findings.

Even if a public health dentist is not in a position to conduct research, he should be prepared to evaluate research findings and interpret them to the public, his co-workers, and dentists in clinical practice. It is particularly important that the public health dentist be in a position to evaluate critically research findings in those areas concerned with the prevention and control of dental disorders—such as the use of fluorides.

Human Behavior

One of the primary objectives of many public dental programs is to modify the attitudes and behavior of individuals so that acceptable health practices will be followed. Instead of the individual relation with a patient that characterizes educational efforts in private practice, public health workers must attempt the more complex task of dealing with large groups of people. Effective action requires both an understanding of the factors which condition and determine individual attitudes and skill in the technics which can be used to educate the public and increase its willingness to seek preventive and corrective services. The social sciences (such as economics, sociology, psychology, and anthropology) provide a background which makes it possible to understand the impact of cultural differences, the influence of social and economic factors, and other important determinants of human behavior. The widespread failure to adopt fluoridation indicates both that the available knowledge has not been applied fully and that more knowledge is needed in this field.

The insights provided by the social sciences give the framework for utilizing skills in communication and health education, subjects that will be outlined in succeeding chapters. These skills, the basis of the separate public health subspecialty of health education, are necessary if effective efforts are to be made to improve oral health conditions. Special technics are available for working with small groups of people, mass audiences, and groups with special cultural or social characteristics.

Administration

The public health dentist needs to possess the skills of an administrator or executive in fields such as professional and public relations, personnel management, establishing minimum standards for performance, organizing and managing, budgeting and planning, and establishing logical and easily understood policies. These skills are not the exclusive domain of the public health dentist but are possessed to some degree by every dentist who organizes and manages a successful dental practice. However, the scope of his responsibility, the magnitude of the problem that he attempts to remedy, and the necessity for integrating his efforts with other professional persons and agencies require that a public health dentist have a broader administrative competency.

The public health dentist cannot be concerned only with relations within his own program. Dental public health programs do not operate in a vacuum, but must be integrated and coordinated with other health department activities in such fields as chronic disease, maternal and child health, health education, and environmental health. The necessity for cooperative efforts means that the dental staff must work effectively with a varied group of other professional individuals and that the objectives and program plans of a dental health program cannot be developed independently. Successful dental public health programs require cooperative planning and effort by such diverse groups as the dental society, parent-teacher associations, the school board, teachers, city council members, state legislators, and physicians and nurses in private practice and public health. A dental health program should avoid overlapping or duplication of effort and should reinforce and support the efforts of others who contribute to the dental program. It also is imperative that the support and, in many instances, the active participation of other groups and agencies be enlisted.

Communication

The effectiveness of the dentist and dental hygienist in public health will depend to a considerable extent on their skills in communication. The ability to convey technical knowledge to co-workers in the health professions will depend upon the ability to write with clarity and precision and to speak effectively. An essential administrative skill is the ability to think a problem through clearly and precisely and to prepare a written presentation, such as a program plan, job description, or annual report, which will communicate these thoughts to others. Education of the public requires skill in public speaking, the ability to preside adroitly at meetings, and ability in interpreting plans and programs orally.

BIBLIOGRAPHY

1. American Board of Dental Public Health. Information concerning certification as a specialist in dental public health. [Ann Arbor], American Board Dental Public Health, 1968. 9 p.
2. American Dental Association. Minutes of house of delegates. Am. Dent. A. Tr., 92: 180, 1951.
3. American Dental Association, Council on Dental Health. State dental division program survey and cost estimate form. Chicago, American Dental Association, (1958). 14 p. mimeog.
4. American Public Health Association, Committee on Professional Education. Criteria and guidelines for accrediting schools of public health. Am. J. Pub. Health, 56:1308-17, Aug. 1966.
5. _____. Educational qualifications of public health dental hygienists. Am. J. Pub. Health, 46:899-905, July 1956.
6. _____. Educational qualifications of public health dentists. Am. J. Pub. Health, 57:682-91, Apr. 1967.
7. Blackerby, P. E. Dental hygiene and dental specialties: public health and dental hygiene. J. Dent. Educ., 31:484-7, Dec. 1967.
8. Cady, F. C. The development of public health services in the United States. Am. Dent. A. J., 28:445-9, Mar. 1941.
9. Davis, W. R. Dentistry and the public health movement. p. 14-23. (In Pelton, W. J., and Wisan, J. M., eds., Dentistry in public health. Philadelphia, Saunders, 1949. XI + 363 p.)
10. Fones, A. C., ed. Mouth hygiene; a course of instruction for dental hygienists; a textbook containing the fundamentals for prophylactic operations. Philadelphia, Lea and Febiger, 1916. XI + 530 p.
11. Gerrie, N. F. Dental public health. Am. Dent. A. J., 40:750-9, June 1950.

12. Gordon, J. E. Dental problems in an epidemiologic perspective. Am. J. Pub. Health, 49:1041-9, Aug. 1959.
13. Kesel, R. G. Dental practice. p. 95-238. (In Hollinshead, B. S., dir. The survey of dentistry; the final report. Washington, American Council Education, c1961. XXXIV + 603 p.)
14. McBride, W. C. The first twenty-five years. J. Dent. Child., 19:144-53, 4th Quar. 1952.
15. Mitchell, G. E., and Campbell, Josephine R. Digest of state dental health programs. Washington, Government Printing Office, 1965. III + 131 p.
16. Mitchell, G. E., Sonken, Selvin, and Connor, Kathryn J. Census of dental programs in local health departments; year ending June 30, 1962. Washington, Government Printing Office, 1964. III + 27 p. (p. 3)
17. Schmeckebier, L. F. The Public Health Service. Baltimore, Johns Hopkins Press, 1923. 298 p. (p. 66-7)
18. Waterman, G. E. School care program; operation and findings give private practice ideas. Ill. Dent. J., 22:351-6, June 1953.
19. Young, W. O. Dental health. p. 5-94. (In Hollinshead, B. S., dir. The survey of dentistry; the final report. Washington, American Council Education, c1961. XXXIV + 603 p.)

Section Two

ASSESSMENT OF THE PROBLEM OF DENTAL DISEASE

CHAPTER 4
Epidemiology and the Rational Bases of Dental Public Health and Dental Practice

CHAPTER 5
The Interpretation of Data and the Evaluation of Scientific Literature

CHAPTER 6
The Epidemiology of Dental Caries and Periodontal Diseases

The use of a phosphate solution as a topical agent to reduce caries attack was reported in a popular magazine. The bold headlines and the flowing words in the article made it easy for the reader to assume that dental caries would soon be a thing of the past. Some patients already were requesting the treatments from their dentist.

One report on the use of the phosphate solution had appeared in an obscure dental journal. The investigator, on the faculty of a well-known dental school, had not previously published research studies. The paper reported a dramatic reduction in caries attack (DMFS) among 225 high school students who had received the treatments in contrast to a control group of 175. No explanation was given, however, for the unusually high prevalence of carious lesions shown in the initial examinations of the experimental group.

It will be some time before other studies of the new procedure may be reported or before evaluations by independent scientific groups such as the Council on Dental Therapeutics will be available. In the meantime, the requests for the treatment by patients force the dentist to make his own evaluation of the claims advanced.

In this situation, as in many others, the intelligent selection of treatment procedures requires a knowledge of the methods of scientific investigation and the patterns of disease attack.

CHAPTER 4

EPIDEMIOLOGY AND THE RATIONAL BASES OF DENTAL PUBLIC HEALTH AND DENTAL PRACTICE

By A. L. RUSSELL, D.D.S., M.P.H.

The basis of scientific investigation is methodical and disciplined observation. The proof of a scientific proposition is predictability. One accepts the laws of gravity as established, for example, because predictions based on these laws inevitably come true; no matter how high a baseball may be driven by a Babe Ruth or a Mickey Mantle it inevitably returns to the earth. Nitrogen, gold, and water inevitably freeze when their temperatures are dropped below a certain critical point. The business of any scientific investigator is to find some basis for estimation of the confidence with which such similar events or reactions may be expected to occur. The disciplined observation which he brings to bear in this task may be the simple observation of a phenomenon without any attempt to modify it or control its end results; or it may take the form of an experiment in which an agent under study is applied to a definite sample of people or things under controlled circumstances.

The philosophy of "try it and see" is ingrained so deeply in the twentieth century mentality that it seems incredible that men ever thought in any other manner. Nevertheless, the Greek philosophers before Aristotle esteemed theory over fact and logic over experimentation. They created concepts which were superb in the abstract but which proved to be utterly unworkable in the real world. Despite the influence of Aristotle (who was an observer of no mean ability), this aversion to observation and experimentation dominated learned men in Western civilization throughout the Middle Ages. That the experiment as a disciplined and reliable means of gaining experience was established as a prime principle in research by artists of the Renaissance was no accident. These men were doing real things with their hands and their brains, under a driving compulsion to do them well.

This same spirit pervades the dental curriculum. The practice of dentistry is a high art based upon sound scientific principles.

The graduate in dentistry or dental hygiene will have had considerable acquaintance with scientific thought and principle as applied in such fundamental areas as chemistry or microbiology. These areas are as basic to public dental practice as to private. In addition to these more familiar disciplines, however, the public health practitioner makes extensive use of the findings and methods of another method of investigation. This science, epidemiology, often receives relatively little attention in the undergraduate dental school. Yet it has a significant contribution to make to dental practice.

Epidemiology, in essence, is the study of the ways in which disease patterns in a population are affected by its way of life. It was practiced after a fashion long before it was named. Peoples as far apart as Burma and Ethiopia had learned, before the advent of written history, that malaria is a disease of the wet lowlands. They and other peoples today continue to make their homes on the higher slopes or plateaus to escape malaria, even at the cost of an arduous daily journey into the valley to work their fields or to draw water. Despite the fact that these customs grew in the most haphazard of fashions, much of this sort of learning led to improvements in the way of life of the peoples themselves. On balance, however, men were wrong much more often than they were right in their speculations about conditions which favored disease. This imbalance continued to be true until a body of rational principle and method was evolved which transformed epidemiology from an occult mysticism into a productive tool in scientific investigation.

The first successes came in the study of acute communicable conditions. The progress of a disease is relatively simple to trace when it cannot occur unless the individual is infected with a specific organism (like the *Rickettsia prowazeki* of classic typhus) with a short incubation period (about two weeks in this case) and with a specific mode of transmission (in typhus ordinarily through lice which have fed upon infected persons). Thorough delousing of individuals is an effective means of control of this category of typhus. Such diseases as cholera, typhoid, yellow fever, plague, and relapsing fever (among many others) are rare in the United States today because their several chains of transmission have been broken through the provision of clean water and food and the control of insects and rodents.

These achievements encouraged epidemiologists to try similar methods in the study of such chronic conditions as rheumatoid arthritis and the periodontal diseases. These disease processes are much more subtle and complex. With most of them, the dividing line between health and disease is not clear-cut, as in smallpox, but is largely a matter of definition on which independent investigators may fail to agree. A given clinical state may be the result of intricate interaction among a number of causative factors, none of which can produce disease acting alone, opposed by a complex of protective factors. Months or years may pass before the effect of an agent becomes obvious in a person or a population. A given agent may produce a variety of clinical effects. The concept of the essential cause and the single, necessary effect must be discarded.

Despite these difficulties and limitations, the epidemiological approach is basic to all public health activity, because it offers the final test of whether any agent or procedure is really useful to people as and where they live. There are many methods for the control of dental caries in laboratory animals, for example, which are quite futile when applied to human beings. The public health dentist discovers and defines the dental problems of his population through epidemiological investigation. He chooses devices for the control of oral disease on the community level which have been tested and proved in people and conducts his own epidemiological evaluation to make certain that they are useful and effective under the specific circumstances. The private practitioner must also turn to epidemiological studies to guide his choice of preventive and treatment procedures. Furthermore, the private practitioner (especially if he has an aptitude for it) is sometimes asked to participate in field studies. He frequently finds it a rewarding and stimulating experience.

A CLASSIC EPIDEMIOLOGICAL STUDY

One of the most brilliant programs ever carried out in the epidemiology of chronic disease was the series of studies which led to the demonstration of the caries-inhibitory properties of a fluoridated water.

It began, as is so frequently the case in scientific progress, with the study of something else. That something was a peculiar condition of dental enamel known along the Continental Divide as Colorado Brown Stain. This was considered to be rather an oddity than a matter of importance; it was usually harmless enough, though it could be disfiguring in some instances. Frederick S. McKay, fresh from dental school in Philadelphia at the turn of the century, had not encountered the condition before he opened a dental office in Colorado Springs. It was distinctly different from the commonplace blotching of enamel found in every fifth to every third person in other areas. As far as McKay knew, it was described nowhere in scientific literature. He determined to find out all about it and in 1908, with the encouragement of and some financial aid from the Colorado Springs Dental Society, began a systematic investigation.

He soon found that the condition was highly prevalent in Colorado Springs and in surrounding El Paso County but that it was to be found only in long-term residents, individuals who had been born there or who had come to the city as infants in arms. The etiological agent, then, was something in the environment which was active during the period of formation of the teeth. Further, its activity was not confined to the vicinity of Colorado Springs; the mottling was endemic in many other communities along the Divide and the plains to the east. It was quite apt to be found where deep artesian wells were the source of water. Within any community the persons affected had almost invariably been users of the same water supply. No other experience nor way of life tended to be shared by all. The conclusion was inescapable; the agent responsible for mottling was some common constituent of the community water supplies. This was the only explanation consistent with the facts.

Yet, *a priori*, this explanation was absurd. Repeated chemical analyses, covering all known elements found in drinking water, failed to discover anything common to all of the waters associated with mottled enamel. Localities were found where mottling occurred in one community but not in another nearby, despite the fact that their waters seemed to be identical in composition. If other explanations were impossible, the concept of a responsible waterborne factor was incredible.

Nevertheless, McKay could reach no other conclusion. In communities like Andover and Britton, South Dakota, where mottling was sometimes so extreme as to be disfiguring, he began to advise mothers to obtain water for use by children from other sources than the community supply. One such place was Oakley, Idaho. McKay found that children living on the outskirts of Oakley, using water from a private spring, were free of mottling. He advised the citizens of Oakley to abandon their old supply and tap this spring for a new source. In 1925 the community voted a bond issue for mains to bring the spring water into the city—the first known instance of community action to improve dental health by an alteration in the domestic water. Children born in Oakley subsequent to the change were free of mottled enamel.[45]

In 1931, about the time that permanent teeth free of mottling were beginning to erupt in Oakley children, McKay sent several samples of suspected waters to H. V. Churchill, an Alcoa chemist who was applying new methods of spectrographic analysis. He identified fluoride in each of them, in amounts ranging up to 14 parts per million.[8] Almost simultaneously, similar findings were announced by Smith, Lantz, and Smith of the University of Arizona, and by Velu and Balozet, who had been studying *le darmous* in Moroccan sheep.[63, 67] The causative agent was identified.[44]

The immediate reaction of the scientific community was one of urgent concern. The discovery touched off a considerable number of studies to determine whether fluorides in the amounts normally found in the water supply, or elsewhere in the environment, were injurious to human health. But McKay had noted something else—something possibly beneficial—in these fluoride communities. As early as 1928 he felt confident enough to publish his opinion that the prevalence of dental caries actually was reduced in amount by these same waters which produced mottled enamel.[46]

Any diligent search of dental literature will uncover the names of many authorities, predating McKay, who speculated that fluorine in tooth enamel might inhibit dental caries. However, these men failed to expand or to develop further an idea which they seem to have set down as an interesting but inconsequential oddity. By contrast, McKay and a brilliant co-worker went on to explore the possibility, and then to demonstrate the fact, that fluoride ingestion could be adjusted to an optimal intake without hazard to the individual, at small cost, and with a consequent sweeping reduction in the mass prevalence of dental caries. This brilliant co-worker was H. Trendley Dean of the United States Public Health Service.

McKay's studies did not end with the advent of Dean. The two men were fast friends and, on occasion, active collaborators. McKay continued to make personal contributions, notably the observation that the caries-inhibitory effect of fluoride water was still discernible in persons as old as 45 years.[43] Neither did Dean's work begin with the fluoride-dental caries hypothesis. He had already shown that "mottled" enamel could be manifest in a wide range of degrees, from fine, lacy markings so faint that they could not be seen except in light of just the proper quality and intensity and coming from just the proper angle, to an extreme hypoplasia in which enamel was pitted, stained, and highly friable. He had devised a community index of fluorosis based on six grades of severity which permitted comparisons among populations on a quantitative basis, and had documented the prevalence of the condition for the United States as a whole.[12, 15] This served as the groundwork for his later investigations of the fluoride-caries relation.

He had examined school children for fluorosis in 51 South Dakota communities in 1938.[18] There was a definite relation between the prevalence of fluorosis in these areas and the prevalence of caries as reported in a survey four years earlier. Similar comparisons between caries prevalence and known fluoride concentrations in four Colorado and eight Wisconsin cities showed the same general pattern.[13] This was presumptive evidence that the relation was a true one. A direct test of the hypothesis was designed.

Experience gained in the study of endemic fluorosis indicated that communities to be surveyed must be chosen with great care when the presence and amount of fluoride in the domestic water was of crucial importance. Sound conclusions could be reached only in those communities with a common water supply from the same source, without alteration during the lifetime of the people to be examined, with a stable fluoride level over a period long enough to establish and define the range of fluctuation.[17] These criteria were satisfied by Galesburg, Monmouth, Macomb, and Quincy—four cities in central Illinois. Galesburg and Monmouth were supplied with waters from wells 2,400 feet deep which averaged, over the course of a year, 1.8 and 1.7 parts per million (ppm) of the fluoride ion. Macomb and Quincy used surface waters averaging 0.2 ppm. Direct examinations were given 319 children in Galesburg, 148 in Monmouth, 112 in Macomb, and 306 in Quincy. Each was 12 to 14 years of age, with lifetime residence in his city. The prevalence of dental caries was found to be about twice as high in the low- as in the high-fluoride cities.[20] At this point, in the words of the investigators, it was

> ... obvious that whatever effect the waters with relatively high fluoride content (over 2.0 p.p.m. of F) have on dental caries is largely one of academic interest; the resultant permanent disfigurement of many of the users far outweighs any advantage that might accrue from the standpoint of partial control of dental caries. On the other hand, the demonstration of such marked dental caries differences as were observed at Galesburg and Quincy made advisable a quantitative study of the influence on dental caries of waters with lower ranges of fluoride concentration. If marked inhibitory influences were operative at concentration levels as low as the minimal threshold of endemic fluorosis (1.0 p.p.m.), the findings would be of considerable import.[20]

Accordingly, a study was made of children aged 12 to 14 years with lifetime residence in eight suburban Chicago communities with various stable fluoride levels in the domestic waters and extended to 13 additional cities in Illinois, Colorado, Ohio, and Indiana.[16, 19] This study is an epidemiological classic. The crucial findings are shown graphically in Figures 1 and 2. Dental caries in these children was related directly to the amount of fluoride in the water they had used from birth:

> Strikingly low dental caries prevalence was found associated with the continuous use of domestic waters whose fluoride (F) content was as low as about 1 part per million, a concentration which under the conditions prevailing in the localities studied produced only sporadic instances of the mildest forms of dental fluorosis of no practical esthetic significance.[16]

This finding did not establish fluoridation of water supplies as a public health measure, but it did make a test of this proposition imperative; provided, of course, that the test could be conducted without hazard to the communities involved.[2] Assurance that this was the case was developed over years of study with people using waters with fluoride levels much higher than the proposed one part per million. Four

EPIDEMIOLOGY AND DENTAL PUBLIC HEALTH 41

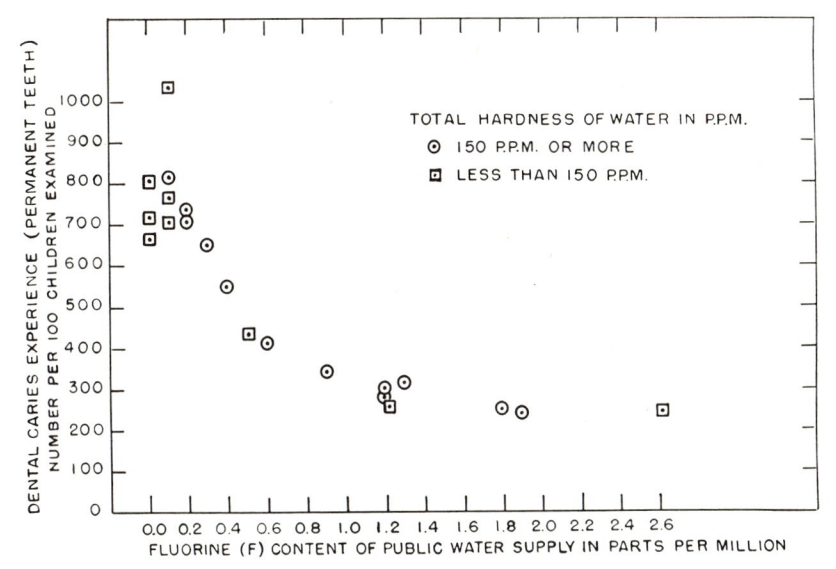

FIGURE 1. Variation in dental caries experience rates observed in 7,257 selected white school children, aged 12-14 years, in 21 cities of four states, according to fluoride concentration and hardness value of the public water supply. (Dean[16])

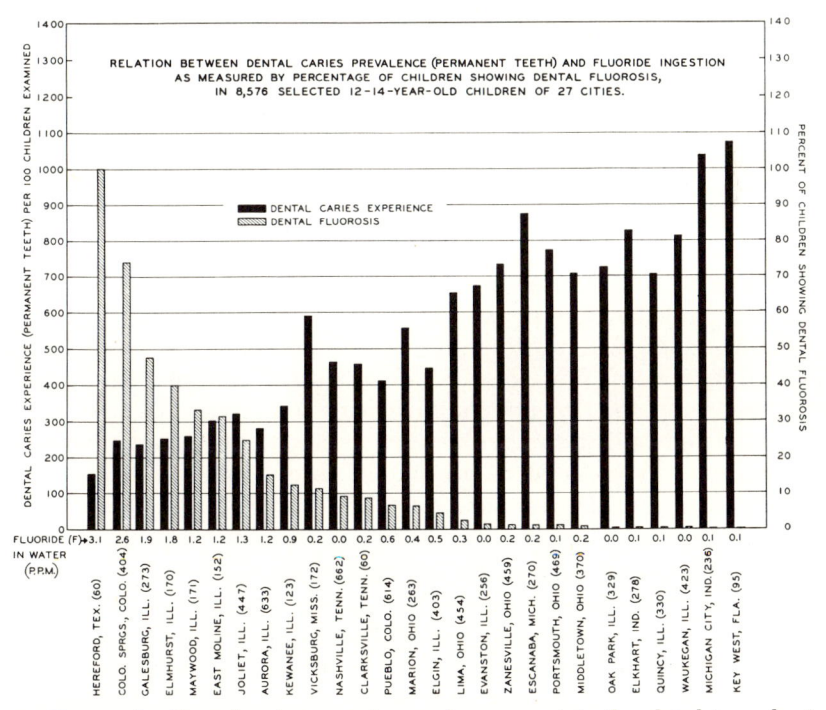

FIGURE 2. Dental caries experience of permanent teeth related to endemic dental fluorosis. (Unpublished data from the files of H. Trendley Dean.)

pioneer studies in controlled fluoridation were begun in 1945 and 1946.

One, under the direction of Dean and his associates, was carried out in Grand Rapids and Muskegon, Michigan.[21] The others, each an independent study, were conducted by Ast and his group in Newburgh and Kingston, New York; by Blayney and his associates in Evanston, Illinois; and by Hutton and his co-workers in Brantford, Ontario.[3, 5, 34] At the end of terms ranging up to 15 years, dental caries prevalence had been sharply reduced in each of the study populations, despite differences in study design and examination technics.[4] Disfiguring fluorosis was not found during specific surveys in Newburgh and Grand Rapids.[56] In the meantime, studies with adults had corroborated McKay's finding that the caries-inhibitory effect was maintained well through middle age.[58] Fluoridation had been established as a practicable and effective public health procedure with benefits far more lasting than caries inhibition through the early years of childhood.

Most of the principles of epidemiological investigation in chronic dental disease are illustrated in this skeleton outline of the development of the caries-fluoride hypothesis. It should be clear that its procedures involve something more than the transfer of office diagnostic procedures to a field situation, and that its objective is something beyond a total inventory of needs for dental care.

In the first place, people were studied as groups, rather than individuals. Individual data were combined into figures representing the typical status of a group or population with some characteristic in common: in this program, use or nonuse of a fluoride water supply. Examination and consideration were not confined to persons considered ill; all of the persons, well and ill alike in the group (or population), contributed to the findings for group status.[15]

Second, no attempt was made in any of the studies to define the absolute prevalence of disease in these populations. The objective in every instance was to determine whether there was more or less dental fluorosis or more or less dental caries in populations using a fluoride water than in populations using a fluoride-free water. The essential determination was the relative prevalence in one population compared with the relative prevalence in one or several contrasting populations. This comparison was valid because care had been taken to apply the same criteria and to follow the same examination procedure throughout each in the series of studies.

The broad goal was to establish an association between the prevalence of a lesion (fluorosis or dental caries) and a way of life (use of a fluoride water). This required two demonstrations: one, that the association itself be dependable and predictable from population to population; and, two, that other factors could not be responsible for the observed patterns. In the study of the 21 cities, for example, it was necessary for Dean and his associates to show that the observed differences in caries prevalence were not due to differences in diet or sunshine, but to some factor in the domestic water; and that this factor could not be total hardness, nor the presence or amount of silica, iron, calcium, magnesium, sodium and potassium, sulfate, nitrate, or chloride.[14]

The successful epidemiological program, like these studies of McKay and Dean, is usually a process of successive elimination of the fortuitous until the cogent factors are revealed, recognized, and established.

The evidence of the 21 cities alone was not enough to show that fluoridation would prove to be a sound public health practice. It was possible that the observed association was purely accidental. Final proof came from the studies at Grand Rapids, Newburgh, Evanston, and Brantford, in these several demonstrations that caries could be inhibited in similar fashion by the simple addition of fluorides in the community water.[4]

Two other conclusions go to the philosophical core of dental epidemiology as a scientific pursuit. In its present stage of development, dental epidemiology is not so much the study of disease as a process as it is a study of the conditions of the people in whom disease occurs. Its immediate goal is the development of methods which might be utilized in disease control. It is a matter of historical record that epidemiological investigation has led to the control of many disease conditions in which etiology was unknown or imperfectly understood. Epidemiology is a very down-to-earth science, with the clear objective of bettering the lives of the peoples it brings under study.

DENTAL EPIDEMIOLOGY

The principal focus of dental epidemiology has been on dental caries and, more recently, the periodontal diseases. The tissues involved in these diseases are readily accessible to direct examination by a variety of methods; visually, by reflected or transmitted light; by probing with an appropriate instrument; by palpation; by x-ray without the interposition of other masses; and so on. Both conditions are chronic and progressive to the point where, lacking treatment, they can be identified in unequivocal fashion by the simplest of diagnostic methods. Each is highly prevalent. Obvious signs of both are easily seen in more than 19 out of 20 United States adults. Even in Ethiopia, with one of the lowest prevalences of dental caries on record, one or more lesions of caries could be demonstrated in about one person in five aged 20 through 29 years on examination with mirror and explorer.[39]

The methods and procedures of dental epidemiology are direct outgrowths of these facts about dental disease. Elaborate case-finding technics, used to build up a study group of persons suffering from a rare disease, are unnecessary; either a whole population or a definable sample is examined. Relative prevalence can usually be established by simple methods of examination.

It is useful, of course, to have some estimate of the absolute prevalence of a condition at the outset of study. An accurate count of cases is theoretically possible with such diseases as smallpox, but dental caries and the chronic periodontal diseases present a more difficult problem in counting. The lesion of dental caries is characterized by a long preclinical course during which it cannot be diagnosed in the living human by any means presently at hand; periodontal disease represents a slow, subtle alteration of tissue from health through imperceptible modifications to an end point, loss of function. An absolute "count" of lesions of these diseases can always be challenged by a new count based on better diagnostic skill, or on an improved diagnostic aid, or on the inclusion of a number of normal areas as lesions (in statistical terms, the inclusion of false positives). But it is helpful where prevalence is wholly unknown, to attempt to count all of the lesions which meet some specific criterion, such as disclosure by a given diagnostic apparatus or technic, or size large enough to require treatment. Findings are most readily understood if reported in clinical terms with descriptive meaning. Excellent examples are the studies of dental caries carried out in children at Hagerstown by Klein, Palmer, and Knutson,[36] with adults by Hollander and Dunning,[33] and of periodontal diseases by Marshall-Day and his associates.[41] Such studies as these have supplied the basic concepts which allow a rational beginning on the determination of the population forces which modify the patterns of disease.

The typical procedure in this phase of investigation starts with a hypothesis—i.e., some such statement as, "If calcium-phosphorus deficiency is an etiological factor in dental caries, then caries activity should be much greater in persons with osteomalacia than in otherwise similar persons without osteomalacia." The proposition is tested by direct observation in an appropriate group of persons with osteomalacia and an appropriate control group of persons without osteomalacia. The crucial point to be determined is whether or not there is more dental caries in the one group than in the other. The difference, if found, is to be tested by professional and statistical logic. This requires a quantitative estimate—i.e., data expressed in meaningful numerical, rather than clinical, terms.

Indices in Dental Epidemiology

This process of quantification of data is fundamental in any scientific analysis. Measures for the quantification of dental epidemiological data are known collectively as indices. An index is a numerical value describing the relative status of a population on a graduated scale with definite upper and lower limits, designed to permit and facilitate comparison with other populations classified by the same criteria and methods.

The simplest index is the proportion of "haves" and "have nots"—the proportions of persons within the population free of the condition, or suffering from it at a given instant of time or in some span of time. The incidence of oral cancer has been reported in terms of the number of new cases per 100,000 persons per year or by the number of deaths per 100,000 persons per year; the incidence of oral clefts has been described by the number of children born with clefts in the total number of live births per year. These are examples of morbidity rates (percent of persons ill), mortality rates (percent of persons dying from the disease), or case rates (frequency of occurrence of the condition), respectively. Rates are invaluable in the study of conditions which occur with relatively low frequency, such as oral cancer.[54] Morbidity rates were adequate to show, for example, that buccal cancer was about four times more prevalent in the male than in the female in one series,[10] and about twice as prevalent in the southern than in the northern United States in 10 metropolitan areas surveyed between 1937 and 1939.[22]

Indices of this type are valuable for diseases which occur with relative infrequency but are difficult to use in measuring conditions which affect nearly everyone in varying degrees of severity. Rates for groups in which the number of persons with evidence of disease approaches 100 percent (as in the case of periodontal diseases or dental caries in susceptible populations) are not particularly discriminatory. In these instances it is valuable to have available an index which weighs the range of severity in individuals against the number of persons affected in the study group. These two values—the number affected plus a measure of severity of involvement—provide what Gordon has called " . . . the biologic gradient of disease."[29]

These measures fall into two distinct types. One type is used to describe irreversible conditions, like the increase in height from infancy through middle age. If it is necessary to determine growth during some specific period, two examinations are necessary, one at the beginning and another at the end of the time span. Most dental caries indices are in this category. The other general type is applied to the study of conditions which may improve or disappear with time, such as a viral gingivitis. With an irreversible or cumulative index such as the average number of teeth or surfaces with signs of caries attack, conclusions in a clinical trial must depend upon the number of new lesions appearing within the time span of the study. This time span can be shortened by any valid device (such as the use of radiographs) which permits detection of the lesion at an earlier stage.

In studies of lifetime caries experience—the total of signs of caries accumulated from the time of eruption to the day of examination—relatively crude indices and methods are frequently ample for the demonstration of relative prevalence. Comparability is greatly enhanced by use of a simple index based upon relatively advanced and unmistakable signs of the condition to be studied.

Within these considerations, the observer should choose the index which will best summarize the evidence he needs and the examination method best suited to return valid evidence.

Indices of Dental Caries. Many indices for dental caries have been proposed, but only three are in general use. These are based on the numbers of persons, or the numbers of teeth, or the numbers of tooth surfaces showing evidence of caries attack. All are measures of irreversible conditions, a total of signs which have been accumulated at any time in the previous lifetime of the individual. These basic signs for permanent teeth are a demonstrable lesion of caries, a filling or other restoration, or a missing permanent tooth.[54] These categories are usually indicated by D (for decayed), M (for missing or indicated for extraction), and F (for filled), usually written as DMF. Analysis may be based on the average number of DMF teeth (sometimes called DMFT) per person or the average number of DMF tooth surfaces (DMFS). When written as shown here, in capital letters, the average is based on permanent teeth only.

This index is relatively objective—that is, it is possible for two examiners to come to agreement as to the presence or absence of any of these signs of dental caries attack. With accurate diagnosis, the lesion of dental caries is only that and can be confused with nothing else; similarly, the filled or missing permanent tooth is almost always an indication of caries attack in young children of Western civilizations. (The principal exceptions are teeth extracted in the course of orthodontic treatment or lost through accident and crowns restored because of fracture.) In adults of middle and later ages a considerable number of teeth may have been lost to periodontal disease rather than to caries. In some primitive cultures teeth may be mutilated or crowned for adornment in such manner that averages are inflated if these teeth are counted as decayed, missing, or filled. When such exceptions are found frequently enough to be of significance in an actual study situation, the investigator will usually try to determine which are due to caries and which to some other and nonpertinent cause. They are most important when contrast is made between two populations of unlike culture and levels of dental care.

When the prevalence of caries is low, or when groups with high and low caries experience are compared, a simple count of persons with and without signs of caries in the permanent teeth may be adequate to establish relative prevalence. This is illustrated in Table 1, which shows dental caries experience of three groups of Alaskan Eskimo males separated according to residence in a relatively urban, intermediate, or relatively remote place (Groups I, II, and III, respectively). It is clear that Group I men would have been rated as highest

TABLE 1. RELATIVE DENTAL CARIES EXPERIENCE OF THREE
GROUPS OF ALASKAN ESKIMOS, BY TWO METHODS OF ESTIMATION

AGES	GROUP I	GROUP II	GROUP III
	percent with one or more DMF teeth		
17-24	97	93	66
25-34	97	87	52
35 and up	97	88	44
	mean DMF teeth per man		
17-24	13.2	7.6	3.5
25-34	14.8	7.0	2.4
35 and up	15.0	6.5	1.3

in caries experience; Group II men, intermediate; and Group III men, lowest—whether the count had been based on the numbers of men with caries experience (one or more decayed, missing, or filled permanent teeth) or the count of DMF teeth.[57] This relation between the number of persons with caries experience and the average number of DMF teeth per person is so exact that, given a sample large enough, the one can be estimated from the other with a considerable degree of precision.

However, with caries prevalence as high as in Group II Eskimos, or higher, very large numbers of people must be examined to establish a valid DMF arithmetic average by estimation from the total with one or more DMF teeth. When this average is needed in such a case, it is usually easier and simpler to make the direct count of DMF teeth for each man. In most instances a smaller sample will suffice when the required count is made directly, rather than inferred from a count of some other characteristic. To show that there was a statistically significant difference in caries experience between the Group I and Group II men aged 17 to 24 years described in Table 1, for example, it would have been necessary to examine about 10 times as many men if the percentage of men with one or more DMF teeth had been selected as the index, than would have been needed for a contrast based on the average number of DMF teeth per man. This may not be an important consideration when the numbers available for examination are unlimited, as inspection of persons for the percentage index can be made swiftly with the tongue blade. Counts of DMF teeth are usually made with mirror and explorer.

These counts describe a single phenomenon—the initial attack of caries per person or per tooth. A count of tooth surfaces is complicated by an additional factor: once initiated anywhere, the lesion of caries will progress until all surfaces are involved and the entire crown is destroyed unless treatment intervenes. Surface counts, hence, reflect two dissimilar phenomena: (a) the intensity of caries attack, and (b) the result of treatment or neglect of care. This fact sometimes creates a difficulty in interpretation when two populations with unlike levels of professional care are compared. Nevertheless, in practice in the United States, the actual behavior of the DMF tooth and surface indices is not as different as this theoretical consideration might lead one to believe. Just as the mean number of DMF teeth can be computed from the proportion of persons in a population with one or more DMF teeth, the average number of DMF tooth surfaces in American children can be computed from the average number of DMF teeth.[38] A typical example is shown in Table 2. This table shows data from a clinical trial during which mirror and bitewing examinations were made for 162 children in a control and 165 children in a study group at the outset of the trial and after six, 12, 18, 24, and 36 months.[48] At each examination, counts were made of the numbers of DMF teeth and DMF surfaces. Also shown in the table are the numbers of DMF surfaces estimated from the numbers of DMF teeth by Knutson's formula.[38] In seven of the 12 comparisons the estimated mean for DMF surfaces differs from the mean based on actual count by less than one percent; in 10 of the 12 cases, by less than two percent. The greatest difference in the whole array is 4.8 percent. About the same quantitative estimates would have resulted, in brief, if DMF surfaces had not been counted at all.

This illustration indicates that the various indices of dental caries, which are simply various ways of estimating the same phenomenon, are highly interrelated. It should not be construed as an argument that it is never necessary to examine for DMF surfaces. The DMF surface increment frequently is the crucial phenomenon under investigation. In the instance just discussed the study had been designed to stand or fall on differences in the increment of DMF surfaces between study and control groups. As a general rule in study design, a valid conclusion can be reached with smaller samples when the crucial phenomenon is observed directly, rather than inferred from

TABLE 2. OBSERVED AND ESTIMATED MEAN NUMBERS OF DMF TOOTH SURFACES IN A TYPICAL CLINICAL TRIAL

TIME OF EXAMINATION	MEAN NUMBERS OF DMF TEETH CONTROL	STUDY	MEAN NUMBERS OF DMF TOOTH SURFACES OBSERVED CONTROL	STUDY	ESTIMATED* CONTROL	STUDY
At outset	6.62	6.64	11.82	11.55	12.08	12.11
After 6 months	7.64	7.24	13.95	13.13	14.04	13.27
After 12 months	8.32	7.79	15.28	14.18	15.35	14.33
After 18 months	9.34	8.39	17.22	15.46	17.32	15.49
After 24 months	10.09	9.14	18.92	16.95	18.77	16.93
After 36 months	11.79	10.66	22.27	19.83	22.04	19.87

*From Knutson's general formula ($y = .19282 \times -.6889$)[38]

another measurement. There is always some error involved when one thing is estimated from another. The same degree of error may be a tiny and inconsequential fraction of the lifetime accumulation of signs such as DMF tooth surfaces, but dangerously large in proportion to the smaller accumulation of DMF tooth surfaces over the short span of the trial. It is sometimes difficult to determine the statistical validity of differences revealed in this indirect fashion. But the example serves as an excellent illustration of the close interdependence of all the cumulative indices of dental caries experience in the permanent teeth.

Where close comparability between several examiners over a considerable time is required, somewhat better agreement can be had with DMF teeth than with DMF surfaces; but reliable and reproducible data cannot be assumed with either index unless examiners have had a period of preexamination training and calibration with each other.[11]

The def index is applied to the deciduous dentition in somewhat the same manner as the DMF index is used in permanent teeth. The letter *d* stands for decayed; *e*, only for extraction indicated because of caries; and *f* for filled; lowercase letters (that is, not capital letters) are used to indicate that the index refers to deciduous teeth.[32] Because the *d* and *e* components of the def index both refer to a carious deciduous tooth, the two categories are sometimes combined into one, indicated by *d*, and reported in terms of *df* teeth or tooth surfaces per child. Missing primary teeth are ignored in this index, because of the uncertainty in determining whether they were extracted because of an attack of caries or exfoliated normally. As a result, a population of children which has received widespread extractions because of dental caries may actually show a lower def average, particularly at the age of seven years or older, than children in another population with fewer carious lesions in primary teeth, but with fewer teeth lost before the normal exfoliation time. This effect can be minimized if use of the def index is restricted to children six or seven years old or younger. Caries prevalence in the primary teeth of older children has been expressed as the mean number of decayed, missing, or filled deciduous molars and cuspids per child, ordinarily described as the dmf index. A deciduous molar or cuspid is presumed to have been lost to caries if it is missing prior to its normal time of exfoliation. This index is useful in groups of children through the ages of 11 or 12 years.[47]

At present there is no morbidity measure for dental caries—that is, no direct method of determining whether or not caries is presently active in a given mouth. Presumptive evidence, from tests for acid-producing potential, has sometimes been considered in epidemiological study. If an unequivocal morbidity measure could be developed, the long term of observation now required for the caries clinical trial might be shortened to weeks or days. All of the measures now in use require the exercise of skilled professional judgment. This judgment can be disciplined (calibrated) through direct training to the point where a team of examiners can return data with negligible between-examiner differences.[11, 54] The evidence is just as conclusive that untrained examiners almost always differ, often to an extreme degree. It follows that quantitative comparisons of data developed in uncoordinated studies are apt to be misleading, even though the same index and apparent method of examination were employed by both teams of examiners.

A true morbidity index for dental caries might evolve from current research in the area of microbiology. If it could be demonstrated that dental caries can occur only in the presence of some specific microorganism or strain of microorganisms, such a measure would follow inevitably. It is clear from studies of germ-free and mono-infected laboratory animals that dental caries is a bacterial disease. So far, the characteristics of the cariogenic oral flora have not been described with sufficient precision to permit their estimation in a practicable study of large numbers of persons living in their usual homes and following their ordinary ways of life.

Indices of Periodontal Disease. Gordon's principle of "the biologic gradient of disease" is even more important in population estimates of periodontal disease status than in estimates of dental caries. The line of demarcation between normal tissue and tissue with the periodontal lesion is more difficult to define and hence much more difficult to judge. Comparability between examiners and comparability throughout a whole series of examinations conducted by a single examiner are much more difficult to achieve and to maintain.

As noted in the preceding section, all field indices ordinarily used to estimate dental caries measure irreversible and cumulative effects. Indices of both reversible and irreversible effects have been devised for the study of the periodontal diseases. Still other periodontal indices are combinations of the two methods.[68]

The unequivocal end result of chronic destructive periodontal disease is loss of alveolar bone. This loss, to all intents and purposes, is irreversible. Most early epidemiological study of the periodontal diseases was based on x-ray surveys of alveolar bone loss, and this method is still extremely useful. Accurate readings of bone loss, as a proportion of root length, can be facilitated through use of the measuring scale devised by Schei, Waerhaug, Lövdal, and Arno.[61] When population rather than individual data are required, a useful estimate of bone loss in a group can be based on the average percentage of teeth per person with gingival recession exposing the cementoenamel junction.[64] Sandler and Stahl have presented findings which may be interpreted as indicating that the average bone score by x-ray used in a study of a hospital population could have been estimated from mean recession scores for the same men about as accurately as mean DMF surfaces can be estimated from mean DMF teeth.[59]

Since bone loss is a relatively late development in destructive disease, these cumulative measures are not very discriminatory in young persons, and a long time span is required for demonstration of a change for the better (following successful treatment, for example). For these reasons several morbidity measures—reversible indices with scores which can diminish as the tissues improve—have been developed.

One reversible index is the PMA index of gingivitis. It is based on the concept that the extent of inflammation serves as an indicator of the severity of the affection. The presence or absence of inflammation is recorded in the papillary tip (P), the marginal (M), or the attached (A) areas of the gingiva around all or part of the teeth in the mouth. Relative severity of inflammation may be scored for each area.[42] Scores have been computed in several ways, some based on the most extreme finding for an area or quadrant. Criteria require positive scoring for any deviation from a stringently defined ideal condition of the tissues, and between-examiner comparability is sometimes difficult to achieve. The index seems most useful in the single-examiner study of gingivitis where it is important to distinguish between the ideal condition and incipient inflammation.

Another index of gingivitis which has gained considerable acceptance is based on the severity of inflammation rather than its extent. This is the Gingival Index (GI) of Löe.[40] Criteria for this estimation are shown in Table 3. These criteria set up clean-cut distinctions between the presence or absence of gingivitis and, if gingivitis is present, the tendency to bleed under several types of examination. Like PMA, GI is an estimate of gingivitis alone and takes no account of deeper periodontal deterioration.

The Periodontal Index (PI) represents an estimate of deeper disease. Each tooth in the mouth is classified on a weighted scale ranging from zero through eight, depending upon freedom from disease, or inflammation, or pocket formation, or ultimate loss of function. The individual's score is the average for the teeth in his mouth. Populations may be divided into groups of persons with or without overt inflammation, or pathological pocket formation, or teeth with too little supporting tissue for efficient function.[53] This index is most useful when it is necessary to distinguish between populations

TABLE 3. CRITERIA FOR THE GINGIVAL INDEX*

0 = Normal gingiva.
1 = Mild inflammation—slight change in color, slight edema. *No bleeding on probing.*
2 = Moderate inflammation—redness, edema, and glazing. *Bleeding on probing.*
3 = Severe inflammation—marked redness and edema. Ulceration. *Tendency to spontaneous bleeding.*

*Löe.[40]

with mild, moderate, and advanced chronic destructive disease. Most of the determinative epidemiological studies (outlined in Chapter Six) made use of the Periodontal Index. Criteria for the Periodontal Index are shown in Table 4. PI is not designed for diagnosis of the individual patient, but there is a general correspondence between the clinical status of a group of persons and the average PI score for the group. Most persons judged to be negative for periodontal disease, for example, have PI scores in the neighborhood of zero or 0.1 or 0.2; most individuals in the terminal stages of disease have scores approaching the upper limit of the scale, 8.0. A summary of the relation between clinical conditions and group PI scores is shown in Table 5.[53]

One of the measures utilizing both reversible and irreversible signs is the Ramfjord Periodontal Disease Index (PDI). Six specified teeth are examined in each mouth: the maxillary right first molar, the maxillary left central incisor, the maxillary left first bicuspid, the mandibular left first molar, the mandibular right central incisor, and the mandibular right first bicuspid. The gingiva surrounding each tooth is scored on a scale running from zero through three. A score of zero indicates absence of signs of inflammation. Scores of one, two, and three are used where there is mild, moderate, or severe gingivitis, respectively. These estimates, being estimates of inflammation, represent a reversible condition. The gingival crevices on the mesial and buccal area of each of the assigned teeth are then probed with a #0 Michigan probe. When the gingival crevice is found to be apical to the cementoenamel junction, the inflammatory condition is ignored, and a score of four, five, or six is assigned, depending upon the distance from the cementoenamel junction to the bottom of the crevice.[52] To all intents and purposes, this is an irreversible measurement. The bottom of the crevice and the height of the adjacent alveolar bone are closely correlated, and bone, once lost, is virtually never restored. There is

TABLE 4. SCORING AND CRITERIA FOR THE PERIODONTAL INDEX[*]

SCORE	CRITERIA
0	*Negative.* There is neither overt inflammation in the investing tissues nor loss of function due to destruction of supporting tissue.
1	*Mild gingivitis.* There is an overt area of inflammation in the free gingivae, but this area does not circumscribe the tooth.
2	*Gingivitis.* Inflammation completely circumscribes the tooth, but there is no apparent break in the epithelial attachment.
6	*Gingivitis with pocket formation.* The epithelial attachment has been broken and there is a pocket (not merely a deepened gingival crevice due to swelling in the free gingivae). There is no interference with normal masticatory function, the tooth is firm in its socket, and has not drifted.
8	*Advanced destruction with loss of masticatory function.* The tooth may be loose; may have drifted; may sound dull on percussion with a metallic instrument; may be depressible in its socket.

[*]Russell.[53]

TABLE 5. RELATION BETWEEN PI SCORES AND
CLINICAL CONDITIONS*

MOST PEOPLE WITH	SCORE IN THE RANGE OF
Clinically normal tissues	0-0.2
Gingivitis	0.1-1.0
Incipient destructive disease	0.5-1.9
Established destructive disease	1.5-5.0
Terminal stages of disease	4.0-8.0

*Russell.[53]

evidence that this measurement is as useful as radiographs in estimating the degree of alveolar bone loss.[37]

An adaptation of the Ramfjord index, known as the Gingival-Periodontal Index (GPI), has been used by O'Leary in screening Air Force personnel to determine which are in need of periodontal treatment. All of the teeth in the mouth are probed, and the highest gingival score or crevice depth for any tooth in each of six segments in the mouth is taken as the score for that segment.[49]

It has been learned by experience that periodontal data, expressed in whatever index, are usually not particularly meaningful unless the state of oral hygiene is taken into account. An index of oral hygiene which has had wide usage in field surveys of periodontal disease is the Simplified Oral Hygiene Index (OHI-S), originated by Greene and Vermillion.[30,31] This index provides a systematic assessment of debris and calculus and has been particularly useful in studying the relation between periodontitis and oral cleanliness. It is applied to six tooth surfaces in the mouth—four posterior and two anterior. The posterior surfaces are located on the first fully erupted tooth distal to the second bicuspid on each side of each arch. The buccal surfaces of the selected upper molars and the lingual surfaces of the lower molars are examined. In the anterior segments, the labial surfaces of the upper right central incisor and the lower left central incisor are appraised. In the absence of either of these anterior teeth, the incisor on the opposite side of the midline is scored. Only fully erupted permanent teeth are included. The scoring system for OHI-S is shown in Table 6.[31]

The score for the individual is the average score for the surfaces examined in his mouth. In general, when applied to children, debris index scores of zero to 0.6 are considered to be good; scores in the range of 0.7 to 1.8, fair; and scores in the range of 1.9 to 3.0, poor. Corresponding ranges for the complete OHI-S score (the sum of the debris and calculus scores) are 0.0 to 1.2, good; 1.3 to 3.0, fair; and 3.1 to 6.0, the highest possible score, poor.

The indices described above were discussed by their originators and demonstrated with clinical patients during the course of a conference on clinical methods in periodontal diseases, held in 1967

TABLE 6. CRITERIA AND SCORING FOR THE OHI-S*

DEBRIS SCORE	CALCULUS SCORE
0 = No debris nor stain present. 1 = Soft debris covering not more than one third of the tooth surface being examined or the presence of extrinsic stains without debris regardless of surface area covered. 2 = Soft debris covering more than one third but not more than two thirds of the exposed tooth surface. 3 = Soft debris covering more than two thirds of the exposed tooth surface.	0 = No calculus present. 1 = Supragingival calculus covering not more than one third of the exposed tooth surface being examined. 2 = Supragingival calculus covering more than one third but not more than two thirds of the exposed tooth surface, or the presence of individual flecks of subgingival calculus around the cervical portion of the tooth. 3 = Supragingival calculus covering more than two thirds of the exposed tooth surface or a continuous band of subgingival calculus around the cervical portion of the tooth.

*Greene and Vermillion.[31]

at the University of Pennsylvania School of Dental Medicine.[9] A series of patients had been selected for the demonstration on the basis of a prior examination in the school's clinic. There were 17 individuals with some evidence of gingival inflammation but without evidence of pocket formation or apical migration of the gingival margin and with neither horizontal nor vertical bone loss on radiographic examination. Each of a second group of 38 individuals had suffered periodontal bone loss as characterized by periodontal pockets with apical migration of the gingival margin, with or without radiographic evidence of bone loss. In short, none of the individuals examined in the demonstration was in an intermediate stage — each exhibited essentially normal periodontal tissues or definite and advanced destructive disease. All of these patients were examined by each examiner. The respective scores within each of the indices, for these two groups of patients, are summarized in Table 7.[62]

The two gingivitis scores, PMA and GI, which were not intended to be measurements of deep disease, made relatively little distinction between the patients with simple gingivitis and those with deeper destructive disease. Each of the three estimates of deeper disease processes — PI, PDI, and GPI — made a clean distinction between the gingivitis group and the periodontitis group, with the sharpest differentiation following the use of PI. Oral Hygiene Index scores (OHI-S) were significantly lower in patients with simple gingivitis, compared with those with one or more periodontal pockets.

Most of the population findings for periodontal disease, to be discussed in a later chapter, have been obtained through use of a com-

TABLE 7. RELATIVE STATES, AS SCORED BY SEVERAL INDICES, OF PATIENTS WITH GINGIVITIS† OR WITH PERIODONTITIS* EXAMINED AT THE PENNSYLVANIA CONFERENCE ON CLINICAL METHODS IN PERIODONTAL DISEASE, 1967**

		MEAN SCORES FOR	
INDEX	EXAMINER	17 PATIENTS WITH GINGIVITIS†	38 PATIENTS WITH PERIODONTITIS*
PMA	Massler	18.00	22.71
GI	Löe	0.75	1.01
PI	Russell	0.07	1.01
PDI	Ramfjord	1.15	3.15
GPI	O'Leary	1.71	3.89
OHI-S	Greene	1.81	2.72

†Patients with evidence of gingival inflammation but without evidence of pocket formation, apical migration of the gingival margin, and with neither horizontal nor vertical bone loss on radiographic examination.
*Patients with periodontal bone loss, characterized by periodontal pockets and/or apical migration of the gingival margin, with or without radiographic evidence of bone loss.
**Ship, Cohen, and Laster.[62]

bination of the Periodontal Index (PI) and the Oral Hygiene Index (OHI-S).

Still other periodontal indices have been suggested. The Gingival Bone Count (GB) of Dunning and Leach is a whole-mouth index which differentiates between gingivitis (measured on a subjective scale of zero to three) and bone loss (measured in quarters of root length on a scale of zero to five). Scores for each characteristic are averaged for all teeth present in the mouth, and the two averages are then combined to give a GB count for the case. Various methods of examination can be used to assemble the data.[25, 26] The Periodontal Disease Rate (PDR) of Sandler and Stahl is analyzed and reported as the average percent of teeth per person showing a positive sign of periodontal disease.[60]

Similarly, there are other methods for the estimation of oral hygiene. Löe uses a system for scoring plaque which emphasizes its occurrence in the area adjacent to the gingival margin. Criteria for this method of scoring are shown in Table 8.[40] Ramfjord scores both plaque and calculus on a scale of zero through three, corresponding to absence of plaque or calculus and its presence in small, moderate, or large amounts.[52] Several systems for scoring of the accumulation of supragingival calculus, usually on the six mandibular incisor and cuspid teeth, have been proposed for use in clinical trials of a possible calculus-inhibitory agent.

In most population studies, much the same conclusions will be drawn whether a reversible or a cumulative index is used to estimate chronic destructive disease. The population with the highest preva-

TABLE 8. CRITERIA FOR THE PLAQUE INDEX OF LOE*

0 = No plaque in the gingival area.
1 = A film of plaque adhering to the free gingival margin and adjacent area of the tooth. The plaque may only be recognized by running a probe across the tooth surface.
2 = Moderate accumulation of soft deposits within the gingival pocket, on the gingival margin and/or adjacent tooth surface, which can be seen by the naked eye.
3 = Abundance of soft matter within the gingival pocket and/or on the margin and adjacent tooth surface.

*Löe.[40]

lence of present and active disease is quite apt to show a comparable degree of accumulated bone loss. As with dental caries, the appropriate index is one which most nearly defines the actual phenomenon the observer wishes to study, yet is practical for the study situation. Similarly, quantitative comparisons of data developed by independent observers should be avoided.

Indices for Other Conditions. Another index which has been widely used is the community fluorosis index originated by Dean. Individual teeth are classified as normal (a category including those with any of the many enamel opacities due to causes other than fluoride ingestion), or as exhibiting questionable, very mild, mild, moderate, or severe fluorosis. Each person's status is determined by the two teeth showing the most advanced stages. A weighted scale running from zero through four is utilized in scoring. The community score is the average of the individual scores for the persons examined. In the continental United States, at least, mean community scores as well as distributions of scores within the community are directly proportional to the level of fluorides in the community water supply. The index was not designed to represent cosmetic values. However, in the series of studies carried out by Dean and his associates, disfiguring mottling was not observed in communities with an index of 0.4 or lower.[15]

Population indices of occlusion have proved to be extremely difficult to develop. Draker's HLD index is based on need for treatment of oral handicapping conditions, including clefts as well as malpositions of the teeth.[7, 23, 24] The OFI developed by Poulton and Aaronson and the Malalignment Index of Van Kirk and Pennell refer to deviations from desirable positions of teeth within the arch.[50, 66] The concept that malocclusion is not one simple condition but rather a series of distinct though related conditions is embodied in a method of assessment proposed by Grainger[51] and modified by Summers.[65]

Field Modifications. At the present time, the World Health Organization is experimenting with some of these indices in the hope that examinations may be carried out with greater ease and rapidity, under primitive field conditions, by relatively unskilled personnel, and without the necessity for sterilization of examination instruments. To these ends examinations for dental caries, periodontal diseases, and oral hygiene are made with the wooden tongue blade. With this technic the examiner's hands are not contaminated, and the examination instrument itself can be discarded or destroyed. For dental caries, the individual patient is classified as having no obvious lesions; or as having lesions of caries in pits and fissures; or in the posterior interproximal areas; or in the upper anterior interproximal areas; or in labial surfaces; or in the lower interproximal areas. This pattern of progression is based upon the relative susceptibility of different tooth types and surfaces.[35] With this method of examination, population contrasts depend upon the proportions of persons classified in each of these stages of disease, rather than an average score.

The PI examination is made according to the same criteria as those followed when mirror and explorer are used, except that mobility is judged by prodding with the end of the wooden tongue blade. The Simplified Oral Hygiene Index (OHI-S) is also estimated by visual means alone, which obviates an estimate of subgingival calculus. The practicability and validity of these modified methods are presently being tested in a number of populations throughout the world.

THE CLINICAL TRIAL

As noted at the outset of this chapter, epidemiological study may consist basically of simple observation of a phenomenon without any attempt to modify it or control its end results, or it may take the form of an experiment in which an agent under study is applied to a definite sample of people under controlled circumstances. Most of the discussion to this point has been couched in terms of the observational study, sometimes termed field epidemiology. The field study is used to uncover and validate relations between one factor and another; the clinical trial is used to determine whether a known or suspected relation is one of cause and effect. There are some essential differences between the two methods of study, despite the facts that similar indices and methods may be employed and that both are concerned with human beings.

It is helpful to discuss the clinical trial in terms of tests of caries-preventive agents, because much work and experience in this area have led to the formulation of standard rules for the design and conduct of such tests.[1, 28, 55]

The basic procedure in the field study is the comparison of findings from studies of two or more independent populations. Comparison is likewise the fundamental objective in the clinical trial, but the comparison here is between two or more segments of a *single* population, theoretically divided in such a way as to be essentially similar in all pertinent characteristics but one—the use or avoidance of the agent under test. Most trials of potential caries-inhibitory agents are carried out with children young enough that the caries process is relatively active. It is clearly necessary to have equal numbers of boys and girls of equivalent ages in the study group and in the control group, but similarity in these two respects is not enough; the groups should be alike in all other characteristics which might affect caries activity. Some of these characteristics are known, but it is suspected that others exist which have not yet been identified. In this type of situation it is impossible to determine with certainty whether the groups are truly equivalent in *all* pertinent factors. To resolve this problem the clinical trial designer resorts to random (not to be confused with haphazard) assignment of children to study and control groups. When carried out properly and thoroughly, randomization sets up favorable odds that study and control groups are as alike as need be in all factors, known or unknown, pertinent or not.

The principle of random assignment is simple; the allotment procedure should be such that each child has an equal chance of being assigned to the study or to the control group. In practice the procedure may be intricate and delicate; it should be left in the hands of a capable statistician. In caries trials the usual method has been to match children for two or three factors of known importance—age, sex, previous caries experience, teeth in eruption, lactobacillus counts, or the like—and then, within each set of children so matched, assign individuals to study and control groups by random means. The sample is built in this way until adequate numbers have been brought into the study. Sample size is another matter which must be determined by the statistician. In general the more effective the agent, the more uniform the individual response, and the longer the period of trial, the smaller the sample may be. The sample must be adequate to ensure that an observed effect is not due to chance, and to ensure that an effective agent will actually be demonstrated as effective.

If a capable statistician is essential to the clinical trial team, the examiner is vital. His role is even more exacting than that of the field-study examiner. In the typical field-study situation, the lesions to be recognized have developed over a relatively long period of risk—most of the lifetime of the individual—so that most of them have become so large and obvious that detection is simple, and comparability in examination is relatively easy to achieve. In the clinical trial the examiner must detect and count lesions which have developed over a relatively short period of time. This requirement forces him to hunt for and count lesions of caries in an early stage of development—at the cost of increased random error in classification of the marginal or doubtful lesion. In the present state of the art, this component of error—reversals in diagnosis—is unavoidable if the length of the trial is to be kept within a practicable span of time. Most tests of caries-inhibitory agents are based on the numbers of new decayed, missing, or filled tooth surfaces which appear during the span of the trial. Because new lesions on proximal surfaces may be detected more quickly with radiography than with visual and tactile examination alone, bitewing films are almost always taken as part of the examination procedure. The true function of the films is not so much to find more lesions as it is to find them at an earlier stage, and hence shorten the time necessary for the trial.

Despite these efforts to shorten the span, an adequate clinical trial of a caries-inhibitory agent requires a considerable length of time. The participants in a workshop convened by the American Dental Association to develop uniform standards and procedures in clinical studies of dental caries recommended a minimum span of two years.[1, 55] The Commission on Classification and Statistics for Oral Conditions of the *Fédération Dentaire Internationale* set up an even more stringent standard:

> When a clinical trial is designed to study the effect of an agent on the prevention of dental caries, a duration of at least three years is necessary to demonstrate a positive effect. These should be regarded as minimal requirements and the results, if favourable, should be regarded not as proving the efficacy of the agent but as indicating the desirability of further long term trials.[28]

Such trials are analyzed by contrasting the caries experience of the control group—the group receiving no treatment or an inert placebo—with the caries experience of the group or groups receiving the agent under test. The difference in caries experience should be statistically significant, and the observer is under the obligation of showing that the difference was due to the influence of the agent under test, and not to some fault in the design and conduct of the study. The difference should be great enough to have clinical as well as statistical significance.

Time is often of lesser importance in trials of therapeutic agents designed for the prevention or treatment of oral conditions other than dental caries. The caries trial is evaluated on the basis of the end product of the disease process—the loss of tooth substance—rather than upon the disease process itself. Cavitation is a slowly developing and irreversible condition and must be appraised with a cumulative and irreversible index. With many conditions other than dental caries, however, the actual mechanisms of disease may be observed more directly and appraised through the use of reversible indices—a change for better or worse can frequently be detected with little delay. A span of eight weeks was ample, for example, to determine the effect of an enzyme chewing gum on the formation of supragingival calculus in human subjects,[27] and a span of 35 days to demonstrate the effect of oral hygiene practices on gingivitis in Norwegian army recruits.[6] With the exception of the time factor, however, trials in areas other than dental caries follow the same philosophy and design. Even in these areas it is sometimes necessary to prolong study until some unequivocal end result—such as the loss of alveolar bone in periodontal disease—can be observed and evaluated.

The material in this chapter is not intended to be an instruction manual for persons who wish to employ these indices and procedures in actual practice. Any individual with these objectives should study the original descriptions and reports cited in this chapter and gain some experience under an experienced investigator before forging out on his own. The intent, rather, has been to equip the reader of scientific literature with some basic tools for evaluation. The subject of discriminatory reading will be considered in detail in the following chapter.

BIBLIOGRAPHY

1. American Dental Association, Councils on Dental Therapeutics, Dental Research, and Dental Health. Clinical testing of dental caries preventives. Chicago, American Dental Association, c1955. 67 p.
2. Ast, D. B. The caries-fluorine hypothesis and a suggested study to test its application. Pub. Health Rep., 58:857-79, June 4, 1943.
3. Ast, D. B., Finn, S. B., and McCaffrey, Isabel. The Newburgh-Kingston caries fluorine study. I. Dental findings after three years of water fluoridation. Am. J. Pub. Health, 40:716-24, June 1950.
4. Ast, D. B., and Fitzgerald, Bernadette. Effectiveness of water fluoridation. Am. Dent. A. J., 65:581-8, Nov. 1962.
5. Blayney, J. R., and Tucker, W. H. The Evanston dental caries study. J. Dent. Res., 27:279-86, June 1948.
6. Brandtzaeg, Per. The significance of oral hygiene in the prevention of dental diseases. Odont. Tskr., 72:460-6, Dec. 1964.
7. Carlos, J. P., and Ast, D. B. An evaluation of the HLD index as a decision-making tool. Pub. Health Rep., 81:621-6, July 1966.
8. Churchill, H. V. Occurrence of fluorides in some waters of the United States. J. Ind. and Eng. Chem., 23:996-8, Apr. 10, 1931.
9. Conference on Clinical Methods in Periodontal Diseases. J. Periodont., 38:580-795, Nov.-Dec. 1967.
10. Connecticut State Dental Society, Tumor Committee. Cancer, a handbook for dentists. Hartford, Connecticut State Dental Society, 1948. VI + 52 p.
11. Davies, G. N., and Cadell, P. B. Four investigations to determine the reliability of caries-recording methods. Arch. Oral Biol., 8:331-48, May-June 1963.
12. Dean, H. T. Distribution of mottled enamel in the United States. Pub. Health Rep., 48:703-34, June 23, 1933.
13. ———. Endemic fluorosis and its relation to dental caries. Pub. Health Rep., 53:1443-52, Aug. 19, 1938.
14. ———. Epidemiological studies in the United States. p. 5-31. (In Moulton, F. R., ed. Dental caries and fluorine. Washington, American Association Advancement Science, 1946. 111 p.)
15. ———. The investigation of physiological effects by the epidemiological method. p. 23-31. (In Moulton, F. R., ed. Fluorine and dental health. Washington, American Association Advancement Science, 1942. 101 p.)
16. Dean, H. T., Arnold, F. A., Jr., and Elvove, Elias. Domestic water and dental caries. V. Additional studies of the relation of fluoride domestic waters to dental caries experience in 4,425 white children, aged 12 to 14 years, of 13 cities in 4 states. Pub. Health Rep., 57:1155-79, Aug. 7, 1942.
17. Dean, H. T., and Elvove, Elias. Some epidemiological aspects of chronic endemic dental fluorosis. Am. J. Pub. Health, 26:567-75, June 1936.

18. Dean, H. T., Elvove, Elias, and Poston, R. F. Mottled enamel in South Dakota. Pub. Health Rep., 54:212-28, Feb. 10, 1939.
19. Dean, H. T., et al. Domestic water and dental caries. II. A study of 2,832 white children, aged 12-14 years, of 8 suburban Chicago communities, including *Lactobacillus acidophilus* studies of 1,761 children. Pub. Health Rep., 56:761-92, Apr. 11, 1941.
20. Dean, H. T., et al. Domestic water and dental caries, including certain epidemiological aspects of oral *L. acidophilus*. Pub. Health Rep., 54:862-88, May 26, 1939.
21. Dean, H. T., et al. Studies on mass control of dental caries through fluoridation of the public water supply. Pub. Health Rep., 65:1403-8, Oct. 27, 1950.
22. Dorn, H. F. Illness from cancer in the United States. Pub. Health Rep., 59:33-48, Jan. 14; 59:65-77, Jan. 21; 59:97-115, Jan. 28, 1944.
23. Draker, H. L. Handicapping labio-lingual deviations: a proposed index for public health purposes. Am. A. Pub. Health Dent. Bul., 18:1-7, Dec. 1958.
24. Draker, H. L., and Allaway, Norman. HLD index of handicapping labio-lingual deviations. Part II. Distribution of index components in two New York state population groups. Pub. Health Dent., 20:67-76, Fall 1960.
25. Dunning, J. M., and Leach, L. B. Gingival-bone count: a method for epidemiological study of periodontal diseases. J. Dent. Res., 39:506-13, May-June 1960.
26. ———. Variations in the measurement of periodontal disease with use of radiographs. Abstr. Internat. A. Dent. Res., 46:73, Mar. 1968.
27. Ennever, J., and Sturzenberger, O. P. Inhibition of dental calculus formation by use of an enzyme chewing gum. J. Periodont., 32:331-3, Oct. 1961.
28. Fédération Dentaire Internationale, Commission on Classification and Statistics for Oral Conditions. Principal requirements for controlled clinical trials. Internat. Dent. J., 17:93-103, Mar. 1967.
29. Gordon, J. E. Dental problems in an epidemiological perspective. Am. J. Pub. Health, 49:1041-9, Aug. 1959.
30. Greene, J. C., and Vermillion, J. R. The oral hygiene index: a method for classifying oral hygiene status. Am. Dent. A. J., 61:172-9, Aug. 1960.
31. ———. The simplified oral hygiene index. Am. Dent. A. J., 68:7-13, Jan. 1964.
32. Gruebbel, A. O. A measurement of dental caries prevalence and treatment service for deciduous teeth. J. Dent. Res., 23:163-8, June 1944.
33. Hollander, Franklin, and Dunning, J. M. A study by age and sex of the incidence of dental caries in over 12,000 persons. J. Dent. Res., 18:43-60, Feb. 1939.
34. Hutton, W. L., Linscott, B. W., and Williams, D. B. The Brantford fluorine experiment. Interim report after five years of water fluoridation. Canad. J. Pub. Health, 42:81-7, Mar. 1951.
35. Klein, Henry, and Palmer, C. E. Studies on dental caries. XII. Comparison of caries susceptibility of various morphological types of permanent teeth. J. Dent. Res., 20:203-16, June 1941.
36. Klein, Henry, Palmer, C. E., and Knutson, J. W. Studies on dental caries. I. Dental status and dental needs of elementary school children. Pub. Health Rep., 53:751-65, May 13, 1938.
37. Knowles, J. W. Estimators of periodontal disease. Abstr. Internat. A. Dent. Res., 46:78, Mar. 1968.
38. Knutson, J. W. Epidemiological trend patterns of dental caries prevalence data. Am. Dent. A. J., 57:821-9, Dec. 1958.
39. Littleton, N. W. Dental caries and periodontal diseases among Ethiopian civilians. Pub. Health Rep., 78:631-40, July 1963.
40. Löe, Harald. The gingival index, the plaque index and the retention index systems. J. Periodont., 38:610-6, Nov.-Dec. 1967.
41. Marshall-Day, C. D., Stephens, R. G., and Quigley, L. F., Jr. Periodontal disease: prevalence and incidence. J. Periodont., 26:185-203, July 1955.
42. Massler, Maury, Schour, Isaac, and Chopra, Baldev. Occurrence of gingivitis in suburban Chicago school children. J. Periodont., 21:146-64, 196, July 1950.
43. McKay, F. S. Mass control of dental caries through the use of domestic water supplies containing fluorine. Am. J. Pub. Health, 38:828-32, June 1948.
44. ———. Mottled enamel: early history and its unique features. p. 1-5. (In Moulton, F. R., ed. Fluorine and dental health. Washington, American Association Advancement Science, 1942. 101 p.)

45. McKay, F. S. Mottled enamel: the prevention of its further production through a change of water supply at Oakley, Idaho. Am. Dent. A. J., 20:1137-49, July 1933.
46. ———. The relation of mottled enamel to caries. Am. Dent. A. J., 15:1429-37, Aug. 1928.
47. Ministry of Health, Scottish Office, and the Ministry of Housing and Local Government. The conduct of the fluoridation studies in the United Kingdom and the results achieved after five years. London, H. M. Stationery Office, 1962. III + 50 p.
48. Muhler, J. C. Effect of a stannous fluoride dentifrice on caries reduction in children during a three-year study period. Am. Dent. A. J., 64:216-24, Feb. 1962.
49. O'Leary, Timothy. The periodontal screening examination. J. Periodont., 38:617-24, Nov.-Dec. 1967.
50. Poulton, D. R., and Aaronson, S. A. The relationship between occlusion and periodontal status. Am. J. Orthodont., 47:690-9, Sept. 1961.
51. Public Health Service, National Center for Health Statistics. Orthodontic treatment priority index. Series 2, No. 25. Washington, Government Printing Office, 1967. VI + 49 p.
52. Ramfjord, S. P. The periodontal disease index (PDI). J. Periodont., 38:602-10, Nov.-Dec. 1967.
53. Russell, A. L. A system of classification and scoring for prevalence surveys of periodontal disease. J. Dent. Res., 35:350-9, June 1956.
54. ———. An appraisal of the value of indices proposed as epidemiologic aids in the practice of dental public health. p. 61-75. (In Easlick, K. A., ed. The practice of dental public health. Rev. ed. Ann Arbor, University Michigan School Public Health, 1960. 198 p.)
55. ———. Clinical testing of dental caries preventives: a summary. Am. Dent. A. J., 54:275-83, Feb. 1957.
56. ———. Dental fluorosis in Grand Rapids during the seventeenth year of fluoridation. Am. Dent. A. J., 65:608-12, Nov. 1962.
57. Russell, A. L., Consolazio, C. F., and White, C. L. Dental caries and nutrition in Eskimo scouts of the Alaska National Guard. J. Dent. Res., 40:594-603, May-June 1961.
58. Russell, A. L., and Elvove, Elias. Domestic water and dental caries. VII. A study of the fluoride-dental caries relationship in an adult population. Pub. Health Rep., 66:1389-1401, Oct. 26, 1951.
59. Sandler, H. C., and Stahl, S. S. The influence of generalized diseases on clinical manifestations of periodontal disease. Am. Dent. A. J., 49:656-67, Dec. 1954.
60. ———. Measurement of periodontal disease prevalence. Am. Dent. A. J., 58:93-7, Mar. 1959.
61. Schei, Olav, et al. Alveolar bone loss as related to oral hygiene and age. J. Periodont., 30:7-16, Jan. 1959.
62. Ship, I. I., Cohen, Walter, and Laster, Larry. A study of gingival, periodontal, and oral hygiene examination methods in a single population. J. Periodont., 38:638-45, Nov.-Dec. 1967.
63. Smith, Margaret C., Lantz, Edith M., and Smith, H. V. The cause of mottled enamel, a defect of human teeth. Tucson, University Arizona College Agriculture, 1931. (Technical Bulletin No. 32)
64. Stahl, S. S., and Morris, A. L. Oral health conditions among army personnel at the Army Engineer Center. J. Periodont., 26:180-5, July 1955.
65. Summers, C. J. Some effects of developmental changes on the indices of malocclusion. J. Pub. Health Dent., 26:212-20, Winter 1966.
66. Van Kirk, L. E., and Pennell, E. H. Assessment of malocclusion in population groups. Am. J. Pub. Health, 49:1157-63, Sept. 1959.
67. Velu, H., and Balozet, L. Darmous (dystrophie dentaire) du mouton et solubilité du principe actif des phosphates naturels qui le provique. Bul. Soc. Path. Exot., 24:848-51, Nov. 12, 1931.
68. World Health Organization. Periodontal disease: report of an expert committee on dental health. Geneva, World Health Organization, 1961. 42 p.

CHAPTER 5

THE INTERPRETATION OF DATA AND THE EVALUATION OF SCIENTIFIC LITERATURE

By A. L. RUSSELL, D.D.S., M.P.H.

It is relatively simple to make accurate observations of phenomena and to compile accurate records of data. This is true because rules have been developed for the guidance of investigators, because the understanding of biological processes has been expanded greatly during the past few decades, and because there are many new and useful aids to diagnosis or to classification. A greater difficulty accompanies the attempt to extract the meaning from such observations, be they one's own or someone else's, perhaps, as reported in a scientific journal. Here, too, a set of rules and procedures has been devised and proven by experience for the interpretation of scientific data. Many of these rules may be lumped together under the heading of statistical analysis. No attempt will be made in this section to discuss formulas nor to give directions for the computation of statistical tests. The object here is simply to equip the reader of scientific literature with enough of the bases of statistical reasoning to help him to read with understanding and discrimination.

INTERPRETATION OF DATA

The central fact about epidemiological data (or any biological data, for that matter) is their inherent variability. When littermate animals are given identical doses of a toxic substance, some may survive while others die. If children in the same school are given two dental examinations on successive days, the results will not be exactly the same. Some of the difference will be due to examiner error, which can be minimized but not eliminated. Some further variation will be due to the fact that some children present on the first day will be absent on the second, and some absent on the first day will be present on the second; the two samples, though taken from the same population (or "universe"), are not identical. Whenever two populations appear to differ in some respect, the first requirement of analysis is to determine whether the difference is a true difference, and not the accidental result of sampling error. Such determinations are estimates, based upon statistical analysis. In this context statistics has been defined as a rigorous way of thinking about variable phenomena, and it has been said that analysis is a powerful aid to thought, but not a substitute for it.

Statistical reasoning is employed throughout the progress of a study, beginning with original design. The first determination is the size of the sample required for a valid conclusion. This must always be computed, because there is no single sample size valid under all or even most conditions. When a single population is surveyed, it is necessary to examine enough people to establish the range and character of variation between one person and another, and to establish a finding valid in itself. When two populations are to be compared, enough people must be examined in both to give reasonable assurance that an observed difference, if one is found, is a true rather than an accidental difference. Conversely, when an inconsequential difference is observed, the samples must have been large enough to give reasonable assurance that a true difference, if it had been present, would have been revealed. The experienced researcher will always follow competent statistical design in any study of whatever type.

The status of the single population is usually described by an arithmetic average, or mean. Other characteristics can be calculated, on the assumptions that any individual finding is as apt to fall above as below the mean and that the probability of chance variation from the true value is expressed by the amount of the deviation squared, rather than by the amount of actual deviation. The standard deviation of a mean is a description of the distribution of individual findings around the average. Given a mean of 10.0 permanent teeth in eruption in a population of children, with a standard deviation of 2.0, about two thirds of the children should show an actual number of teeth equal to the mean plus or minus its standard deviation—that is, between eight and 12 teeth. Further analysis can produce a statistic called the standard error of the mean. Given a mean of 10.0 with a standard error of 0.2 (usually written 10.0 ±0.2), it can be predicted that about two out of three means taken from successive samples of this same population will fall within the value of the mean plus or minus its standard error, or within the range of 9.8 through 10.2. About 19 out of 20 means taken from successive samples from the same universe will fall within the range of the mean plus or minus two standard errors—in this instance, from 9.6 through 10.4.

In analogous fashion, a standard error can be calculated for the difference between two means. In essence this is a determination as to whether there is a tighter cluster of findings around the two individual means under test than around the single mean for the two populations combined and considered as one. When the difference between two means is twice as great as the standard error of the difference, the probability is about 19 to one that the difference is due to something beyond chance. This statistic is called the t test, and the ratio between the difference and its standard error is called the t value. The basic procedure can be expanded for the simultaneous consideration of any number of means. This analysis takes a multiplicity of forms, described generally as the analysis of variance. Its result is usually expressed as an F ratio. Like the t value, the F ratio is an expression of probability. When two means are compared by both methods of analysis, the F ratio will be found to be equal to the square of the t value. The significance of the F value varies with the number of comparisons and the sizes of the various samples.

With either of these two approaches (or several others not so frequently used), the test gives an estimate of the odds that the observed result may have been due to accident. This estimate is expressed as probability of chance, or P. If a coin is tossed, it is certain to drop with the head or tail face uppermost; this certainty is expressed numerically as 1.0. There is an even chance that heads or tails will appear; the probability of either can be expressed as $P = 0.50$. An estimate that chance could account for the result only about once in 20 trials is expressed as $P = 0.05$; about once in 100 trials, as $P = 0.01$; and about once in 1,000 trials, as $P = 0.001$. The results of any test for chance may be expressed in terms of P, and this value has the same meaning regardless of the type of analysis used.

The t test and F test rest on the assumption that there is a "normal" distribution of individual values about their means. When such a distribution is plotted, it takes a characteristic bell shape with the highest peak in the center and about as many values above as below the average, dropping off in such fashion that fewer and fewer values are found as the distance from the mean is increased. Unfortunately, distributions like these are rarely found in epidemiological studies of dental disease. While the t test is a robust test—that is, quite apt to detect a difference under conditions not ideal for its use—there are situations where the error due to a nonnormal distribution may be great enough to raise doubts as to the validity of such analyses. When the difficulty is due to a few extreme values, it may be resolved by use of the median (the middle value) rather than the average. In such cases the median is usually more descriptive than the mean; buying habits, for example, are apt to correspond more closely with the median than the mean income in a group composed of 98 poor people and two millionaires.

Still another family of tests is used to compare two or more distributions directly rather than through the mean, or mode, or similar statistic. One senses intuitively, for example, that there is a difference between two populations, in the first of which 75 percent of the people are rich and 25 percent of the people are poor, and in the second of which 90 percent of the people are poor and 10 percent of the people are rich. It is not always so obvious that two distributions are different. To test these differences, a family of statistics, commonly called nonparametric statistics, has been developed. The simplest example of a nonparametric statistic is Chi square. Through the use of Chi square or similar analyses it is possible to estimate the odds that two distributions differ by more than chance. The results of a Chi square test are ordinarily expressed in terms of P or probability.

As pointed out earlier, P has the same meaning and value regardless of the statistical test on which it is based. In most situations, a difference with a P of 0.05 is considered to be significant; a difference with a P of 0.01, highly significant; and a P of 0.001 or less is considered to be very highly significant. This is purely statistical significance. Statistical significance is an arbitrary figure which is, in part, a function of sample size. Any difference, no matter how trifling, can be made statistically significant if the sample is made large enough. The determination of statistical significance, then, is simply a prelude and an aid to the professional decision on whether the difference has practical meaning.

A consistent and predictable finding may set up odds against chance even though no one of the observed results is significant in itself. The probability of throwing heads (or tails) on any single coin toss is 0.50 and this probability is not altered by any sequence of results preceding the throw in question; but the odds against throwing 10 successive heads or tails are about 500 to one (P = approximately 0.002). This principle is the basis for a group of tests known collectively as sequential analysis.

The object of determinative epidemiological research is to discover relations between the way of life or the environment of a population and the prevalence or severity of disease. For this reason considerable use is made of correlation analyses in epidemiology. In the simplest form these involve determination of the relation between one population factor (such as the amount of fluorides in the community water) and some one other factor (such as caries experience of the population). When this relation is straight-line (for example, when a given rise in temperature is always followed by the same change in the column height of a fluid thermometer), the relation can be expressed as the coefficient of correlation (r) which may vary in value between zero and $+1.00$ or zero and -1.00. When the relation is

INTERPRETATION OF DATA AND OF SCIENTIFIC LITERATURE 67

curvilinear rather than straight-line (when, for example, the application of further amounts of an agent produces a smaller and smaller added result), the relation may be expressed as the correlation ratio (eta, or η) with a single positive range of values between zero and 1.00. Situations in which a single and necessary cause produces a specific and invariable effect are rare in biology. Hence, much use is made of analyses more nearly parallel to the facts of living, in which the total effect of a variety of factors, working simultaneously, some beneficial and some perhaps inimical, is estimated. Such analyses are usually called multiple correlations or multiple regressions.

It is difficult to discuss correlation technics, even superficially, without leaving some false implication, because the whole jargon of correlation statistics is couched in terms of cause and effect. *It is vital to remember that no correlation estimate can prove that one factor is the cause of another, no matter how suggestive the words nor how logical the inference.* Hence, causation is not implied when it is said that about one sixth of the variance (the individual fluctuations squared) in one factor "can be explained by" the effect of the other when a value of +0.40 or −0.40 is computed for a simple correlation. Lower orders of correlation are less noteworthy. About 99 percent of the variance is left "unexplained" with a correlation of +0.10 or −0.10, and the correlation must be greater than 0.70 to "explain" as much as half of the observed variance. Multiple correlation analyses permit the observer to consider the total effect of a number of independent factors, or the effect of a single factor or combination of factors as it might have been exerted if the influence of still other factors had been nullified, or held constant.

These and other statistical technics are of prime importance in the interpretation of epidemiological evidence, despite the fact that the resulting estimates fall short of the unequivocal precision which might be inferred from the preceding paragraphs. This is due to no fault in design of the tests, but rather to the fact that the basic requirements upon which the tests are predicated can rarely be met in the field study. Essentially all assume randomness—a sample, for example, in which any person in a population is as likely as any other to be selected for examination or, when two groups are contrasted, a situation in which any person in the entire study is as apt to be assigned to one group as to the other. Some others assume that measurements will be infallible, a condition approachable only in some physical experiments. In the usual field study with large numbers, the t test or F test is apt to emphasize a difference too small to be important, whereas nonparametric methods such as Chi square may be too weak to expose a difference with real meaning. Correlation analyses, potentially the most valuable in epidemiology, are particularly apt to be misleading. The correlation model requires strictly random samples and normal universes, and the higher the number of independent variables in a multiple correlation, the greater the chance of a falsely high estimate. Technics which combine correlation or regression technics with analyses of variance (a series of tests known as covariance) are the more demanding in that the requirements for each of the elements in the statistical analysis must be met. In the typical covariance model, for example, the correlations must be linear and the distributions must be normal or bell-shaped. These requirements are extremely difficult to meet with typical dental epidemiological data. Interpretation of epidemiological data calls for a high degree of statistical common sense, and the statistical treatment is only the beginning point in analysis. Conclusions of even the best study are greatly strengthened when corroborated by another, and still another, especially those conducted by independent observers with other populations.

FALLACIES AND LIMITATIONS OF EPIDEMIOLOGICAL STUDY

Most of the pitfalls in epidemiological study are due to failures in logic. It is neither logical nor scientific to pick and choose evidence, accepting that which supports some preconceived notion and discarding all that points in some other direction. Almost anything can be "proved" by this procedure; it has been a favorite method of the scientific crank and the antifluoridationist. All of the valid evidence adduced in a study must be considered in reaching a conclusion.

More subtle is a general class of error which can be described loosely as the comparison based on noncomparable data. It should be obvious that the dental caries experience of two populations cannot be compared if one was examined with the tongue blade and the other with mirror and explorer plus bitewings. Study and control groups in the clinical trial (or other contrast) should be free of known bias—i.e., of factors other than the one under study affecting the one population more than the other, so that a false conclusion is reached. A very useful degree of protection against bias from unknown factors is assured by random assignments to study and control groups in the clinical trial. When this is done, unknown factors usually cancel out by exerting equivalent influence on both sides of the contrast. When time at risk is a factor, it is hazardous to associate a transient condition (such as gingivitis) with a lifelong accumulation of signs (such as decayed, missing, and filled teeth). The inclusion of false-positive cases for consideration as though they were genuine is a similar error, illustrated most clearly in the series of field studies by observers who were unable to distinguish common enamel opacities from dental fluorosis and reported "fluoride effects" in areas where fluoride intake was actually deficient rather than excessive.

Even more tenuous are the errors arising from the misinterpretation of valid evidence. One of the commonest of these is the *post hoc, ergo propter hoc* fallacy—the conclusion that A is the cause of B because A preceded B in time. Patent as this trap may seem to be, it is probably the basis for most of the superstitions of mankind. In scientific thought, error of this type is frequently the result of generalizing too broadly from some specific finding of fact. The findings in any given study have been established only as true for the conditions of that particular situation. The standard error of a mean gives an estimate of the values of means taken from future samples from that universe, but that universe may be no broader than the children in public school number one who were present on the day of examination because they were immune to mumps. The results of a correlation analysis are applicable only to the group from which the data were taken. In the early stages of study the experienced scientist will usually let his facts speak for themselves, with a minimum of generalization. Firm conclusions are usually reserved until the general findings have been verified by at least one (and preferably two or more) investigations by independent observers.

There are obvious limitations on any study of human beings. An agent known or suspected to be harmful cannot be introduced into a human population for any purpose. Hence, study of an inimical agent is restricted to contrasts between populations with and without the factor, or to the reaction when the agent is withdrawn. Associations developed in this manner may be cause-and-effect relations, but this last determination must be established by specific clinical trial.

THE EVALUATION OF SCIENTIFIC LITERATURE

A few decades ago the physician or dentist—or the chemist, physicist, mathematician, or biologist—could keep abreast of developments in his profession by discriminate reading in a few well-chosen journals. Since then a fantastic expansion of human knowledge has led to a point where no single man can be expert or even competent in the whole of any specific field in science, or the whole spectrum of professional practice. Scientific publication has kept pace, or nearly so, with scientific discovery. Mrs. Irene Campbell and her staff in the library of the Kettering Laboratory have abstracted more than 8,000 scientific reports on a single subject—the effect of fluoride—through 1958.[2] But this has, as well, been the era of the cancer quack, the food faddist, flying saucers, and the antifluoridationist; a physician has published a book which proves (he says) that the earth's rotation is occasionally slowed or stopped by the tail of a comet, and there is a book by a university president which proves (to him, at least) that Einstein was an idiot; a Flat Earth Society has proved (to its own satisfaction) from the orbital flights of the astronauts that the world cannot possibly be round. It is still necessary to read with a critical eye.

Most of the responsible journals are published by a professional organization or a learned society; examples of these are the *Journal of the American Dental Association,* the *Journal of Dental Research,* or the *International Dental Journal.* Manuscripts submitted to these publications, and others of their type, must pass scrutiny by a jury of scientists before publication. This eliminates a great deal of rubbish. Nonetheless, when considering a report, it is prudent to weigh the record of the author and the character of the institution he represents. There is keen competition for qualified scientists, and no able man need go it alone. Nearly all are associated with a university or an institute of proved standing which can provide adequate facilities and opportunities for sound research.

A good scientific report must meet some rather rigid requirements. The material used and the methods of study must be described in enough detail to permit the reader to judge whether the sample was adequate and whether the procedures were sound. There must be a clear exposition of the facts developed. There should be sufficient detail so that the reader may decide for himself whether the interpretation is logical and the conclusions amply supported by the evidence. A demonstration of statistical significance is not enough to support a conclusion; it simply establishes some degree of probability that the difference described is a real rather than an accidental difference. It remains the obligation of the author to show that this real difference is due to the factor under study and not to some unknown influence or some force beyond his control. It is reasonable to ask whether some other, and possibly different, conclusion might be better supported by the evidence as presented. It is always wise to ask whether the author has generalized too widely from a narrow and specific observation. In the strictest sense the facts developed in a scientific investigation are certainly true only under the conditions of that study. A caries-inhibitory agent which seems effective in a given group of animals may be ineffective in the next; and an agent with uniform and predictable potency in animals may prove useless in man.

The reader who will accept nothing is, of course, quite as gullible as the uncritical reader who will accept anything. It would probably be possible to raise some meaningless quibble or other on any paper ever written about a study based on observation. If a report is to be questioned, it should be on solid grounds, such as some defect in method extreme enough to invalidate the evidence or some error in logic grave enough to vitiate the conclusion. Where there are limitations on his evidence, the careful author is apt to point them out in his discussion, and to restrict his conclusions as indicated.

For the professional man with adequate training and background, however, the problem of finding the significant report may overshadow the difficulty in interpreting it once it is located. Even if all of the publications were readily available, no one person could read all of the papers on studies of possible significance in the practice of dentistry. Librarians have developed ingenious automatic methods for the classification and retrieval of subject material. The reader with a specific objective should, first of all, enlist the help of a good librarian who will be able to identify and locate source material or suggest review articles and collections of pertinent data.

Data from many and sometimes obscure sources may be brought together in such compilations, thus saving the reader the time and effort necessary to assemble the material for himself or translate it from a foreign language, and interpretation may be furnished by someone considered expert in the specific field in question. These publications take many forms. All research papers on fluorides between 1901 and 1962 by officers of the United States Public Health Service have been published in a single volume edited by F. J. McClure.[3] These are presented without alteration and in full. A few scores of the most significant papers in the Kettering Library listing have been listed and published with a short description of the data and conclusions of each.[1] A certain amount of interpretation is implicit in the acceptance or rejection of individual papers for inclusion in such a listing. Finally, there is the typical review article by a recognized authority, in which evidence is summarized and put into perspective. This involves a high degree of interpretation, but can be of great value. The conclusions of the single, unconfirmed study may be misleading. Conclusions reached and confirmed in a series of independent studies are apt to be sound. The summary article which evaluates the series as a whole is, when well done, useful beyond the obvious utility of condensing a mass of detail into simpler and more readable form.

The reader of such material must, perforce, place great confidence in the integrity of the compiler. His best safeguard is the standing and competence of the sponsoring body itself. When reviews are published by such organizations as the American Dental Association, the American Medical Association, the American Public Health Association, the American Association for the Advancement of Science, the National Research Council, or an outstanding university, great care will have been taken in the selection of reviewers, and their contributions will have had the closest scrutiny before publication. Popular articles in lay periodicals are sometimes shallow, sketchy, and misleading.

If too little reading is bad, reading restricted to a narrow field of interest can lead to loss of perspective and discrimination. Along with the journals of his national and state societies, or his speciality organization, the practitioner may read some such journal as *Science* with enjoyment and with profit. There is very little in the broad field of scientific knowledge which is wholly without application to the theory and practice of dentistry.

Bibliography

1. Campbell, Irene R. The role of fluoride in public health. Cincinnati, Kettering Laboratory College Medicine University Cincinnati, 1963. V + 108 p.
2. Campbell, Irene R., and Widner, Evelyn M., with the assistance of Kukainis, Irene P. The occurrence and biological effects of fluorine compounds. Vol. I. The inorganic compounds. Cincinnati, Kettering Laboratory College Medicine University Cincinnati, 1958. IV + 955 p.
3. McClure, F. J., ed. Fluoride drinking waters. Washington, Public Health Service, 1962. VI + 636 p.

Additional Readings

Chilton, N. W. Design and analysis in dental and oral research. Philadelphia, Lippincott, c1967. 365 p.

Easlick, K. A., ed. Report-writing in dentistry; a teaching outline. 9th ed. Ann Arbor, Overbeck, 1960. 70 p.

Ezekial, Mordecai, and Fox, K. A. Methods of correlation and regression analysis. 3rd ed. New York, Wiley, c1959. XV + 548 p.

Hill, B. A. Principles of medical statistics. 8th rev. New York, Oxford University Press, 1966. IX + 381 p.

Mainland, Donald. Elementary medical statistics. 2nd ed. Philadelphia, Saunders, c1963. XIII + 381 p.

Snedecor, G. W., and Cochran, W. G. Statistical methods. 6th ed. Ames, Iowa, State University Press, 1967. 593 p.

Wallis, W. A. Statistics, a new approach. Glencoe, Ill., Free Press, c1956. XXXVIII + 646 p.

CHAPTER 6

THE EPIDEMIOLOGY OF DENTAL CARIES AND PERIODONTAL DISEASES

By A. L. RUSSELL, D.D.S., M.P.H.

While the dentist is concerned with the treatment of many other conditions, he has the primary professional responsibility for the control of periodontal conditions and dental caries, and his chair-time is usually monopolized by treatment for these conditions.

Dental Caries. Dental caries seems to be a fairly recent disease in the history of man. Lesions of caries are rare in the teeth of ancient skulls (and, when found, usually occur in cementum), despite the fact that the teeth are no more favorable in form, and the enamel no more perfect, than the teeth and enamel of contemporary civilized populations.[9] It remains a relatively rare disease in some areas of the world. In others, including western Europe and most of North and South America, virtually every person is attacked at some time during his lifetime. Some findings for mean numbers of decayed, missing, and filled permanent teeth, reported by a single research team, for persons aged 20 to 24 years, are shown in Figure 3.[36] Most Ethiopians in this age group had escaped attack. Nearly all of the people seen in Baltimore exhibited one or more lesions. It has been estimated that the cost of treatment for dental caries in the United States exceeds the cost of treatment for any other single disease.

Such estimates of the gravity of dental disease in the United States have been reinforced by the findings of the National Health Examination Survey, which, during the years 1960, 1961, and 1962, was carried out with a random sample of the entire United States popu-

74 ASSESSMENT OF THE PROBLEM OF DENTAL DISEASE

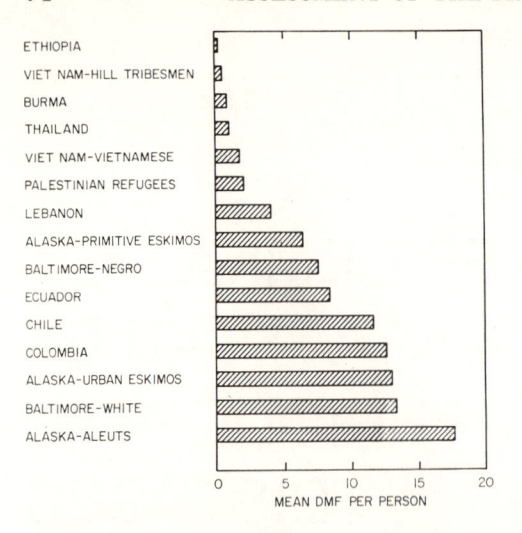

FIGURE 3. Mean DMF per person for civilian groups aged 20-24 years. (Russell[36])

lation of persons aged 18 through 79 years. Because this was a random sample, the results of the survey may be applied to persons of these ages in the United States as a whole. Mean numbers of decayed, missing, and filled permanent teeth for white and Negro persons, as determined by the survey, are shown in Table 9. Interpreted broadly, it is obvious from the data in Table 9 that more than half of the teeth in the average white man or woman have become decayed, missing, or filled by the age of 25 through 34 years and that DMF means are uniformly higher in white than in Negro persons, sex for sex and age for age.[15] At the younger ages – up through about 44 years – missing teeth in these DMF findings are due principally to teeth lost from dental caries. After that age, loss of teeth from periodontal disease must have contributed a significant number of missing teeth to the DMF totals, for reasons to be considered later in this chapter.

The National Health Examination Survey sample was too small for definition of regional disease prevalences within the United States. There are apparent variations in caries prevalence within the nation, though these differences are hard to evaluate because much of the data has been obtained by noncomparable methods. Reports from examinations of entrants into the armed forces during World War II are in general agreement that the highest prevalence of dental caries was seen in recruits from New England, the Pacific Northwest, and the Great Lakes area, with distinctly lesser prevalences in young men from the South, the Southwest, and the Mountain states.[28, 42, 43] Natural fluoride waters may have accounted for some of the discrepancies in the latter two areas, but there is some indication that factors other than fluoride are responsible for at least some of these differences. At present the reasons for this pattern are unexplained.

Females seem to be slightly more susceptible than males in some populations, though the difference is sometimes small enough to be explained by the earlier eruption of teeth in females;[17] in some

TABLE 9. DECAYED, MISSING, AND FILLED PERMANENT TEETH IN A RANDOM SAMPLE OF UNITED STATES ADULTS, 1960-1962*

SEX AND AGE	WHITE	NEGRO
Both sexes		
Total, 18-79 years	21.2	14.5
Men		
Total, 18-79 years	20.6	12.9
18-24 years	14.4	8.3
25-34 years	17.3	8.4
35-44 years	19.3	9.4
45-54 years	21.6	14.9
55-64 years	25.4	18.4
65-74 years	26.9	23.7
75-79 years	28.8	26.6
Women		
Total, 18-79 years	21.9	15.7
18-24 years	15.1	9.2
25-34 years	19.2	13.6
35-44 years	20.8	15.1
45-54 years	22.8	15.8
55-64 years	26.2	21.2
65-74 years	27.9	25.2
75-79 years	29.8	30.1

*Johnson, Kelly, and Van Kirk.[15]

other studies no differences can be seen. Onset is early in susceptible populations, with the first lesions appearing very soon after the eruption of the first deciduous or permanent teeth. Pits and fissures are more susceptible than smooth surfaces of teeth. The first attack is almost always in the occlusal fissures, or buccal pit, or both, of the mandibular first molar. The mandibular incisors are ordinarily the last to succumb.[18, 20] The order of attack in low-susceptibility populations is very much the same, except that the first lesion may occur on the occlusal of any second molar.

The association between the use of refined sugar and caries prevalence is one of the salient relations observed in a series of international surveys conducted, over the past decade, by the organization then known as the Interdepartmental Committee on Nutrition for National Defense (ICNND). The Committee was constituted to coordinate nutrition studies in armed forces friendly to the United States; later its activity was expanded to include surveys of the nutrition of civilian groups as well. On request from a host nation, the Committee provided teams including specialists in nutrition, medicine, dentistry, biochemistry, food technology, agriculture, and other disciplines as determined by the needs and wishes of the host nation.[5] The dental data developed in these surveys are particularly valuable because of their comparability—most of the dental examiners have come from a single research group—and because of the associated information about the populations developed at the same time.

Mean numbers of decayed, missing, and filled permanent teeth in some of these areas are shown in Figure 4. The lowest prevalence of caries was noted in Ethiopia and the Far East; an intermediate experience in Lebanon, representing the Near East; and the highest experience, paralleling that in the United States, in Central and South America.[32] Sugar consumption, as determined by ICNND dietary teams, followed the same pattern. Consumption in the Far East ranged from six to 16 kg. per person per year, in the Near East from 13 to 19 kg., and in tropical South America from 23 to 44 kg., about the same as in western Europe and North America. Thai families studied used an average of 0.2 gram of sugar per person per day; families in Lebanon, 26 grams; families in Chile, 50 grams; and families in Ecuador, from 45 to 58 grams per day.[13] Sugar was used daily by fewer than half of the families studied in Ethiopia, and caries prevalence was significantly lower in the families with the lesser sugar consumption.[21]

High-carbohydrate diets were not necessarily associated with high caries prevalence unless sugar was a prominent factor. The principal food in Ethiopia is a cereal called teff, and rice is the staple in South Vietnam, Thailand, and Burma.[32]

There is no suggestion anywhere in the ICNND data that any particular nutritional factor (except fluorine) is caries-inhibitory or that caries is lessened by adequate nutrition. There is always some hazard in correlating food intake or nutritional status on some specific day with signs of dental caries which have accumulated over the

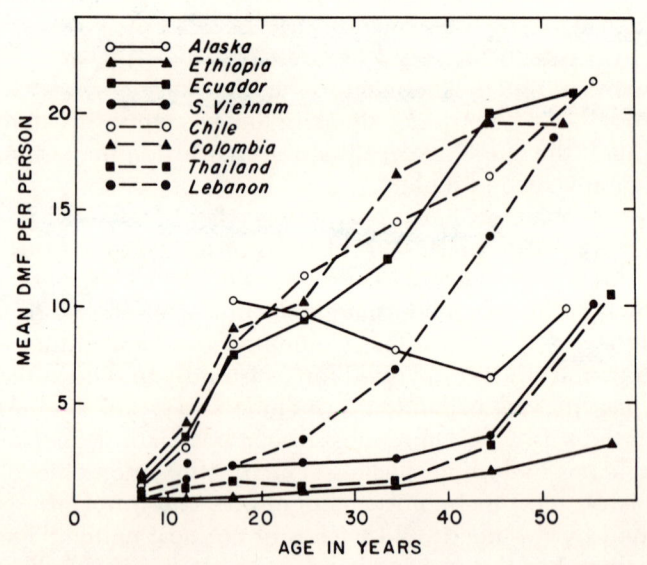

FIGURE 4. DMF teeth in 8 countries. *Solid line: open circle* = Alaska, *solid triangle* = Ethiopia, *solid square* = Ecuador, *solid circle* = South Vietnam. *Broken line: open circle* = Chile, *solid triangle* = Colombia, *solid square* = Thailand, *solid circle* = Lebanon. (Russell[32])

lifetime of the individual up to that day of examination, but these peoples were, in most instances, subsisting on a traditional diet limited for centuries by custom and opportunity, so that the food taken on the day of examination was probably representative of the diet over the lifetime of the people.

Each population initially had been chosen for study because some grave nutritional deficiency was known or suspected. These deficiencies were found to exist. The Ethiopian diet as a whole was deficient in vitamin A and caloric intake, and critically low in ascorbic acid. The diets in Burma, Thailand, and South Vietnam depend heavily upon highly polished rice. Thiamine was dangerously low in South Vietnam, and riboflavin was also deficient. This was the pattern in the other Asian nations, though thiamine was adequate in military personnel in Thailand. The principal deficiency in Lebanon was riboflavin. The Alaskan diet was low in vitamin A and very low in ascorbic acid, particularly in the more remote villages which were the homes of most of the older men with low caries experience. In some of these villages, at some times, caloric intake for an able-bodied adult male fell as low as 700 per man per day. It is clear that a traditional diet deficient in these basic nutrients has not proved cariogenic in these populations.

Nutritional deficiencies were not confined to the low-caries populations. The intake of ascorbic acid was high in Ecuador, but riboflavin, calcium, and thiamine were low and there was a high incidence of goiter. In Chile 29 percent of civilians were low or deficient in vitamin A. About half of the military personnel examined in Colombia were low or deficient in thiamine and riboflavin.[32]

This failure to demonstrate an effect of "protective" nutrients (excepting fluorine) on dental caries is the usual finding in studies with human beings. Very low caries incidence has been reported in populations suffering from osteomalacia, rickets, or pellagra from various areas of the world.[7, 24, 25, 44] It may be said that, in general, caries prevalence tends to be lowest in groups most ill-fed. It does not follow that starvation or deprivation is necessarily caries-inhibitory; if so, one would expect that within malnourished populations people with caries would be better fed than people without caries; but it is not so. Vietnamese children who were caries-free and who had experienced caries attack showed very similar levels of serum ascorbic acid, vitamin A and carotene, urinary thiamine, riboflavin, and N'-Methylnicotinamide, hemoglobin and hematocrit, and height and weight.[40] Quite similar findings had been returned from a series of five Guatemalan villages where children with and free of caries had about the same average values for serum protein, riboflavin, ascorbic acid, carotene, vitamin A, vitamin E, and alkaline phosphatase. Their customary diets were deficient in vitamin A, riboflavin, and animal protein.[14] In one United States study about the same order and magnitude of dietary deficiencies were found in a group of college students with rampant caries as in another group virtually free of decay.[6]

It is difficult to determine whether caries prevalence is increasing in the United States. Enlistment records for the Civil War show that loss of teeth was a major cause for rejection of recruits, suggesting that the disease may have posed as great a problem a century ago as it does today.[28] There is presumptive evidence that prevalence is growing in some areas, such as parts of South Vietnam, Alaska, and New Guinea, where adults now exhibit few signs of caries attack.[38, 40] Children in these areas have already accumulated significantly more decayed, missing, and filled permanent teeth than have their elders.

The single factor with the most profound effect upon the prevalence and pattern of dental caries, in this and many other series of studies, is the ingestion of adequate amounts of fluorides. In North America optimum ingestion is ensured most easily by fluoridation of the community water supply. Individuals with optimum fluoride intake over a lifetime enjoy a marked and lasting inhibition of caries, particularly in the smooth surfaces of teeth.[31, 39] The efficacy, safety, and practicability of fluoridation are discussed at some length in Chapter Seven, "Measures Available for the Prevention and Control of Dental Caries."

From the standpoint of a citizen of the United States, then, the principal epidemiological characteristics of dental caries are (a) the first lesions occur very soon after eruption of the first teeth; (b) nearly every person is attacked, most of them early in life; (c) there is a definite relation between the use of sugar and caries attack; and (d) caries attack is inhibited sharply by ingestion of optimum amounts of fluoride from birth throughout life.

Periodontal Diseases. The principal features of the epidemiology of periodontal diseases have been described elsewhere.[30] Whereas dental caries is a relatively recent disease in human history and is most prevalent in peoples of the Western civilizations, destructive disease of the periodontal tissues is usually demonstrable in prehistoric human jaws, and the condition is much more prevalent and severe in such other areas as Asia than in the United States.[8] Mean periodontal (PI) scores for a series of groups aged 40 to 49 years, all civil populations, are shown in Figure 5. Like the data previously shown for dental caries, these were developed by members of one research team in the course of ICNND studies between 1958 and 1961.[36]

The National Health Examination Survey teams considered periodontal diseases as well as dental caries. Periodontal Index scores for the random sample of the United States examined during the years 1960, 1961, and 1962 are shown in Table 10.[16] These findings for the United States, as a whole, were very similar to the findings for individuals in Baltimore cited in Figure 5. Unlike the pattern in dental caries, Negroes showed higher periodontal scores than white persons

EPIDEMIOLOGY OF CARIES AND PERIODONTAL DISEASES

FIGURE 5. Mean Periodontal Index scores for civilian groups aged 40-49 years. (Russell[36])

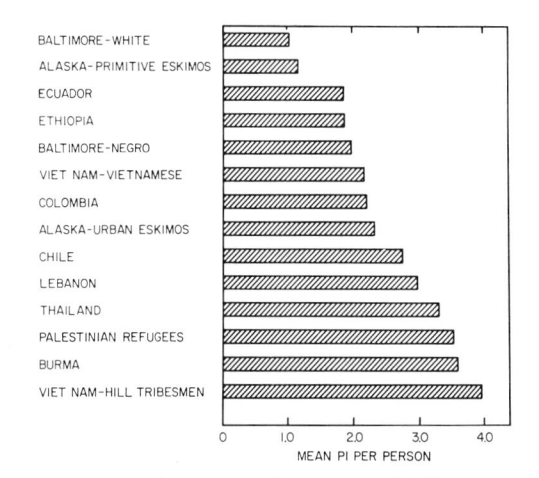

through the entire age range except in the case of men aged 75 to 79 years, where the sample of Negro males was small.

The Periodontal Index may also be used as a device for separating persons into groups without obvious periodontal disease, with periodontal disease which has not proceeded to pocket formation, or with established disease. These percentages, as elicited by the National Health Examination Survey, are shown in Table 11.[16] In the entire age range of 18 through 79 years, only about one man in five and about one woman in three were free of obvious periodontal de-

TABLE 10. AVERAGE PERIODONTAL INDEX OF WHITE AND NEGRO ADULTS, BY SEX AND AGE: UNITED STATES, 1960-1962*

SEX AND AGE	ALL RACES	WHITE	NEGRO
	Average Periodontal Index		
Both sexes			
Total, 18-79 years	1.13	1.06	1.60
Men			
Total, 18-79 years	1.34	1.28	1.79
18-24 years	0.62	0.58	0.78
25-34 years	0.92	0.87	1.30
35-44 years	1.27	1.22	1.67
45-54 years	1.62	1.55	2.06
55-64 years	2.15	2.00	3.13
65-74 years	2.50	2.47	2.83
75-79 years	2.91	3.01	2.16
Women			
Total, 18-79 years	0.93	0.85	1.43
18-24 years	0.48	0.46	0.62
25-34 years	0.60	0.53	0.95
35-44 years	0.82	0.74	1.30
45-54 years	1.23	1.11	1.92
55-64 years	1.56	1.39	2.90
65-74 years	1.62	1.51	2.03
75-79 years	2.94	2.41	5.53

*Kelly and Van Kirk.[16]

TABLE 11. PERCENT DISTRIBUTION OF ADULTS, BY STATUS OF PERIODONTAL DISEASE ACCORDING TO SEX AND AGE: UNITED STATES, 1960-1962*

SEX AND AGE	WITHOUT PERIODONTAL DISEASE	WITH PERIODONTAL DISEASE — WITHOUT POCKETS	WITH PERIODONTAL DISEASE — WITH POCKETS
Both sexes			
Total, 18-79 years	26.1	48.5	25.4
Men			
Total, 18-79 years	20.9	49.0	30.1
18-24 years	29.0	60.6	10.3
25-34 years	26.3	51.7	22.0
35-44 years	22.1	48.1	29.7
45-54 years	15.0	48.1	36.9
55-64 years	15.3	39.1	45.6
65-74 years	5.6	36.0	58.4
75-79 years	6.2	33.7	60.0
Women			
Total, 18-79 years	31.0	47.9	21.0
18-24 years	36.8	53.6	9.6
25-34 years	37.6	50.2	12.3
35-44 years	33.3	46.2	20.5
45-54 years	26.6	43.7	29.6
55-64 years	20.8	43.6	35.5
65-74 years	15.2	52.0	32.8
75-79 years	11.0	35.3	53.8

*Kelly and Van Kirk.[16]

terioration. By the ages of 45 to 54 years, roughly one third of the individuals who had retained teeth exhibited established disease. This was true of more than half of the dentulous persons in the ultimate ages, 75 to 79 years.

Despite its relatively lower prevalence (and lesser severity in young adults) in the United States, periodontal disease leads to a considerable loss of teeth in American adults in the middle and older age groups. When the American Dental Association surveyed the needs for dental care among patients reporting to practitioners in 1952, it was found that periodontal treatment was needed by 9.5 percent of males and 9.7 percent of females aged 15 years and over, with an average of 13.8 and 13.6 diseased teeth per patient, respectively. Extractions for periodontal disease were needed by 11.2 percent of males in the same age range, for an average of 8.2 teeth per case, and by 8.3 percent of females, for an average of 7.1 per patient. For patients aged 35 years and over in males, and 40 years and older in females, periodontal disease was the reason for between two and three times as many extractions as dental decay.[1] A needs survey on a slightly different basis was conducted by the Association in

December of 1965. The average patient in 1965 required about half as many tooth extractions as the average patient in 1952.[3] Nevertheless, in all persons over 39 years old, periodontal disease was the reason for many more extractions than was dental caries.[2] Similarly, analysis of a sample of the records of patients receiving treatment in Public Health Service installations indicated that after the age of 34 periodontal disease was the dominant reason for the loss of teeth (Figure 6).[29] It is clear that periodontal disease constitutes a grave public health problem which must grow in relative importance as the damaging effects of dental caries are prevented or controlled.

Though the condition is often associated with physical maturity or middle age, onset may be early in susceptible individuals, at or shortly after puberty. Advanced destructive disease has been reported

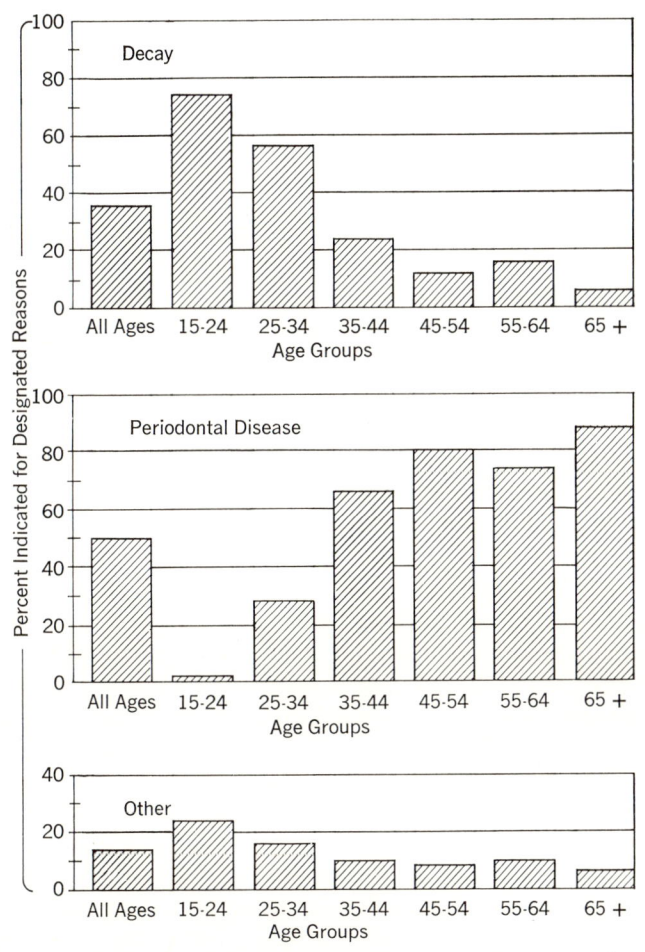

FIGURE 6. Teeth indicated for extraction because of decay, periodontal disease, and other reasons. (Pelton, Pennell, and Druzina.[29] Graph from: Young, W. O. Dental health. p. 5-94. [In Hollinshead, B. S., dir. The survey of dentistry; the final report. Washington, American Council Education, c1961. XXXIV + 603 p.])

in about 1.6 and about 1.0 percent of children aged 11 to 13 years in Great Britain and the United States, respectively.[27, 35] Attack is usually earliest, and most severe, in the mandibular incisor and maxillary molar teeth. Some pathologic loss of bone can be demonstrated in most persons aged 20 to 29 years,[26] and loss of teeth from the disease becomes a factor of importance in this decade of life. The disease tends to be more prevalent, and extractions for this cause are somewhat more common, in males than in females.[1, 2]

Early in the course of the determinative phase of epidemiological study of the disease, it was noted that both the prevalence and the severity of the condition were associated with some factor which could be described vaguely as social. Children who needed but did not receive fillings or extractions over the course of 12 months exhibited considerably more disease than children whose needs were fully met.[33] Disease was usually more prevalent, or severe, or both, in Negroes than in whites living in the same communities. There was usually less disease in men in the favored occupations, as compared with men in work with a lower social status and income.[37] Patients from a middle economic group in a private oral surgery practice lost about as many teeth from caries as from periodontal disease at ages over 40 years; indigent patients in the same city lost from nearly three to over seven times as many teeth to periodontal disease in the same age range.[4, 19]

Rural children showed more gingival disease than urban children of comparable age. Disease in these rural children was most prevalent in those counties where the educational level of adults was relatively low. Differences between urban and rural children disappeared when comparisons were restricted to localities with similar median school years completed by persons 25 years of age or older.[34] Negroes and whites in Birmingham were found to have had quite similar experience with periodontal disease when groups with like education, professional dental care, and mouth cleanliness were compared. Oral debris seemed to be the most deleterious factor of the several studied.[37] These findings were reported by the epidemiology staff of the National Institute of Dental Research, United States Public Health Service. Studies by other observers in Bombay, Atlanta, Ecuador, Montana, and Ceylon demonstrated consistent and strong associations between oral cleanliness and periodontal health.[10, 11, 46] Very similar conclusions were reached by workers from the Norwegian Institute of Dental Research, who carried out a painstaking and detailed clinical study of workers in a manufacturing plant in Oslo.[22]

Profound changes can be induced in the periodontal tissues of some laboratory animals by altering their nutritive status or dietary patterns. The periodontal studies carried out in connection with the ICNND nutrition surveys were designed specifically to determine relations between particular nutritive states and disease, on the hypothesis that any deficiency of etiologic importance would be found associated consistently with increased prevalence or severity. There was every reason to expect that such an association, if one existed, would be revealed. Wide variations in disease prevalence were found, as illustrated in Figure 5, and one or more grave deficiencies in the traditional dietary were discovered in each of the populations. Nevertheless, no consistent association between disease and the nutritive items studied could be established in the series of surveys; the correlation which did emerge in each was an overwhelming association between disease and lack of mouth cleanliness.

The findings in South Vietnam are reasonably representative of the findings for the entire series.[41] Active periodontal disease was appraised (using the Periodontal Index), gingival recession was scored, and oral hygiene estimated (according to the Simplified Oral Hygiene Index of Greene and Vermillion) for 752 individuals 15 years of age or older. The combined effects of age, oral debris, and calculus were sufficient, statistically, to account for about two thirds of the total variance in PI scores; the coefficient of multiple correlation was +0.82. The correlation was not improved when a number of other factors were considered simultaneously for the smaller subsample of people who received biochemical as well as physical examinations. About two thirds of the variance was still referable to the effects of age and hygiene. With the statistical effect of these factors held constant, there were slight but significant residual associations between disease and deficiency in serum vitamin A and hematocrit, but little or no effect could be ascribed to hemoglobin levels, serum ascorbic acid, serum carotene, serum protein, thiamine, riboflavin or N'Methylnicotinamide in urine, physical signs of malnutrition (such as cheilosis or loss of the ankle or knee jerk), height-weight ratios, skin thickness, or ethnic grouping. About the same result was found when these factors were correlated with recession scores. There were slight residual correlations, significant statistically, between recession scores and hematocrit and serum vitamin A. Neither vitamin A nor hematocrit levels were found to be associated with periodontal disease in other studies in the ICNND series.

Both age and oral hygiene are importantly associated with both PI and recession scores when either is considered with the effect of the other held constant. Hygiene is more closely associated with present disease than age; the reverse is true with recession.[41]

Some of the limitations of this type of analysis were pointed out in a previous chapter, and the Vietnam data would have only limited value if they were not quite consistent with results from other populations. About the same patterns are seen in the other ICNND surveys so far analyzed in this manner, and in such independent studies as that carried out in Ceylon by Waerhaug of the Norwegian Institute of Dental Research.[46] Calculus and oral debris are always found to be the dominant factors associated with disease, and the association becomes stronger as age of the people advances. The slight associations with deficiency in vitamin A or low hematocrit levels, seen in Vietnam, did not appear in Lebanon or Chile, where deficiency in the vitamins had no relation with disease. There was a slight advantage in favor of persons with adequate serum ascorbic acid in Ethiopia, but Alaskan Eskimos with zero levels of ascorbic acid in blood serum did not differ from their fellows with adequate levels of the vitamin. These results do not rule out diet or nutrition as contributory factors in periodontal disease, though they do set up formidable odds against a primary etiologic role for dietary vitamin A, ascorbic acid, thiamine, riboflavin, or niacin.[32] They do establish an association between mouth cleanliness and periodontal disease in population groups, which is as definite and predictable as the association between waterborne fluorides and dental caries. Widespread clinical experience and formal clinical trials have shown that periodontal disease is virtually halted in groups with controlled oral hygiene and kept free of calculus.[23] It is possible that the socially oriented differences in prevalence which perplexed early epidemiological investigators were largely or even wholly due to systematic group differences in personal oral hygiene and the utilization of professional dental prophylaxis.

An excellent review paper, describing in depth the epidemiological characteristics of periodontal disease, has been presented by Waerhaug.[45]

The principal epidemiological characteristics of periodontal disease, then, are these: (a) onset of the destructive process may occur as early as puberty; (b) virtually all adults show some signs of disease; (c) in a high proportion of persons gross destruction of supportive tissue leads to substantial loss of function and teeth in middle and later life; and (d) active disease is rarely found in the absence of oral debris or calculus.

A simple catalog of population findings in dental caries and periodontal disease would fill a book larger than this one. The findings outlined here are those which seem, at present, to offer the greatest utility toward the ultimate objective of epidemiological study—the control of disease. It is obvious that a useful measure of control could be had if these findings were applied and utilized to their fullest extent. It is equally clear that the control program must reach all individuals in the population at the earliest practicable age. The control measures available and their application will be the subject of the next three chapters.

Bibliography

1. American Dental Association, Bureau of Economic Research and Statistics. Survey of needs for dental care. II. Dental needs according to age and sex of patients. Am. Dent. A. J., 46:200-11, Feb. 1953.

2. American Dental Association, Bureau of Economic Research and Statistics. Survey of needs for dental care, 1965. II. Dental needs according to age and sex of patients. Am. Dent. A. J., 73:1355-65, Dec. 1966.
3. ———. Survey of needs for dental care, 1965. VIII. Summary and comparison with previous surveys. Am. Dent. A. J., 74:1561-2, June 1967.
4. Andrews, George, and Krogh, H. W. Permanent tooth mortality. Dent. Progress, 1:130-4, Jan. 1961.
5. Berry, F. B., and Schaefer, A. E. Program of the Interdepartmental Committee on Nutrition for National Defense. Am. Med. A. J., 166:775-7, Feb. 15, 1958.
6. Collins, R. O., Jensen, A. L., and Becks, Hermann. Study of caries-free individuals. II. Is an optimum diet or a reduced carbohydrate intake required to arrest dental caries? Am. Dent. A. J., 29:1169-78, July 1, 1942.
7. Dreizen, Samuel, et al. Prevalence of dental caries in malnourished children. Am. J. Dis. Child., 74:265-73, Sept. 1947.
8. Dummett, C. O. The relation of periodontal diseases to public health. Am. Dent. A. J., 54:49-56, Jan. 1957.
9. Falin, L. I. Histological and histochemical studies of human teeth of the bronze and stone ages. Arch. Oral Biol., 5:5-13, Sept. 1961.
10. Greene, J. C. Oral hygiene and periodontal disease. Am. J. Pub. Health, 53:913-22, June 1963.
11. ———. Periodontal disease in India: report of an epidemiological study. J. Dent. Res., 39:302-12, Mar.-Apr. 1960.
12. Griffith, C. A., Hall, A. B., and Simon, W. J. An analysis of the oral surgery records of the University of Minnesota school of dentistry. Am. Dent. A. J., 28:1930-7, Dec. 1941.
13. Hand, D. B., Schaefer, A. E., and Wilson, Christine S. A comparative study of food consumption patterns in Latin America, Middle Eastern and Far Eastern countries. Paper presented before the First International Congress of Food Science and Technology, London, Sept. 18-21, 1962.
14. Hurtarte E., Augusto, and Scrimshaw, N. S. Dental findings in a nutritional study of school children in five Guatemalan highland villages. J. Dent. Res., 34:390-6, June 1955.
15. Johnson, Elizabeth S., Kelly, J. E., and Van Kirk, L. E. Selected dental findings in adults by age, race, and sex; United States — 1960-1962. U.S. Department of Health, Education and Welfare, Public Health Service (National Center for Health Statistics, Series 11, No. 7). Washington, Government Printing Office, Feb. 1965. 35 p.
16. Kelly, J. E., and Van Kirk, L. E. Periodontal disease in adults; United States — 1960-1962. U.S. Department of Health, Education and Welfare, Public Health Service (National Center for Health Statistics, Series 11, No. 12). Washington, Government Printing Office, Nov. 1965. 30 p.
17. Klein, Henry, and Palmer, C. E. Studies on dental caries. VII. Sex differences in dental caries experience of elementary school children. Pub. Health Rep., 53:1685-90, Sept. 23, 1938.
18. Knutson, J. W., Klein, Henry, and Palmer, C. E. Studies on dental caries. VIII. Relative incidence of caries in the different permanent teeth. Am. Dent. A. J. and Dent. Cosmos, 25:1923-34, Dec. 1938.
19. Krogh, H. W. Permanent tooth mortality: a clinical study of causes of loss. Am. Dent. A. J., 57:670-5, Nov. 1958.
20. Leigh, R. W. Incidence of caries in the different teeth and their respective surfaces. Mil. Dent. J., 6:183-94, Dec. 1923.
21. Littleton, N. W. Dental caries and periodontal diseases among Ethiopian civilians. Pub. Health Rep., 78:631-40, July 1963.
22. Lövdal, Arne, Arno, Arnulf, and Waerhaug, Jens. Incidence of clinical manifestations of periodontal disease in light of oral hygiene and calculus formation. Am. Dent. A. J., 56:21-33, Jan. 1958.
23. Lövdal, Arne, et al. Combined effect of subgingival scaling and controlled oral hygiene on the incidence of gingivitis. Acta Odont. Scandinav., 19:537-55, Dec. 1961.
24. Mann, A. W., et al. A comparison of dental caries activity in malnourished and well-nourished patients. Am. Dent. A. J., 34:244-52, Feb. 15, 1947.
25. Marshall-Day, C. D. Nutritional deficiencies and dental caries in Northern India. Brit. Dent. J., 76:115-22, Mar. 1944.

26. Marshall-Day, C. D., Stephens, R. G., and Quigley, L. F. Periodontal disease:prevalence and incidence. J. Periodont., 26:185-203, July 1955.
27. Medical Research Council (Great Britain). Reports of the committee for the investigation of dental disease. II. The incidence of dental disease in children. London, H. M. Stationery Office, 1925. 48 p.
28. Nizel, A. E., and Bibby, B. G. Geographic variations in caries prevalence in soldiers. Am. Dent. A. J., 31:1619-26, Dec. 1, 1944.
29. Pelton, W. J., Pennell, E. H., and Druzina, Anton. Tooth morbidity experience of adults. Am. Dent. A. J., 49:439-45, Oct. 1954.
30. Russell, A. L. Epidemiology of periodontal disease. Internat. Dent. J., 17:282-96, June 1967.
31. _____. The inhibition of approximal caries in adults with lifelong fluoride exposure. J. Dent. Res., 32:138-43, Feb. 1953.
32. _____. International nutrition surveys: a summary of preliminary dental findings. J. Dent. Res., 42:233-44, Jan.-Feb. 1963.
33. _____. Longitudinal technics in the study of oral disease. Am. J. Pub. Health, 46:728-35, June 1956.
34. _____. A social factor associated with the severity of periodontal disease. J. Dent. Res., 36:922-6, Dec. 1957.
35. _____. Some epidemiological characteristics of periodontal disease in a series of urban populations. J. Periodont., 28:286-93, Oct. 1957.
36. _____. World epidemiology and oral health. p. 21-39. (In Kreshover, S. J., and McClure, F. J., eds. Environmental variables in oral disease. Washington, American Association Advancement Science, 1966. XII + 312 p.)
37. Russell, A. L., and Ayers, Polly. Periodontal disease and socioeconomic status in Birmingham, Ala. Am. J. Pub. Health, 50:206-14, Feb. 1960.
38. Russell, A. L., Consolazio, C. F., and White, C. L. Dental caries and nutrition in Eskimo scouts of the Alaska National Guard. J. Dent. Res., 40:594-603, May-June 1961.
39. Russell, A. L., and Elvove, Elias. Domestic water and dental caries. VII. A study of the fluoride-dental caries relationship in an adult population. Pub. Health Rep., 66:1389-401, Oct. 26, 1951.
40. Russell, A. L., et al. Dental caries and nutrition in South Vietnam. J. Dent. Res., 44:102-11, Jan.-Feb. 1965.
41. Russell, A. L., et al. Periodontal disease and nutrition in South Vietnam. J. Dent. Res., 44:775-82, July-Aug. 1965.
42. Schlack, C. A., Restarske, J. S., and Dochterman, E. F. Dental status of 71,015 naval personnel at first examination in 1942. Am. Dent. A. J., 33:1141-6, Sept. 1, 1946.
43. Senn, W. W. Incidence of dental caries among aviation cadets. Mil. Surg., 93:461-4, Dec. 1943.
44. Taylor, G. F., and Marshall-Day, C. D. Osteomalacia and dental caries. Brit. Dent. J., 69:316, Nov. 1940.
45. Waerhaug, Jens. Epidemiology of periodontal disease—review of literature. p. 181-211. (In Ramfjord, S. P., Kerr, D. A., and Ash, M. M., eds. World workshop in periodontics, 1966. Ann Arbor, University Michigan, c1966. XX + 458 p.)
46. _____. Preliminary report on WHO periodontal survey in Ceylon, October-December 1960. Geneva, World Health Organization, WHO/PA/175.62, (1962). IV + 47 p.

Section Three

PREVENTION AND CONTROL OF DENTAL DISEASES

CHAPTER 7

Measures Available for the Prevention and Control of Dental Caries

CHAPTER 8

Measures Available for the Prevention and Control of Periodontal and Other Oral Diseases

CHAPTER 9

The Application of Preventive and Control Measures

Although the prevention of disease should be the ultimate objective of all health professions, curative and restorative procedures often overshadow preventive measures in professional education, in clinical practice, and in public appreciation. Over four decades ago Dr. Joseph Mountin* made a charge to the medical profession which is still valid and which, when paraphrased, applies with equal relevance to dentistry:

Unfortunately, preventive dentistry immediately calls to mind the activities of public and private agencies requiring added philanthropy on the part of the private dentist. The idea is erroneous, since prevention should be an integral part of the dentist's activities,

---

*Mountin, J. W. Preventive medicine in private practice. Nat. Eclectic Med. A. Quar., 17:46-52, June 1925.

equally as deserving of recompense as his more dramatic or tangible services. This presupposes that we understand the real purpose of our profession, measure up to its responsibilities, and embrace our true place and function. However, before we, as dentists, can embrace this role, we must change our attitude towards our patients, and we must bring them to see the services that we are capable of giving. . . . This does not necessitate our re-entering dental school; in fact, practically all of us are equipped with sufficient knowledge. All we need is a change of attitude.

CHAPTER 7

MEASURES AVAILABLE FOR THE PREVENTION AND CONTROL OF DENTAL CARIES

By A. L. RUSSELL, D.D.S., M.P.H.

In most Western civilizations, dental caries attacks virtually all of the people early in childhood and continues to harass most of them throughout life or until teeth are wholly lost. As a consequence, control of dental caries is a major concern of all of the people and not merely of a few. Nevertheless, the fact that it is not considered to be a fatal disease imposes constraints upon the methods which may be applied in its control. The Pasteur treatment for rabies, for example, is acceptable despite the definite hazard accompanying its application, because this hazard is slight compared to the much greater danger of death from untreated rabies; but a control measure for dental caries must be quite devoid of hazard to life or function if it is to be so much as considered for practical application. It must, of course, be effective. Its potency must be maintained for a substantial span of time, preferably for the lifetime of the individual. It should take effect immediately upon application, and it should reach all of the people in the population. Its cost should fall within the means of the community, whether cost is measured in dollars or as a requirement for skilled personnel or facilities. The ideal control measure for dental caries, in short, must have immediate, high, and lasting effectiveness, be innocuous, and reach all of the people at a cost in money and facilities well within the economic capabilities of the community.

Some of these requirements are met by timely and competent restorative care. Restorative care, however, misses the ideal by not reaching all or most of the people at a cost in money and facilities within the economic capabilities of a community.

From some points of view the distinction between preventive and treatment measures is an artificial one. Some disease entities, like typhoid fever and smallpox, have been controlled largely through preventive measures; others, like scarlet fever, largely through individual treatment. A practical control program usually represents a fine balance between the two methods, and the caries control program is no exception. But dentists and facilities in the United States are presently too few and too little to cope with the demand for dental care, much less the total need, and there is little indication that this situation will improve in the immediate future. Care facilities are even less adequate in other areas, such as parts of South America, where the prevalence of oral disease is quite as high and the numbers of professional personnel even smaller. It is obvious that treatment efforts must be augmented by powerful preventive measures if dental caries is to be controlled.

The preventive agent which has so far proved most potent and practicable is the fluoride ion.

FLUORIDATION

As this is written, the United States is well into the third decade of experience with controlled fluoridation. The measure has proved itself fully in practice. No hazard to health has resulted. It has been adapted readily in a variety of water systems, large and small. In each case it has been followed by the expected improvement in oral health. In the light of this experience it seems incredible that the proposal should have been challenged. This challenge is understandable only if one remembers the intense, emotionally charged opposition that fought the adoption of vaccination for smallpox, or the introduction of anesthesia into surgical practice. In the words of the editor of the Washington *Post*:

> Remember the noisy rumble a decade ago when Washington began adding sodium silicofluoride to the water supply? Some otherwise sober citizens saw this as little short of a Bolshevik plot to seep from within and turn our drinking water into a potion of deviltry. But time has borne out the experiment, and the final reply has come from the most definitive of sources — literally, from the mouths of children ... fluoridation offers a signal example of what science can do to improve our natural environment. Our children are being given an advantage hitherto available only to those who lived in areas where natural fluoridation of the water combats decay. Why can't more be done to use the tools of science to make our cities habitable ...?[154]

Despite this uniformly favorable experience, and the fact that virtually all practitioners in the recognized health professions support the measure, opposition has not ended. The motivations of antifluoridationists have been a matter of considerable interest to social scientists.[108] Open opposition to fluoridation is usually based on two contentions: that community fluoridation is a violation of personal rights, and that it is hazardous for the people who use fluoridated water. Every court of last resort in the country has ruled that the addition of fluoride ion to public water supplies is a legal and proper exercise of governmental power and that it does not constitute an infringement of individual constitutional rights.[29] On the matter of alleged hazards, the usual tactic of the antifluoridationist is an attempt to confuse and frighten the uninformed citizen so that he will vote against fluoridation when the issue is brought to referendum. This aspect of the question is discussed more fully in Chapter Nine.

Possibly no other public health measure has received as much competent research as that which has been devoted to fluoridation. Of the tens of thousands of scientific reports dealing with this subject, Irene Campbell of the Kettering Laboratory, College of Medicine, University of Cincinnati, has selected 158 of the most important and has combined them in a single publication[30] for the convenience of individuals who want the basic facts in the matter. Every professional person should be familiar with these basics, so that he may meet his obligation to those open-minded and concerned persons who want to know what is fact and what is fancy about one of the most important public health developments in recent years.

The field studies which established a correlation between waterborne fluorides and dental caries in children and adults have been outlined in Chapter Four. As pointed out in that section, the correlation itself was insufficient to prove that the same inhibition of caries would follow if a fluoride-deficient community water were to be adjusted to a desirable level; it was necessary to make a direct test of the proposition.[7] But a study of this sort, utilizing a human population, could not be considered seriously until it could be established that there was little or no danger that the people would be harmed as a result. To appreciate the position of the dental scientist at that point it is necessary to review the evidence available to the designers of the first fluoridation studies. To understand the status of the question today, it is necessary to review the information which has accumulated since that time.

Physiology and Metabolism of Fluorides

Fluorine is one of the most ubiquitous of the elements. There was an average of 292 parts per million of the fluoride ion (ppm F) in the 137 samples from 30 profiles of soil examined by Robinson and Edgington, and the fluoride content increased with depth from the surface.[115] Barth has estimated that the earth's crust contains, on the average, about 800 grams per ton (about 880 ppm).[16] It is present in nearly all fresh ground waters, though the concentration in some surface water is very low—less than 0.1 ppm F. Deep well waters in the United States have carried as much as 27 ppm F. It occurs in sea water generally, as well as in the oceans off the shores of the United States, in concentrations ranging from 1.0 to 1.4 ppm.[147] Hence, it is difficult to understand how any form of life, on land or in the sea, could have evolved and survived unless it was fully able to cope with a continuous intake of fluorides from its environment, including feast or surge periods during which the amounts ingested would reach peaks many times higher than the average over a longer period of time. All of the evidence is fully consistent with this proposition. Species for species, the fluoride content of plants remains remarkably constant whether they are grown in soil with much or with little fluoride. There is no consistent difference in the fluoride content of the soft tissues of freshwater and saltwater fish; very little fluoride appears in cows' milk and the amount is increased only slightly, if at all, by the addition of large amounts of fluorides to the drinking water or the grain ration.[97] Negligible amounts of fluoride are stored in human soft tissues, and these concentrations do not rise with increased levels of fluoride in the individual's domestic water.[2, 138] It is clear that no serious imbalance can or does exist between the life processes and ordinary amounts of fluoride acquired from the environment.

But there was no certainty about the upper limits of these innocuous "ordinary amounts" when traces of fluoride were first shown to be constituents of some domestic water supplies. Most previous reports of effects in humans had been concerned with such massive intakes of fluoride as those experienced by the cryolite workers studied by Roholm. Some of these men and women had been exposed to heavy concentrations of dust which averaged about 97 percent cryolite (a sodium-aluminum fluoride, Na_3AlF_6). Their daily absorption was estimated at 0.2 to 1.0 milligram of fluoride per kilogram of body weight (in the case of a man weighing 150 pounds, from about 14 to about 68 milligrams of fluoride per day). Some had been employed as long as 31 years. Under these conditions a number of toxic effects were observed, principally gastric complaints and osteosclerosis.[116] But the amounts inhaled by these workers far exceeded the amounts available from potable waters. F. J. McClure, working closely with Dean, set out to determine whether any other undesirable physiological effect beyond mottling might be produced by the relatively minute levels of the ion carried by domestic water supplies.

It was known that reduced breaking strength in the long bones of dairy cattle and swine might follow long-continued ingestion of massive amounts of fluorides. If increased bone fragility were a hazard in human beings using a fluoride water, McClure reasoned, native residents of fluoride areas should have had more fractures than persons using a low-fluoride water. Accordingly, he obtained histories of fracture experience from 2,529 young adult men reporting for physical examination at induction centers in Texas, Oklahoma, Indiana, Virginia, and New Hampshire, and from 1,458 high school boys in Illinois and the District of Columbia. There was no relation between fracture experience and the lifetime use of waters containing from none to as much as 6.0 parts per million of fluorides. Neither was there any association with height or weight of the men.[95]

Further, a second study of equal significance demonstrated that fluorine in urine was "strikingly proportional" to the amount of fluoride in domestic water supplies ranging from 0.5 to 5.1 ppm of the element. This finding was based on determinations on samples of urine from about 1,900 young men with lifetime residence in such nonfluoride areas as the District of Columbia, Indianapolis, Chicago, and New Hampshire, against samples of urine from men in the fluoride areas in Texas and Illinois. Within this range of fluoride waters, it was concluded, "The metabolism of fluorine under these conditions seems to be a normal function of the human body and seems characterized by a condition approaching metabolic equilibrium, at least in the adult organism." Urine specimens from 394 men from the low-fluoride areas and for 101 men from the high-fluoride areas of the Texas Panhandle were further examined for occult blood, albumin, and glucose. No differences between these groups were found.[99]

Balance studies, in which young men lived in rooms controlled for comfortable or "hot moist" conditions and were challenged with varying amounts of fluoride in food or water, led to the conclusion that

> ... the elimination of absorbed fluorine via the urine and perspiration is practically complete when the quantities absorbed do not exceed 4.0 to 5.0 mg. daily. There was no significant retention of fluorine in the bodies of these young adult men, when total daily fluorine ingested did not exceed 4.0 to 5.0 mg. daily. The data suggest that these may be the limits of fluorine which may be ingested daily without an appreciable hazard of body storage of fluorine.[100]

But intakes higher than this could occur in such communities as Bartlett, Texas, where the community water carried about eight parts per million of fluoride. Accordingly, in 1943, a Public Health Service team gave detailed physical and oral examinations to a random sample of persons who had lived in Bartlett for 15 years or more. There was no indication that this fluoride exposure had had any adverse effect, other than mottling of dental enamel, upon health or well-being of these people.[86] These and other studies on human population groups were supported by a large body of evidence obtained by direct experimentation with large animals—sheep, swine, and dairy cattle—as well as from numerous experimental laboratory animals, particularly with the white rat.

This, in summary, was the state of information at the time the first fluoridation trials were begun in 1945. The studies outlined, amplified by numerous others, had established these basic facts:

1. that the human body possessed a prompt and efficient excretory mechanism for fluorides which minimized the danger of long-term accumulation,

2. that skeletal damage, the usual first sign of chronic intoxication from large doses of fluorides, could not be demonstrated in users of fluoride-bearing domestic waters,

3. that large groups of people had used waters carrying up to eight parts per million of fluorides for long periods of time without impairment of general health, and

4. that caries-inhibitory benefits might be expected at a fluoride level around one part per million, a concentration too low to produce objectionable mottling in the teeth of children.

Since that time the physiology of trace amounts of fluorides has been documented in great detail.

When a small amount—five milligrams or less—of a soluble fluoride is ingested by the human adult, it is rapidly removed from circulating body fluids. A portion appears promptly in urine; from 20 to 25 percent is eliminated by this route within three to five hours.[137] Balance studies have indicated that nearly all is eliminated via urine, feces, and perspiration when the quantities ingested do not exceed four to five milligrams over an entire day. Where the domestic water is free of fluoride, the fluorine present in the urine of persons in the United States averages from 0.3 to 0.5 ppm and has been obtained from foodstuffs. With a fluoride-containing domestic water, the level of fluoride in urine rises in proportion, as outlined earlier in this section.[99] The excretory mechanism in the kidney is strikingly selective for fluoride, which does not enter the "halogen pool"—that is, its elimination is not modified by the numbers, or proportions, of chlorine and bromine ions present. In fact, though fluorine belongs to the chemical family of halogens, along with chlorine, iodine, and bromine, its metabolism and physical effects in no way parallel those of other members of this group.[33, 66]

This prompt and efficient excretory mechanism, however, is insufficient in itself to explain the rapid disappearance of the fluoride ion from circulating body fluids after ingestion. The rhythm of excretion suggests that the larger portion of the ingested fluoride is very quickly placed in inert storage in some body site where it can be immobilized and retained until disposed of by the routine processes of elimination. This actually happens; the storage site is the inorganic portion of skeletal bone.[35, 137]

The hydroxyapatite crystals of bone and teeth have a strong physical chemical affinity for fluoride. The fluoride content of fossil bone increases with time, and more rapidly in soils or ground waters with the higher concentrations of F.[107] Fluoride in living human bone builds up slowly with age of the individual even though his domestic water is fluoride-free, because of absorption from food. A stabilized dynamic equilibrium is developed between the amount of fluoride ingested from all sources and the amount stored in bone; little is retained by an adult living in the temperate zone of the United States who uses a water containing about one part per million of F. There is more storage in the skeleton as water levels are increased, and an increased bone density to x-ray can sometimes be demonstrated with waters carrying four or five parts per million or more. At these levels the increase in bone fluorine content can be demonstrated only by x-ray or chemical analysis; there is no interference with normal function, nor alteration in the physiology of the tissue.[137] From this point of view bone may be considered as a convenient bin in which an excess of ingested fluoride can be stored to await orderly elimination.

The relation of fluoride to the chemistry and physiological properties of bone is more complex than simple storage. If formed during a period when the individual receives adequate fluoride, the size of the hydroxyapatite crystal is increased, a change which adds to the stability of bone.[111] There is some indication that osteoporosis may be less frequent in elderly persons who have used a fluoride water than in those whose water has been fluoride-deficient.[19, 86]

Nevertheless, the principal protective mechanism is provided by the parallel processes of rapid elimination by urine plus inert storage in the nonliving portion of bone. This mechanism is remarkably effective against either the sudden, accidental high-level dose or the prolonged intake of lesser but still excessive amounts. Hodge and Smith have estimated that an adult of average body weight must ingest and retain at least five to 10 grams of fluoride within two to four hours to endanger life, and must take in 20 to 80 mg. of fluoride daily for from 10 to 20 years to run the risk of chronic poisoning.[66] To obtain these amounts from a water fluoridated to one part per million, life might be endangered only if the adult could drink about 660 gallons of the water (or the average child about 165 gallons) *within two to four hours*. The hazard of chronic poisoning might ensue only after the consumption of from five to 20 gallons of the fluoridated water every day for more than 3,000 consecutive days. On these bases Hodge and Smith have concluded:

> The possibility of acute fatal poisoning is nil. Children drinking fluoridated water will grow normally. No detectable alterations will occur in bone structure; such changes have been found in a small fraction of a population taking 8 times the recommended 1 ppm but there is no evidence that the alterations will be harmful.[66]

Fluorides are not stored in soft tissues and do not accumulate there. The trace amounts found on analysis are due principally or wholly to levels in circulating body fluids. The amount of fluoride in blood plasma remains about the same in persons using waters with fluorides in the range of 0.15 to 2.5 ppm F, with individual values ranging from 0.14 to 0.19 ppm.[132] Relatively new and delicate technics based upon measure of the radioactive isotope of fluorine,[18]F, have indicated that the apparent accumulation of fluoride in the placenta with time is due to absorption by the small islands of calcification which often develop late in term.[45] Evidence is equivocal as to whether the very slight elevation of fluoride in umbilical circulation following fluoride ingestion by the mother is great enough to have any effect on the fetus.[54]

Other possibilities, predicated upon the known enzyme-inhibiting properties *in vitro* of fluorides in high concentrations, have failed to materialize in human populations using a water with a level of about one part per million of the ion. Carpal growth is not inhibited, nor growth in height or weight. Renal function is not altered.[94, 98, 126] The incidence of goiter is not affected, nor is there any interference with the usefulness of iodine in controlling goiter.[84, 137] There is, in short, no indication of acute or chronic damage to any of the systems of the human body as the result of usage of a water fluoridated to recommended levels.

At these low levels of concentration, the fluoride present in the water occurs in ionic form—dissociated from the particular cation to which it was bonded in concentrated form. The result is the same, whether the fluoride is introduced to the water as sodium fluoride, calcium fluoride, a fluorosilicate, or as hydrofluoric acid.

Some of this information about the physiology of fluoride has been accumulated as the result of direct observation during the course of fluoridation studies. When the Newburgh-Kingston study was proposed, for example:

> There was no reason to believe that fluoride, when added to the drinking water as a routine part of the water treatment process, would act differently from fluoride present in the water at the source. Nevertheless, it was considered desirable to test this remote possibility by periodic medical examination of groups of children under carefully controlled conditions.[126]

Accordingly, large groups of children—the numbers eventually totaled 817 in Newburgh and 711 in Kingston—were examined annually. Excellent cooperation was obtained; 88 percent of the Newburgh children and 74 percent of the Kingston children who remained in the cities as residents at the end of the study term returned for the final examination. This examination was unusually thorough, including a careful history, a complete physical examination, selected physical measurements, and laboratory and radiographic studies. No significant difference in general health between children in the two cities was seen at annual or final examinations. Height and weight were the same, and the onset of menstruation in girls came at equivalent ages. No differences in bone density could be demonstrated in radiographs of the right hand, knees, and the lumbar spine. There was essential similarity in findings for skeletal maturation, hemoglobin level, erythrocyte and leukocyte counts, quantity of sugar, albumin, red blood cells, and casts in urine, and in vision and hearing. On the final examination 19 of 476 children in Newburgh (4.0 percent) and 20 of 405 children in Kingston (4.9 percent) were referred to the family physician for conditions including such minor ailments as a plantar wart or ringworm. Long-term downward trends in stillbirth and maternal and infant mortality rates continued in each of the cities. Each had about the same experience with deaths from cancer and from cardiovascular-renal disease. The overall conclusion reached was, "No differences of medical significance could be found between the two groups of children; thus further evidence was added to that already available on the safety of water fluoridation."[125, 126]

Meanwhile, investigations by health departments within such states as Illinois had shown no differences in health between persons living in fluoride and nonfluoride areas. For the United States as a whole no differences could be found in death rates for 1949-1950 between the 32 cities with established water-fluoride levels of 0.7 ppm or more and 32 randomly selected nearby cities with valid histories of 0.25 ppm F or less in the domestic supply. Mortality rates were about the same for cancer, heart disease, intracranial lesions, nephritis, and cirrhosis of the liver. No untoward results developed in the other fluoridation study centers.[64]

The consensus of United States workers has been summarized by Heyroth:

> ...the prolonged intake of quantities of fluoride too small to induce dental fluorosis does not give rise to any of the nondental manifestations of chronic intoxication by fluorides. Epidemiologic data and clinical and radiographic examinations of exposed industrial workers indicate that only when the fluoride content of a water supply exceeds 5 or 6 ppm will its prolonged usage give rise to detectable osseous changes and then only in the most susceptible persons. The evidence as a whole is consistent in offering assurance that bringing the fluoride concentration in communal water supplies to that known to be optimal for dental health is a prophylactic public health procedure which has an ample margin of safety.[65]

During the same period of time Great Britain instituted its own investigation, designed to test whether fluoridation might be efficacious and safe under the conditions of life in the United Kingdom. Particular attention was paid to possible influences of such British characteristics as high consumption of tea by adults,* and to conditions for which uniquely valid information might be obtained from the complete data kept for each person under the national health plan. Controlled fluoridation studies were begun in three areas, and particular attention was paid to the few localities with natural fluorides at

---
*Dry tea contains more fluoride than most other plant sources. Ten to 12 cups of tea, taken daily, could add as much as 1.0 mg. of fluoride to the diet.

optimum levels. The research teams concluded that fluoride, at the levels encountered in British waters, did not affect mortality rates, did not cause osteochondritis of the spine, and did not result in harmful accumulations of fluorides in bone; did not cause objectionable mottling, even in conjunction with malnutrition; did not relate to mongol births, peptic ulcer, or absenteeism from school; and had no association with thyroid enlargement. The report ends:

> After detailing the more important evidence the World Health Organization's Expert Committee concludes "All these findings fit together in a consonant whole that constitutes a great guarantee of safety—a body of evidence without precedent in public health procedures."
>
> The Ministry's Research Committee agrees with these conclusions. In its opinion the raising of the fluoride content of drinking water to a level of 1 p.p.m. is safe.[102]

Efficacy of Fluoridation

The pioneer fluoridation studies were carried out in Grand Rapids, Michigan; Newburgh, New York; Brantford, Ontario; and Evanston, Illinois. Their success has already been noted, but little attention has been paid to the patterns or degree of caries inhibition which resulted. Some understanding of these patterns is essential in any consideration of the effects of fluoridation upon dental practice, private and public.

The principal findings in these studies have been reviewed by Ast and Fitzgerald,[8] and full-term reports have been issued for each of them.[5, 9, 24, 26]

A general summary, as computed by Ast and Fitzgerald, is shown in Table 12. After terms ranging up through 15 years of fluoridation, DMF teeth in children aged 12 to 14 or 13 to 14 years were lower by 48, 56, 57, and 70 percent to a level of three or four DMF teeth per child. These were independent studies, utilizing different procedures. The Grand Rapids and Brantford data were based on mirror and explorer examinations. Mirror and explorer examinations were supplemented with radiographs in Newburgh, and radiographic examination was supplemented with mirror and explorer examinations in Evanston. Similar results have been observed consistently in other studies, quite independent of these, including several in continental Europe.

The first fluoridation studies were designed on the hypothesis that no caries inhibition would be seen in children born prior to the time of fluoridation. Instead there was an almost immediate downward trend in DMF permanent teeth, demonstrable in most instances after two years of study. In younger children this effect was due almost entirely to a saving of occlusal caries in permanent first molars which had been in eruption at the time of fluoridation. This

TABLE 12. GENERAL COMPARISON OF DMF TEETH PER CHILD, AND MISSING TEETH PER CHILD, AT THE END OF THE STUDY TERM IN FOUR PIONEER FLUORIDATION COMMUNITIES.*

		DMF TEETH PER CHILD	PERCENT DIFFERENCE	MISSING TEETH PER CHILD	PERCENT DIFFERENCE
Grand Rapids (F)	1944-45	9.58		0.84	
Ages 12-14	1959	4.26	-55.5	0.29	-65.5
Evanston (F)	1946	9.03		0.19	
Ages 12-14	1959	4.66	-48.4	0.06	-68.4
Sarnia (No F)	1959	7.46		0.75	
Brantford (F) Ages 12-14	1959	3.23	-56.7	0.22	-70.7
Kingston (No F)	1960	12.46		0.92	
Newburgh (F) Ages 13-14	1960	3.73	-70.1	0.10	-89.1

*Adapted from Ast and Fitzgerald.[8] Grand Rapids, Brantford, and Newburgh started fluoridation in 1945. Evanston started fluoridation in 1947. Sarnia and Kingston are fluoride-deficient.

advantage was largely lost within the next few years, though important protection for smooth surfaces of these teeth was demonstrable eight years later.[13, 123] But principal benefits are enjoyed by children born at the time of fluoridation of the community supply or shortly thereafter.[31, 50, 59, 69, 80, 113] It became clear that findings from populations using a natural fluoride water might be applied directly to communities using water which is fluoridated by controlled methods.

An additional benefit of fluoride ingestion at optimal levels during the period of tooth formation is a marked improvement in the appearance of the teeth. Forrest, on the basis of studies with English children, has described her findings as follows:

> The benefit derived from fluoride did not seem to be merely a freedom from caries .... The appearance of the teeth was striking and can be described as excellent. They were well formed and of particularly good colour and structure in contrast to those in the nonfluoride areas which frequently showed evidence of poor calcification.[49]

and adds:

> ...it is misleading to use the term "mottling" to describe the condition of the teeth found with a concentration of 1 p.p.m. of fluoride in the water. The milder forms of fluorosis which may occur among a very few people at this level are not detectable by the ordinary observer.[50]

Her observations are consistent with experience in the United States.[39, 118]

It also may be expected that children born in a community with a fluoridated water can expect a lifelong protective effect, provided they continue to use a water with optimum fluoride.

In Colorado Springs, Colorado, it was possible to demonstrate that the physical characteristics of the water system had not varied in any essential manner for the 70 years prior to 1950.[122] Nor had there been any important fluctuation in fluoride levels for the period between 1906 and 1930, because groups of native residents aged 20 through 44 years in 1950 showed essentially the same degree of dental fluorosis throughout that age range. It was likewise possible to demonstrate that the city water of nearby Boulder, Colorado, had been essentially fluoride-free over this same span of time. Dental caries status of lifelong residents of the two cities, aged 20 through 44 years is shown in Figure 7. Differences in tooth mortality are shown in Figure 8. Throughout the age range studied, Colorado Springs natives showed about 60 percent fewer decayed, missing, and filled permanent teeth than did natives of Boulder who had lost three or four times as many permanent teeth. The oldest Colorado Springs group (aged 40 to 44 years) had fewer DMF teeth per person than the youngest Boulder group (aged 20 to 24 years); and Colorado Springs na-

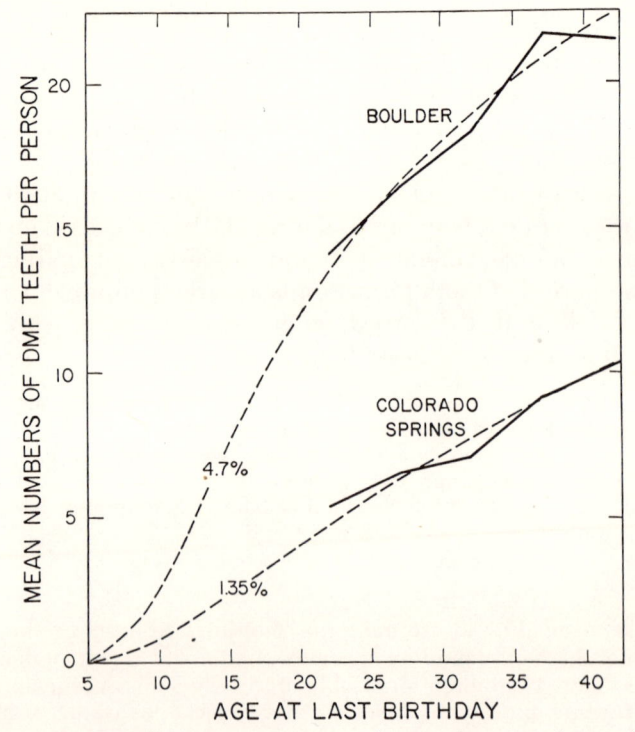

FIGURE 7. Dental caries experience of native-born residents of Colorado Springs, Colorado, with lifetime use of a fluoride-bearing water, and of Boulder, Colorado, with lifetime use of a fluoride-free water.[122] The dotted lines represent estimates of the permanent tooth attack rate per year in each population.

PREVENTION AND CONTROL OF DENTAL CARIES

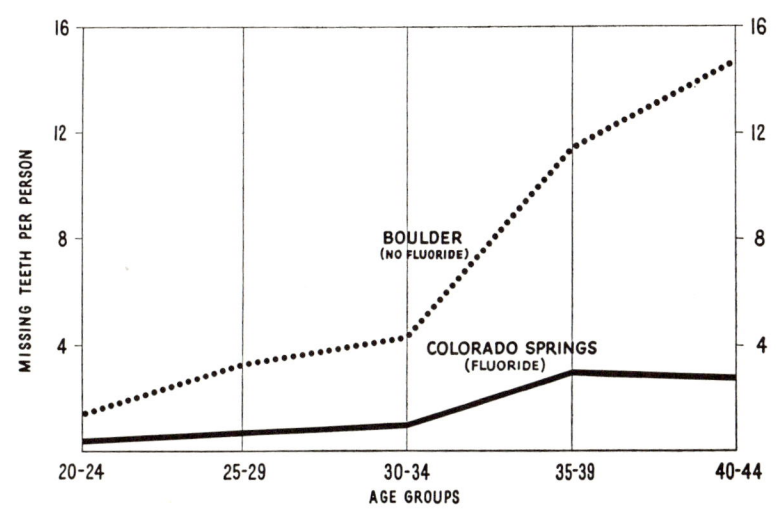

FIGURE 8. Permanent tooth mortality from all causes in adult natives of a fluoride-free community (Boulder, Colorado) and of a community with 2.5 ppm F in the water supply (Colorado Springs, Colorado). (Russell and Elvove[122])

tives up to the age of 34 years averaged fewer DMF teeth than children aged 12 to 14 years in the 11 of the 21 cities with 0.4 ppm or less of fluorides in their community waters. The magnitude of inhibition was about the same as Dean found in 12- to 14-year-old children in natural-fluoride Kewanee compared with the low-fluoride group in the 21 cities, or in Grand Rapids or Brantford children the same ages at the end of those study terms. These findings are consistent with an attack rate of 4.7 percent (the proportion of teeth free of caries at the beginning of a year which becomes carious during the year) in natives of Boulder, and an attack rate of 1.35 percent in permanent teeth in Colorado Springs. Lifetime caries experience resulting from these attack rates are plotted in Figure 7 as broken lines. The average fluoride level at Colorado Springs—2.5 ppm—is above optimum, and the people examined there had used the water for essentially their entire lives. Under these circumstances the caries-inhibitory effect, so similar to that previously demonstrated in children, persisted without apparent diminution through the age of 44 years, with no suggestion that it might be lost after that time.[119, 122]

Arnold, analyzing data from native children of Aurora (a community with natural fluorides), had noted that these children had about 95 percent fewer carious lesions in the proximal surfaces of their four upper incisors than children using a fluoride-free water.[3] A high order of protection for these and other approximal surfaces had been maintained in the Colorado Springs group. Comparisons in older persons were difficult because of the high tooth mortality in Boulder, but at the age of 25 to 34 years there were from 85 to 90 percent fewer carious approximal surfaces in the maxillary incisors of people examined in Colorado Springs. The advantage in approximal surfaces ranged from 62 percent in the distal surfaces of maxillary molars upwards to essentially complete inhibition of caries in the mandibular incisors. These comparisons are shown graphically in Figure 9.[119] A similar persistence of the caries-inhibitory effect of a fluoride-bearing water has been reported from such diverse areas as Illinois, Ecuador, and Czechoslovakia.[43, 73, 78]

The inhibitory effect was not limited to smooth surfaces nor to teeth relatively insusceptible to caries. Table 13 is a summary of the caries experience of the most susceptible teeth, the permanent first molars, in these two populations. In the oldest group in Colorado Springs (aged 40 to 44 years) about eight out of 10 mandibular first molars and about seven out of 10 maxillary first molars were still present and functional. About 60 percent of all first molar surfaces remained free of decay after periods at risk in the mouth ranging from 34 to 38 years. This is markedly less than the caries experience of the Boulder group. This degree of inhibition could not have been attained without a considerable lessening of caries susceptibility in pit and fissure as well as in smooth surfaces.

Patterns of caries activity in children born after fluoridation suggest that they may expect a very similar benefit. Table 14 lists first molar attack rates observed during the eighth year of fluoridation in children of suburban Washington, D.C.[123] Prior to fluoridation about one mandibular first molar occlusal surface in five (22.34 percent), free of caries at the outset, might be expected to become carious

TABLE 13. STATUS OF PERMANENT FIRST MOLAR SURFACES IN LIFELONG RESIDENTS OF BOULDER, COLORADO (WITH NEGLIGIBLE FLUORIDE IN THE COMMUNITY WATER), AND OF COLORADO SPRINGS, COLORADO (WITH AN AVERAGE FLUORIDE CONTENT OF 2.5 PPM IN THE COMMUNITY WATER).*

| | | AVERAGE NUMBERS OF FIRST MOLAR SURFACES PER PERSON ||||||
| | | MANDIBULAR ||| MAXILLARY |||
AGES	NUMBERS EXAMINED	MISSING	DECAYED OR FILLED	PRESENT AND SOUND	MISSING	DECAYED OR FILLED	PRESENT AND SOUND
Boulder (no fluoride)								
20-24	51	1.08	3.98	4.94	1.47	3.47	5.06
25-29	41	3.17	3.80	3.03	1.10	4.37	4.53
30-34	29	3.28	3.90	2.82	2.41	3.21	4.38
35-44	34	6.62	2.21	1.17	5.15	2.65	2.20
Colorado Springs (2.5 ppm F)								
20-24	72	.42	1.80	7.78	.28	1.04	8.68
25-29	101	.89	1.74	7.37	.64	1.28	8.08
30-34	82	.98	2.00	7.02	.61	1.69	7.70
35-39	75	1.86	1.62	6.52	1.40	1.56	7.04
40-44	55	1.91	2.06	6.03	2.73	1.56	5.71

*Russell. Unpublished data.

PREVENTION AND CONTROL OF DENTAL CARIES

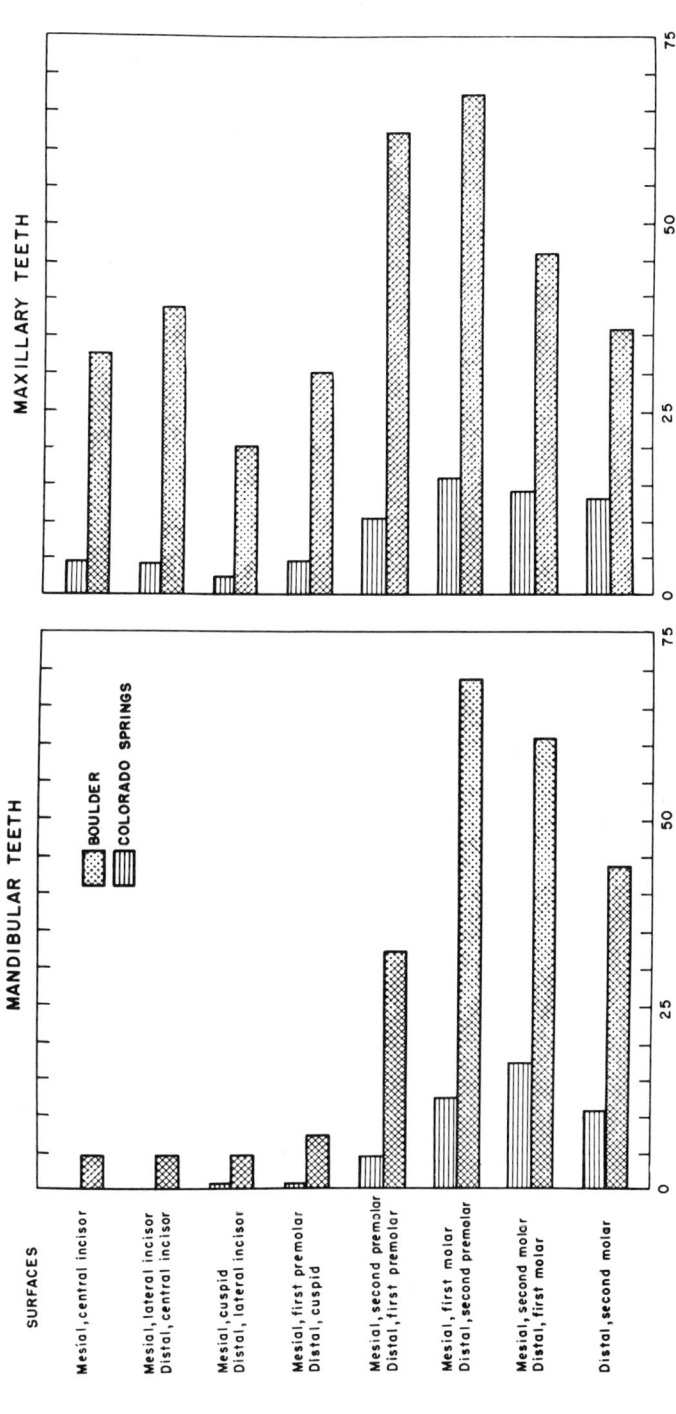

FIGURE 9. Percentages of approximal surfaces which are decayed, filled, or missing because of dental caries in adults aged 25 to 34 years in Boulder, Colorado (using a fluoride-free drinking water) and in Colorado Springs, Colorado (using a water with 2.5 ppm of fluorine). (Russell[119])

TABLE 14. CARIES ATTACK RATES IN PERMANENT FIRST MOLARS OF CHILDREN AGED 5 TO 8 YEARS, PRIOR TO AND DURING THE EIGHTH YEAR OF FLUORIDATION, MONTGOMERY AND PRINCE GEORGES COUNTIES, MARYLAND.*

	PERCENTAGE OF CARIES-FREE FIRST MOLAR SURFACES BECOMING CARIOUS DURING THE YEAR		
	PRIOR TO FLUORIDATION	DURING EIGHTH YEAR OF FLUORIDATION	DIFFERENCE, PERCENT
Maxillary first molar			
All surfaces	4.02	0.92	- 77
Occlusal surfaces	16.54	3.89	- 76
Mandibular first molar			
All surfaces	5.56	1.84	- 67
Occlusal surfaces	22.34	5.19	- 77

*Russell and Hamilton.[123]

during a 12-month period in children of these ages. During the year of observation only about one occlusal surface in 20 (5.19 percent) actually decayed. This attack rate is quite consistent with the experience of Colorado Springs adults outlined above. Of the restorations still required by these children, about 19 out of 20 were for pits and fissures in the enamel.[123]

Fewer cases of dental fluorosis (and these of the near-invisible borderline type) developed in Newburgh and in Grand Rapids than had been expected on the basis of findings in the 21 cities.[9, 118]

New drinking water standards were adopted by the Public Health Service in 1961, based on the findings of Galagan that children drink more fluid in a warm climate than in a cool one.[51, 52] These standards are shown in Table 15.[151] The values have been corroborated by a five-year study carried out by Richards and his associates in the California State Health Department.[113] The evidence from Grand Rapids and Newburgh suggests that fluoridation to the upper limits shown in the table would probably result in little or no objectionable mottling of teeth.

Early results from studies of a fluoridated school water supply indicate that this measure may have some value in rural areas.[70, 71] Higher levels than one part per million have been considered, since school-age children are too old for mottling of enamel (except third molars); no other adverse effect follows use of waters with fluoride levels as high as five parts per million, and, in any event, children take only a portion of their daily fluid intake during the hours they are in school.

Compared with the requirements for the ideal caries control measure outlined earlier in this section, water fluoridation fares very

TABLE 15. FLUORIDE LEVELS RECOMMENDED FOR COOL AND WARM CLIMATES.*

| | RECOMMENDED CONTROL LIMITS |||
ANNUAL AVERAGE OF MAXIMUM DAILY AIR TEMPERATURES[†]	F CONCENTRATIONS IN PARTS PER MILLION		
	LOWER	OPTIMUM	UPPER
50.0 - 53.7	0.9	1.2	1.7
53.8 - 58.3	0.8	1.1	1.5
58.4 - 63.8	0.8	1.0	1.3
63.9 - 70.6	0.7	0.9	1.2
70.7 - 79.2	0.7	0.8	1.0
79.3 - 90.5	0.6	0.7	0.8

*Public Health Service.[151]
†Based on temperature data obtained for a minimum of five years.

well. It is an effective caries inhibitor with long-lasting benefits, safe in use, which reaches all of the people of the community without effort on their part and without demands upon the efforts of professionally trained dental personnel.[14] The effect, however, is not instantaneous; the principal benefits accrue to people yet unborn at the time fluoridation begins. Fluoridation is a partial answer to the problems of tomorrow rather than to the problems of today.

The skills required of waterworks personnel are of the same nature as required without fluoridation: "Fluoridation has presented no new or unusual problems to the water works superintendent and his operators."[23] Costs in money are trifling; depending upon method, the usual estimate in the United States is from seven to 14 cents per person per year. Costs in England were found to be about half a shilling per person per year.[102] By whatever estimate, the lifetime cost of fluoridation per person ordinarily is less than the fee for restoration of a single carious tooth.

OTHER VEHICLES FOR SYSTEMIC FLUORIDES

Much thought has been given to methods for making the benefits of fluoride available to people who cannot use a community water supply. Though fluoride intake from a normal North American diet is uniform enough to be considered as a constant factor,[96] most community waters in the United States contain some fluoride, and the actual amount tends to fluctuate from season to season. Hence, fluoride intake from any other source must be kept in constant adjustment to the fluoride supplied in the domestic water. Intakes from such sources as milk or table salt are difficult to control, because individual consumption of these items varies much more widely than individual requirements for water.

Nevertheless, these vehicles offer promise in areas where there are few or no public water supplies, where the water actually used is consistently virtually free of fluorides, and where distribution and utilization of the vehicle is under effective control.[91] Such areas are found more frequently in other parts of the world than in the United States. A 1966-67 Commission of the *Fédération Dentaire Internationale* issued a policy statement which, in part, read as follows:

> In general the staple foods, such as salt, flour, bread and rice, are the preferable alternative vehicles for the systemic administration of fluorides because they give most promise of simulating the effects of water-borne fluoride. Among these salt is the universal nutrient; it has been most extensively tested and is the current choice. . . .[110]

There have been some difficulties in determining the proper amount of fluoride to be incorporated in salt.[103]

An independent study is presently underway in Colombia. In that nation, four isolated mountain villages have been selected for study. In two of these, domestic salt is being fluoridated to a level where the fluoride content of the urine of children is consistent with that of children observed in fluoride areas. The domestic water of a third village is being fluoridated to a level of 1.0 ppm. The fourth village is being utilized as a control. Salt fluoridation can be controlled readily in Colombia because the processing and distribution of salt is a government monopoly.[112]

On the basis of studies in Switzerland, Marthaler and König have concluded that fluoride tablets, distributed about 200 days a year for eight years or longer, have some value in the inhibition of dental caries. Children six to 15 years old who had received the tablets had mean percentage reductions in caries of 36 percent for teeth and 47 percent for tooth surfaces when compared with children of the same ages who had not received fluoride.[92]

American children who had used a tablet containing 2.21 mg. of sodium fluoride (yielding one mg. of the fluoride ion) for one year or more were found to have about the same dental caries experience as children using a fluoridated water. When taken daily these tablets supplied about twice as much fluoride as the fluoridated salt used in Switzerland. The American observers concluded:

> It seems highly probable from this study that fluoride taken daily in tablet form has a beneficial effect on the teeth . . . it is doubtful, however, whether any large-scale or community-wide program of caries control would be successful if tablets were used. Although the persons involved in this study were, on the whole, a highly educated group, only about half of them actually continued to give their children tablets for the necessary number of years. . . .[6]

The Council on Dental Therapeutics of the American Dental Association has decided that ". . . some potential benefit from fluoride containing vitamin preparations must be acknowledged."[1] An investigation has been made of the caries-inhibiting effect of acidulated phosphate-fluoride tablets chewed by children in school.[38] It is not known, however, how long such supplementation must be continued to maintain the caries-inhibitory effect throughout life.

Each of these alternatives is more costly in terms of money or effort than fluoridation of a community water supply, and some are decidedly less effective, but such measures are worth careful consideration when a fluoridated community supply is not available.

TOPICAL APPLICATION OF FLUORIDES

A considerable inhibition of dental caries can be attained through the direct application of fluoride solutions to young teeth. This method antedates the fluoridation of community waters. A summary of findings in the series of studies completed by Knutson and Scholz appears in Tables 16 and 17.[83] A standard technic was used throughout this series. The teeth were cleaned with pumice, isolated with cotton rolls, and dried with compressed air. A two percent solution of sodium fluoride in distilled water was applied to the dried crowns with a cotton applicator or spray so that all surfaces became visibly wet. The applied solution was then allowed to dry in air for about three minutes. Four such applications were given at intervals of about one week. Optimal application ages were estimated as three, seven, 10, and 13 years, on the theory that fluoride should be applied

TABLE 16. NUMBER OF INITIALLY NONCARIOUS TEETH, AND PERCENT ATTACKED BY CARIES IN FLUORIDE-TREATED AND UNTREATED TEETH OF 1,032 CHILDREN, BY SPECIFIC TOOTH.*

TEETH	UPPER INITIALLY NONCARIOUS TEETH TREATED	UPPER INITIALLY NONCARIOUS TEETH UNTREATED	UPPER PERCENT ATTACKED BY CARIES TREATED	UPPER PERCENT ATTACKED BY CARIES UNTREATED	LOWER INITIALLY NONCARIOUS TEETH TREATED	LOWER INITIALLY NONCARIOUS TEETH UNTREATED	LOWER PERCENT ATTACKED BY CARIES TREATED	LOWER PERCENT ATTACKED BY CARIES UNTREATED	BOTH INITIALLY NONCARIOUS TEETH TREATED	BOTH INITIALLY NONCARIOUS TEETH UNTREATED	BOTH PERCENT ATTACKED BY CARIES TREATED	BOTH PERCENT ATTACKED BY CARIES UNTREATED
Central incisor	810	803	4.2	5.5	1,001	998	0.5	0.9	1,811	1,801	2.2	2.9
Lateral incisor	720	729	4.7	9.5	967	969	.7	.8	1,687	1,698	2.4	4.5
Cuspid	473	461	1.3	2.0	613	615	.2	.5	1,086	1,076	.6	1.1
First bicuspid	532	539	4.7	8.7	586	592	2.0	4.2	1,118	1,131	3.3	6.4
Second bicuspid	422	449	6.4	12.2	431	419	7.4	11.7	853	868	6.9	12.0
First molar	294	293	21.8	33.4	199	199	35.2	45.2	493	492	27.2	38.2
Second molar	215	218	22.7	42.2	167	176	29.2	55.1	382	394	25.7	48.0
All teeth	3,466	3,492	6.9	11.9	3,964	3,968	4.4	7.1	7,430	7,460	5.6	9.3

*Knutson and Scholz.[83]

TABLE 17. NUMBER OF INITIALLY NONCARIOUS TOOTH SURFACES, AND PERCENT ATTACKED BY CARIES IN FLUORIDE-TREATED AND UNTREATED TEETH OF 1,032 CHILDREN, BY SPECIFIC TOOTH SURFACE.[*]

TOOTH SURFACES	UPPER SURFACES INITIALLY NONCARIOUS TREATED	UPPER SURFACES INITIALLY NONCARIOUS UNTREATED	UPPER PERCENT ATTACKED BY CARIES TREATED	UPPER PERCENT ATTACKED BY CARIES UNTREATED	LOWER SURFACES INITIALLY NONCARIOUS TREATED	LOWER SURFACES INITIALLY NONCARIOUS UNTREATED	LOWER PERCENT ATTACKED BY CARIES TREATED	LOWER PERCENT ATTACKED BY CARIES UNTREATED	BOTH SURFACES INITIALLY NONCARIOUS TREATED	BOTH SURFACES INITIALLY NONCARIOUS UNTREATED	BOTH PERCENT ATTACKED BY CARIES TREATED	BOTH PERCENT ATTACKED BY CARIES UNTREATED
Occlusal	3,466	3,492	3.9	6.8	3,964	3,968	3.4	5.5	7,430	7,460	3.7	6.1
Mesial	3,466	3,492	1.8	3.0	3,964	3,968	.8	.7	7,430	7,460	1.2	1.8
Distal	3,466	3,492	1.1	2.0	3,964	3,968	.5	.6	7,430	7,460	.8	1.2
Lingual	3,466	3,492	.7	.8	3,964	3,968	.0	.1	7,430	7,460	.3	.4
Buccal and labial	3,466	3,492	.1	.2	3,964	3,968	.6	1.1	7,430	7,460	.4	.7
All tooth surfaces	17,330	17,460	1.5	2.6	19,820	19,840	1.1	1.6	37,150	37,300	1.3	2.1

[*]Knutson and Scholz.[83]

as soon as practicable after eruption of groups of teeth, to minimize the period of time at risk from caries before application.

The success of topical application with sodium fluoride solutions led investigators to search for other fluoride vehicles and other methods of administration in the hope of developing methods which were less time-consuming and, possibly, more effective. Of these new agents one of the most widely used has been an aqueous solution of stannous fluoride. Stannous fluoride is more soluble than sodium fluoride; thus higher concentrations of the salt can be employed. The concentration most usually employed is eight percent. With solutions of this strength it was thought that one rather than four applications might suffice. The technic of applications was essentially the same as that employed for sodium fluoride solutions, except that solutions for use in the mouth should be prepared fresh each day, preferably just before each application. Nearly all trials with this agent have shown a definite inhibition of caries experience in children receiving the applications. General findings have been summarized by Horowitz.[67] However, well-conducted trials have been reported in which there was little or no apparent caries-inhibitory effect after application with aqueous sodium fluoride solution, stannous fluoride solution, a phosphate-fluoride gel, or an acidulated sodium fluoride solution.[10, 145]

Research in this general area has been vigorous over the past few years. Other complexes, such as that of fluoride-aluminum, have been studied in animals,[93] and electrophoretic technics have likewise been explored with animals as subjects.[152] It has been suggested that the time of application in the average trial is inadequate,[140] and that better results might be had if the fluoride were bound to the tooth enamel for two hours or more by means of an adhesive bandage.[89] Englander has reported excellent results with fluoride gels applied via mouthguard tray during each day of the school year to children in Cheektowaga, New York.[42] Stannous hexafluorozirconate has been employed in preliminary trials with some promise of success.[104, 105] Advantages have been claimed for acidic fluoride and phosphate solutions.[27] Fluoride solutions have been employed on the toothbrush or as a mouth rinse.[18, 25]

There is some question as to the duration of caries inhibition following topically applied fluoride. Gish, Muhler, and Howell have reported on a group of 157 Indiana children, given a yearly application of eight percent stannous fluoride solution and followed for five years, during which time there was no apparent loss of protective effect.[56] However, Syrrist has reported that the inhibitory effect which followed two years of topical applications of sodium fluoride in 78 children was entirely lost during the following five-year period.[144] Further, there is a growing consensus that reported differences between one fluoride solution and another may be more apparent than real. Some studies have shown stannous fluoride, sodium fluoride, and acidulated fluoride solutions to be of approximately equal value.[10] The words of Torell and Ericsson, applied to one type of topical agent, seem applicable to all: "The laboratory data and earlier clinical results were very promising. The results published later, however, were less dramatic."[148]

This should not be interpreted as evidence that these agents are worthless, but that they are probably less effective than was hoped at the outset. The clinical trial of a caries-inhibitory agent is difficult to carry out, and it must be remembered that the results of a single trial can never be accepted as final and definitive. The most significant evidence comes from a consistent series of trials over which the performance of an agent is uniformly beneficial or uniformly a failure. From this point of view, it seems probable that topical applications are of value, but on a plane of effectiveness well below that of lifetime use of a fluoridated water.

One important advantage of topical application is immediacy of effect. Caries inhibition presumably begins as soon as treatment is initiated.

CARIES-INHIBITORY DENTIFRICES

There are three serious drawbacks to the program of topical application: (1) it is not as effective as water fluoridation; (2) it is costly in terms of dollars; and (3) it requires the services of trained people who may be in short supply. These last two objections might be overcome with an effective caries-inhibitory dentifrice, purchased by the individual and applied by himself. As Wallace has pointed out in a thoughtful and comprehensive review, there is reason to believe that any of a number of therapeutic ingredients, incorporated into the proper vehicle and used under the proper conditions, might prove to be a useful caries-inhibitory agent.[153] However, field trials with such agents as dibasic ammonium phosphate and urea, the antibiotics, or enzyme inhibitors such as N-lauroyl sarcosinate have yielded equivocal results.

Caries-inhibitory dentifrices employing fluorides as the essential agent have been approved by the American Dental Association's Council on Dental Therapeutics. A typical set of clinical findings from a clinical trial of one of these dentifrices is shown in Table 18. Two comparable groups of grade-school children used the test or a placebo dentifrice according to their normal habits. They were examined by Muhler at the outset and after six, 12, 18, 24, and 36 months. The table shows the results observed in children who were present at each examination in the series. Over this span (36 months)

TABLE 18. INCREMENTS OVER A THREE-YEAR PERIOD OF NEW DMF TEETH AND SURFACES, CHILDREN USING A STANNOUS FLUORIDE OR A PLACEBO DENTIFRICE, WHO WERE PRESENT AT EVERY EXAMINATION.*

GROUP	MEAN INCREMENT, DMF TEETH	P	PERCENT DIFFERENCE	MEAN INCREMENT, DMF SURFACES	P	PERCENT DIFFERENCE	95% CONFIDENCE INTERVAL IN PERCENT REDUCTION
6 month data							
Control	1.02 (.11)	.009	42.2	1.90 (.17)	.048	25.8	5.0–46.6
SnF$_2$ dentifrice	.59 (.10)			1.41 (.16)			
12 month data							
Control	1.56 (.14)	.031	28.2	3.02 (.22)	.078	18.5	0.6–36.4
SnF$_2$ dentifrice	1.12 (.13)			2.46 (.21)			
18 month data							
Control	2.55 (.19)	.003	31.4	4.82 (.30)	.008	24.3	10.0–38.6
SnF$_2$ dentifrice	1.75 (.15)			3.65 (.27)			
24 month data							
Control	3.31 (.24)	.016	24.5	6.57 (.43)	.035	19.2	4.5–33.9
SnF$_2$ dentifrice	2.50 (.19)			5.31 (.35)			
36 month data							
Control	5.14 (.30)	.006	23.7	10.35 (.59)	.006	22.4	9.8–35.0
SnF$_2$ dentifrice	3.92 (.26)			8.03 (.48)			

*Muhler, J. C. Effect of a stannous fluoride dentifrice on caries reduction in children during a three-year study period. Am. Dent. A. J., 64:216-24, Feb. 1962. There were 162 subjects in the control dentifrice group, and 165 subjects in the stannous fluoride dentifrice group. P is the probability that a difference as large as or larger than the observed difference between means could have occurred by chance alone. Confidence intervals so determined will contain the true percent reduction 95 percent of the time. Figures in parentheses are the standard error of the mean.

children using the stannous fluoride dentifrice accumulated an average of about one fewer new DMF teeth, and slightly more than two fewer new DMF surfaces, than children using the placebo dentifrice. The 95 percent confidence interval is an estimate, based upon the result of this trial, that might be made of the results of other trials conducted with children from this same universe. In a series of 40 such trials, the difference might be expected to exceed 35 percent on one occasion, and to be less than 9.8 percent on one other test.

The data shown in Table 18 were reported in 1962. Since that time a number of clinical trials have been reported with similar dentifrices, with results generally within the confidence limits shown—that is to say, with differences in caries experience ranging from 9.8 to 35 percent less in the study groups of children than in the controls.[55, 68, 79, 135] One group of studies, begun with children 11 or 12 years old in Yorkshire, Buckinghamshire, London, Essex, and Kent, Great Britain, may be analyzed as a series because similar criteria and procedures were followed throughout. Children 11 or 12 years of age were randomly assigned to study or control groups, were examined by mirror and explorer plus posterior bitewings, and were followed for two years. At the end of that time, caries experience in terms of new decayed and filled teeth ranged from two to 18.7 percent less in the stannous-fluoride children than in the controls, with a median value of 8.4 percent; differences in new decayed, missing, and filled tooth surfaces ranged from −0.1 percent to 24 percent with a median difference of 13.8 percent. In general, ordinary clinical examination failed to show an appreciable difference between study and control children in this series of trials. The principal difference was found in proximal surfaces newly erupted during the period of the trial. It should be noted here that a very slight delay in onset of caries after the eruption of a tooth can appear as a very large percentage difference unless the period of observation is much longer than the two-year span covered in this series of studies.[48, 74–76, 106, 133, 134]

The results of a few trials have suggested that a combination of agents—such, for example, as a fluoride prophylaxis paste, topical application, and a fluoride dentifrice—may prove to be more effective than a single agent.[22, 37, 128]

Among research workers the opinion seems to be growing that one fluoride compound is about as effective as another in a dentifrice, provided that it is used in conjunction with a compatible polishing agent—one which does not bind the fluoride ion.[61] About the same degree of caries inhibition was seen in two clinical trials in which a sodium fluoride paste was compared with a stannous fluoride paste, each employing a suitable abrasive.[109, 155]

In general, although the apparent effect is sometimes slight, clinical trials with fluoride dentifrices or combinations of topically applied fluoride agents have tended to be on the positive side. When used singly, topical applications seem to be somewhat more effective than dentifrices. Wallace has said: "... the most effective combination of therapeutic agent and vehicle has probably not yet been conceived, much less evaluated."[153]

OTHER VEHICLES

Vehicles or agents other than the fluorides have been tested as possible caries-inhibitory agents. Among these are the inorganic phosphates. These salts, in almost any form, have inhibited dental caries in laboratory animals when added to the diet in adequate amounts.[44] When incorporated into the diets of humans, a positive caries-inhibitory effect in four proximal surfaces of the maxillary incisors and cuspid has been reported in one instance,[142] and negative results were observed in three studies based on examination of the entire dentition.[11, 21, 130] The addition of six percent of calcium phosphate to the flour used for baking bread did not check rising caries attack rates in Greenland Eskimos, during a period in which the per capita consumption of sugar rose from 11 to 88 pounds and the per capita consumption of cereals from 74 pounds to 205 pounds.[12] It has been suggested that these human trials might have been more successful if a phosphate more soluble than the calcium salts had been employed. Preliminary trials with such a salt (NaH_2PO_4) have indicated that it may have some effect in curbing the cariogenic potential of sugar-coated cereals.[32, 141] In one trial, caries increments over 30 months were about the same in a group of children supplied with a sugar-dicalcium phosphate chewing gum as in a second group chewing a gum which was sugar-free.[46] At this stage it is difficult to forecast whether the inorganic phosphates, in any form or any vehicle, will actually prove to be of value in the control of dental caries in human beings.

A new and intriguing method of preventing caries in pits and fissures by sealing them with an adhesive resin is presently under investigation.[36]

Another agent currently under study is dextranase, an enzyme which attacks the polysaccharide, dextran. Dextran forms the capsule, or slime layer, which envelops certain lactic acid bacteria and may be an essential factor in the gumminess of the dental plaque. In addition, the capsule of a bacterium frequently has another function essential to the survival of the organism in that it may enable it to resist the defense mechanisms of the host. Hence, an agent which inhibits or prevents the formation of long-chain, insoluble dextrans might inhibit the process of dental caries by interdiction of cariogenic plaque formation or by exposing the bacteria to antibodies in saliva.

Dextrans are polysaccharides composed of glucose units, produced by an enzyme in dextran-forming organisms which attacks sucrose (and only sucrose), breaking it down into fructose and dextran.

Neither free fructose nor free glucose can be converted to dextran by this enzyme. It should be noted that caries may be induced in experimental animals on diets nominally free of sucrose, but including other carbohydrates.

Preliminary studies with dextranase have involved its application to small numbers of hamsters inoculated with cariogenic dextran-producing streptococci. Both plaque and dental caries have been inhibited in such animals treated with dextranase.[47] Further study is needed to determine whether the agent is effective in animals with a heterogeneous caries-producing flora, safe for use by humans, and effective against human dental caries.

Destruction of a protective capsule might enhance the effectiveness of a vaccine against cariogenic bacteria, if such a vaccine can be developed. There is some evidence that the saliva of caries-immune individuals contains a normal antibody,[41, 60] although attempts at passive immunization of susceptible rats with gamma globulins from caries-resistant animals have failed.[143] Interest in vaccines against caries has been renewed by (among other things) a recent demonstration of antibody titers in humans after inoculation with vaccines produced from the "M" proteins of at least three types of streptococci. "M" proteins are not only antigenic in nature but also seem to have a role in determining the virulence of the organism. They are protective by virtue of their opsonic capacity, i.e., that immune factor which stimulates phagocytosis.[117]

One of the earliest observations in dental caries research was the finding that lactobacilli could not be implanted in the mouths or in the intestinal tracts of individuals who did not harbor the organisms at the outset, and that such individuals exhibited a high agglutinin titer for the organisms. Such workers as Jay and Williams were able to detect antibodies in the sera of individuals inoculated subcutaneously with lactobacilli of the types which form rough colonies on Hadley tomato agar. The occurrence of tissue reactions—abscesses—at the site of inoculation discouraged these early efforts at vaccination.

Much work remains to be done before an effective vaccine can be produced. Many different strains of bacteria have been implicated in caries of experimental animals, and the same condition may obtain in human caries. Polyvalent vaccines have been effective against other disease entities, however, and the possibility exists that the organisms of human caries may be so closely related that an antigen from one strain could be effective against other strains. There may be difficulties with mutation of organisms.[15] Rapid mutation is one of the reasons that such vaccines as those against influenza may be ineffective in any given year, even though they are based on viruses of the same types which produced disease in the previous season.

Direct attacks on the oral flora, through such agencies as mouthwashes or toothpastes containing bacitracin or penicillin, or through penicillin administered as a prophylactic in children with rheumatic fever, have led to little or to partial success in caries control. At best the results seem too meager to offset the dangers attending indiscriminate lay use of a wide-spectrum antibiotic.[85, 88, 156]

It has proved to be well-nigh impossible to evaluate reports of this nature as they appear in scientific literature. A hypothetical caries-inhibitory agent may appear to be effective, with both clinical and statistical significance, in one trial, and seem to be quite ineffective in the next. It is not always possible to explain such disparities on the basis that one or the other of the studies was poorly planned or executed. These discrepancies may be due to the influence of factors not now recognized, or it may be that something analogous to the "uncertainty principle" of physics must be applied to the interpretation of studies of this type. Whatever the reason, experience has shown that no one clinical trial is sufficient to demonstrate the value of a caries-inhibitory agent. The value can be determined only after corroboration has been furnished through a series of independent trials, conducted by scientists working independently of each other.

These problems of evaluation are the reason for being of the Council on Dental Therapeutics of the American Dental Association. The Council conducts studies of new products as they are announced, determines whether they are safe and efficacious, and grants its seal of acceptance to those "... of recognized value in dentistry which are labeled and advertised to dentists in accordance with the Council's *Provisions for Acceptance of Products*."[1] Evaluatory reports appear periodically in the *Journal of the American Dental Association* and have been summarized in the Association's publication entitled *Accepted Dental Remedies* in editions dated 1967 and earlier, to be superseded by a publication with the same general aims which will be called *Accepted Dental Therapeutics*. These evaluations have proved to be fair and adequate. The practitioner would be wise to wait for the Council's report before advocating a new product or procedure, no matter how optimistic its first reports in journal or press.

NUTRITION AND DIET

Alterations in the nutrition of laboratory animals can result in profound changes in their dental caries experience. There is very little evidence that human dental caries can be controlled in parallel fashion. As Robinson has said:

> Good nutrition is important for general well-being and health, but neither good nutrition nor freedom from systemic disease offers any substantial assistance in prevention of dental caries.[114]

There are obvious difficulties in relating the nutritional status of a human population to its experience with dental caries. Field

PREVENTION AND CONTROL OF DENTAL CARIES 115

dental caries measures are counts of the total attack of caries over the lifetime of the individual, from the time of eruption of teeth to the day of examination. Nutritional studies usually appraise the status of the person, or his dietary intake, on the day, or the week, of the field examination. The most significant study is one which relates traditional nutritional practice of a whole population with its dental caries experience. Some of these findings have been discussed in Chapter Six (The Epidemiology of Dental Caries and Periodontal Diseases), and it is obvious from a glance at Figure 4 (page 76) that dental caries experience is very low in many countries where the traditional diet, followed with little change for centuries, is and has been grossly inadequate in one or more of the essential nutrients. Conversely, dental caries is most prevalent and destructive in precisely those countries—Great Britain, the Scandinavian nations, New Zealand, the United States of America—with the highest nutritional standards.

There is a convincing uniformity in findings for human population groups.

Caries activity was lower in a group of malnourished children living in the vicinity of Birmingham, Alabama, than in their well-nourished neighbors.[40, 90] Similarly, differences in nutritional status seem to have had little effect upon caries at higher levels of subsistence. Children in a private school in Manhattan had no less decay than children in a public school, although nearly one third of the children in the public school were in families receiving relief assistance, and the private school children enjoyed diets of better quantity and quality.[82] Collins, Jensen, and Becks determined that essential food elements were no more deficient in 122 college students with rampant caries than they were in a group virtually free of decay.[34] Klatsky and, independently, Siegel, Waugh, and Karshan concluded that the relative freedom from caries commonly seen in primitive peoples could not be attributed to superior nutrition.[81, 131]

The same general pattern was seen throughout the series of ICNND nutrition surveys mentioned in an earlier chapter. Dental caries was very low in primitive Eskimos and in Ethiopia despite traditional diets low in ascorbic acid, in vitamin A, and (from time to time) in calories.[87, 121] Caries experience was minimal in Burma, Thailand, and South Vietnam where there were long standing deficiencies in thiamine and riboflavin.[120] But it does not follow that malnutrition in itself is a caries-inhibitory factor. Within such populations as these, malnourished individuals show no more freedom from caries than persons more adequately fed.[72, 124]

There was a consistent and substantial lowering of dental caries prevalence in children of European countries where foodstuffs were rationed during the second World War. Some observers concluded that the common factor—a drastic reduction in sugar consumption—improved the balance of the diet by raising the proportions of "protective" foods.[149] More probably the effective factor was the withdrawal of sugar in itself.[139] Caries incidence was lowered in populations of children with reduced sugar consumption, even when, as with children in French foundling institutions, the wartime diet was "a deficient ration"; "unbalanced notably to the disadvantage of animal proteins, fats, calcium, etc."[58] The single common factor, where caries prevalence was lowered, was the withdrawal of sugar, "independent of dark or white bread, or independent of whether the diet as a whole is satisfactory or not."[127] Caries prevalences gradually rose to prewar levels with the resumption of the traditional diets.[150]

The converse has been observed in the many instances when sugars have been introduced to native diets with a subsequent increase in dental caries levels, whether the quality of the native diet was improved or degraded. Typical examples are the experience of Eskimos in Greenland and in Alaska.[12, 129]

The caries-enhancing effect of sugar in the diet is not wholly determined by the amount in food.[20] A classic study of the direct influence of carbohydrate ingestion in caries-susceptible persons was carried out in the Vipeholm Hospital, Lund, Sweden by a group of scientists that included such distinguished men as Gustafsson, Quensel, Swenander Lanke, Lundqvist, Grahnén, Bonow, and Krasse. After four years of observation they concluded that sugar consumption increases caries activity, which decreases again when sugar is withdrawn; that the risk is greatest if the sugar is sticky and retentive in form and when it is eaten frequently—that is, between as well as with meals. There were individual exceptions to these general rules; responses varied widely from one person to another, and there were individuals in whom "carious lesions may continue to appear despite the avoidance of refined sugar, maximum restriction of natural sugars and total dietary carbohydrates." This report is worth careful study by any person interested in the management of dental caries, whether in the public program or in the individual patient. It is available in English.[63] The principal findings have been summarized and evaluated by the senior investigator.[62]

Dietary Control of Caries

If caries can be accelerated by sugars in the mouth, then caries should be inhibited if these substances are withdrawn from the diet. This is the basis for a control program developed, decades ago, by Bunting and his associates at The University of Michigan. "Diet, it seems," he reported, "controls dental caries through the determination of the environment of the teeth, rather than through changes in the resistance of the tooth itself."[28] A practicable control program was developed which proceeds through three phases: (1) an initial period of two weeks during which the patient's carbohydrate intake is limited to 100 grams per day, excluding such items as potatoes and bread as well as sugars; (2) a second period on the same regime except that potatoes are permitted at one meal and up to six slices of whole wheat bread may be eaten per day; and (3) a final period in which the patient may eat moderate amounts of sugar at any one meal during the day. During this span of six weeks it is thought to be "very likely that a bacterial flora becomes established . . . which creates an environment unfavorable to the growth requirements of lactobacilli and other important acid-producing bacteria."[77]

An independent, wide-scale test of the efficacy of carbohydrate restriction was carried out by Becks and his associates at the University of California. Studies were made with 1,250 individuals with rampant caries. In about two out of three of these patients no new carious lesions developed in the year following carbohydrate restriction; only one or two new lesions appeared in an additional one sixth of the cases.

This is a hardship regime for most individuals, and tends to fail unless there is a high degree of motivation in the patient (and his parents, if the patient is a child). Becks has summarized his experience as follows:

> The reduction of refined sugars is strictly an individual control or prevention program and naturally a difficult one. It is quite obvious that any attempt on the part of dentists to reduce refined carbohydrates and sugars in the daily food intake of their patients requires that they have a thorough understanding of foods and the many problems of nutrition. On the other hand it does not seem reasonable to apply this somewhat complicated procedure to patients who develop only one, two or three cavities per annum. In fact, it is our belief that this procedure should apply only to rampant dental caries cases in which the life expectancy of the denture, because of the development of many cavities, is greatly endangered.[17]

If carbohydrates can enhance caries by their simple presence in the mouth, then it should be possible to inhibit caries by the prompt removal of carbohydrates after eating—that is, by quick and effective use of the toothbrush. The proposition may be true, but there is surprisingly little evidence to this point in scientific literature.[136] Also, despite the theoretical possibility of control by immediate toothbrushing, practically, it is almost impossible. Such brushing would have to take place within minutes if not seconds of ingestion of each meal or snack containing sweets.

SUMMARY

Of all the caries-inhibitory measures presently in use, water fluoridation most nearly meets the requirements for the perfect agent, as outlined at the beginning of this chapter. Its principal disadvantage lies in the long latent period between the time of fluoridation and the growth of an adult population with teeth showing the full inhibitory effect. It is safe, long lasting, and reaches all of the people in the community, at the lowest cost per person and with the highest degree of effectiveness of any of the measures discussed in this section.

Some estimate of the relative effectiveness and cost of these other control measures, as contrasted with fluoridation of the central water supply, can be based on the 10-year study by Jordan and his associates with the 300 children in the schools of Askov, Minnesota. Every known control measure, with the exception of fluoridation, was applied to these children. There was classroom instruction in dental health for both children and parents. Topical applications of sodium fluoride or stannous fluoride were given to children aged three, seven, 10, and 13 years. Teeth were brushed twice a day, under classroom supervision, in grades one through six; an ammoniated dentifrice was used at the beginning, followed by a penicillin paste, and (for the last three years) a stannous fluoride dentifrice. Toothbrushes and pastes were supplied to preschool and high-school children. Clinical and radiographic examinations and restorative care were available. Lactobacillus counts were made where indicated. Considerable emphasis was put on revising dietary habits and restricting the intake of sweets. At the end of the 10-year term, caries experience had been reduced by about 28 percent in children aged three to five years, by about 34 percent in children aged six to 12 years, and by about 14 percent in children aged 13 to 17 years.[146]

Caries-prevalence means were comparable in Askov and at Grand Rapids at the beginning of the respective terms of study. Ten years after fluoridation Grand Rapids children aged four or five years had about 53 percent fewer deciduous teeth with caries experience, and children aged six to 12 years had about 55 percent fewer permanent teeth with caries experience. The difference was about 36 percent in children aged 13 to 16 years.[4] Fluoridation alone, in Grand Rapids, was about twice as effective as the sum total of all other caries-inhibitory methods known and applicable in Askov during the term of that study. As summarized in the *Journal of the American Dental Association*, the Askov study:

> ... to put it in a nutshell, tends to show that if a community combines all the approved dental health practices but omits fluoridating the community water supply, the benefits that accrue are only moderate. They are much less than the benefits received from fluoridated water, and the cost is many times greater.... The ten year Askov program cost 57 times as much as water fluoridation will cost, and was less than half as effective as water fluoridation has proved to be in comparable communities.[146]

Fluoridation, despite its overwhelming advantages, is no cure-all. By the time they had reached middle age—mid-forties—nine out of 10 Colorado Springs natives reared using fluoride waters had required professional care for dental caries for the treatment of about 20 decayed, missing, or filled tooth surfaces per person. The British

Fluoridation Commission, which explored the subject in the United States in 1952, concluded that optimal results were achieved by "a combination of fluoridation and a high standard of conservative dentistry."[101] Nevertheless, given fluoridation and adequate care, it is clear that more and more of our increasing proportion of older people can expect to retain more and more of their teeth for longer and longer spans of life.

Alternative methods of dental caries control, less efficacious than fluoridation of community water, are well worthwhile where the water cannot be fluoridated, provided, of course, that the individual or community can afford their cost in money and manpower.

Half a century ago medical care was concentrated principally upon the communicable diseases which killed children; today it is concerned, more and more, with the preservation of health and function in the middle and older ages. An analogous shift in emphasis may be predicted for dental practice over the next few decades. It is not at all certain that this change will result in any reduction in the total professional work load; conquest of the communicable diseases of childhood has led to an increased, rather than a diminished, need for medical care. But the true benefit from the control of any disease is not found in lessened dollar costs or a reduced need for professional care; it is found in a longer, fuller, and richer life for the people of the community.

Bibliography

1. American Dental Association, Council on Dental Therapeutics. Accepted dental remedies 1967. Chicago, American Dental Association, 1966. XVI + 287 p.
2. Armstrong, W. D. Mechanisms of fluoride homeostasis. Arch. Oral Biol., 4:156-9, Aug. 1961.
3. Arnold, F. A., Jr. Fluorine in drinking water; its effect on dental caries. Am. Dent. A. J., 36:28-36, Jan. 1948.
4. Arnold, F. A., Jr., et al. Effect of fluoridated public water supplies on dental caries prevalence. Tenth year of the Grand Rapids-Muskegon study. Pub. Health Rep., 71:652-8, July 1956.
5. ———. Fifteenth year of the Grand Rapids fluoridation study. Am. Dent. A. J., 65:780-5, Dec. 1962.
6. Arnold, F. A., Jr., McClure, F. J., and White, C. L. Sodium fluoride tablets for children. Dent. Progress, 1:8-12, Oct. 1960.
7. Ast, D. B. A plan to determine the practicability, efficacy, and safety of fluoridating a communal water supply, deficient in fluorine, to control dental caries. p. 40-5 (In McKay, F. S., et al. Fluorine and dental public health. New York, New York Institute Clinical Oral Pathology, 1945. 62 p.)
8. Ast, D. B., and Fitzgerald, Bernadette. Effectiveness of water fluoridation. Am. Dent. A. J., 65:581-8, Nov. 1962.
9. Ast, D. B., et al. Newburgh-Kingston caries-fluorine study. XIV. Combined clinical and roentgenographic dental findings after ten years of fluoride experience. Am. Dent. A. J., 52:314-25, Mar. 1956.
10. Averill, H. M., Averill, Jeanne E., and Ritz, Angeline G. A 2-year comparison of three topical fluoride agents. Am. Dent. A. J., 74:996-1001, Apr. 1967.
11. Averill, H. M., Freire, P. S., and Bibby, B. G. The effect of dietary phosphate supplements on dental caries incidence in tropical Brazil. Arch. Oral Biol., 11:315-22, Mar. 1966.

12. Baarregaard, Anker. Dental conditions and nutrition among natives in Greenland. Oral Surg., Oral Med. and Oral Path., 2:995-1007, Aug. 1949.
13. Backer Dirks, O. The assessment of fluoridation as a preventive measure in relation to dental caries. Brit. Dent. J., 114:211-6, Mar. 19, 1963.
14. ———. The relation between the fluoridation of water and dental caries experience. Internat. Dent. J., 17:582-605, Sept. 1967.
15. Bartels, H. A., Blechman, Harry, and Pokowitz, Walter. Failure to demonstrate the anti-lactobacillus factor with streptomycin-resistant lactobacilli. J. Dent. Res., 45:1227, July-Aug. 1966.
16. Barth, T. F. W. The geochemical cycle of fluorine. J. Geol., 55:420-6, 1947. Chem. Abstr., 42:1536, 1948.
17. Becks, Hermann. The physical consistency of food and refined carbohydrate restrictions—their effects on caries. p. 187-92. (In Easlick K. A., ed. Dental caries; mechanism and present control technics as evaluated at the University of Michigan workshop. St. Louis, Mosby, 1948. 234 p.)
18. Berggren, H. Topical fluorides (including dentifrices). Internat. Dent. J., 17:40-6, Mar. 1967.
19. Bernstein, D. S., et al. Prevalence of osteoporosis in high- and low-fluoride areas in North Dakota. Am. Med. A. J., 198:499, Oct. 31, 1966.
20. Bibby, B. G. Effect of sugar content of foodstuffs on their caries-producing potentialities. Am. Dent. A. J., 51:293-306, Sept. 1955.
21. Bibby, B. G., and Averill, H. M. Caries control through phosphates. J. Dent. Res., 42:477-87, Jan.-Feb. 1963.
22. Bixler, David, and Muhler, J. C. Combined use of three agents containing stannous fluoride: a prophylactic paste, a solution and a dentifrice. Am. Dent. A. J., 68:792-800, June 1964.
23. Black, A. P. Feasibility of water fluoridation. Am. Dent. A. J., 65:588-94, Nov. 1962.
24. Blayney, J. R. A report on thirteen years of water fluoridation in Evanston, Ill. Am. Dent. A. J., 61:76-9, July 1960.
25. Brams, N. U. Preventive dentistry in the Scandinavian school dental health service. Internat. Dent. J., 17:384-92, June 1967.
26. Brown, H. K. The Brantford-Stratford fluoridation caries study—1961 report. Canad. J. Pub. Health, 53:401, Oct. 1962.
27. Brudevold, F. Caries control by topical treatments and by the use of fluoride dentifrices. Internat. Dent. J., 17:31-9, Mar. 1967.
28. Bunting, R. W. Diet and dental caries. Am. Dent. A. J., 22:114-22, Jan. 1935.
29. Butler, H. W. Legal aspects of fluoridating community water supplies. Am. Dent. A. J., 65:653-8, Nov. 1962.
30. Campbell, Irene R. The role of fluoride in public health: a selected bibliography. Cincinnati, Kettering Laboratory College Medicine, University Cincinnati, 1963. V + 108 p.
31. Carlos, J. P., Gittelsohn, A. M., and Waddon, William, Jr. Caries in deciduous teeth in relation to maternal ingestion of fluoride. Pub. Health Rep., 77:658-60, Aug. 1962.
32. Carroll, R. A., Stookey, G. K., and Muhler, J. C. The clinical effectiveness of phosphate-enriched breakfast cereals on the incidence of dental caries in adults: results after one year. Am. Dent. A. J., 76:564-7, Mar. 1968.
33. Chen, P. S., Jr., et al. Renal clearance of fluoride. Proc. Soc. Exp. Biol. and Med., 92:879-83, Aug.-Sept. 1956.
34. Collins, R. O., Jensen, A. L., and Becks, Hermann. Study of caries-free individuals. II. Is an optimum diet or a reduced carbohydrate intake required to arrest dental caries? Am. Dent. A. J., 29:1169-78, July 1, 1942.
35. Copp, D. H., and Shim, S. S. The homeostatic function of bone as a mineral reservoir. Oral Surg., Oral Med. and Oral Path., 16:738-44, June 1963.
36. Cueto, E. I., and Buonocore, M. G. Sealing of pits and fissures with an adhesive resin: its use in caries prevention. Am. Dent. A. J., 75:121-8, July 1967.
37. DePaola, P. F. Combined use of a sodium fluoride prophylaxis paste and a spray containing acidulated sodium fluoride solution. Am. Dent. A. J., 75:1407-11, Dec. 1967.
38. DePaola, P. F., and Lax, Martin. The caries-inhibiting effect of acidulated phosphate-fluoride chewable tablets: a two-year double-blind study. Am. Dent. A. J., 76:554-7, Mar. 1968.

39. Diefenbach, V. L., Nevitt, G. A., and Frankel, J. M. Fluoridation and the appearance of teeth. Am. Dent. A. J., 71:1129-37, Nov. 1965.
40. Dreizen, Samuel, et al. Prevalence of dental caries in malnourished children. Am. J. Dis. Child., 74:265-73, Sept. 1947.
41. Ellison, S. A. Salivary antigens. J. Dent. Res., 45:644-54, May-June 1966.
42. Englander, H. R. Views on the rationale of topical fluoride therapy. Am. Col. Dent. J., 35:15-21, Jan. 1968.
43. Englander, H. R., and Wallace, D. A. Effects of naturally fluoridated water on dental caries in adults. Pub. Health Rep., 77:887-93, Oct. 1962.
44. Ericsson, Y. Phosphates in relation to caries. Internat. Dent. J., 15:311-7, Sept. 1965.
45. Ericsson, Y., and Malmnas, C. Placental transfer of fluorine investigated with F^{18} in man and rabbit. Acta Obs. and Gyn. Scand., 41:144-58, 1962.
46. Finn, S. B., and Jamison, H. C. The effect of a dicalcium phosphate chewing gum on caries incidence in children: 30-month results. Am. Dent. A. J., 74:987-95, Apr. 1967.
47. Fitzgerald, R. J., et al. The effects of a dextranase preparation on plaque and caries in hamsters, a preliminary report. Am. Dent. A. J., 76:301-4, Feb. 1968.
48. Fluoridated toothpaste trials. Edit. Brit. Dent. J., 123:1, July 4, 1967.
49. Forrest, Jean R. Caries incidence and enamel defects in areas with different levels of fluoride in the drinking water. Brit. Dent. J., 100:195-200, Apr. 17, 1956.
50. Forrest, Jean R., and James, P. M. C. A blind study of enamel opacities and dental caries prevalence after eight years of fluoridation of water. Brit. Dent. J., 119:319-22, Oct. 5, 1965.
51. Galagan, D. J., and Lamson, G. G., Jr. Climate and endemic dental fluorosis. Pub. Health Rep., 68:497-508, May 1953.
52. Galagan, D. J., and Vermillion, J. R. Determining optimum fluoride concentrations. Pub. Health Rep., 72:491-3, June 1957.
53. Galagan, D. J., et al. Climate and fluid intake. Pub. Health Rep., 72:484-90, June 1957.
54. Gedalia, I., Zukerman, H., and Leventhal, H. Fluoride content of teeth and bones of human fetuses: in areas with about 1 ppm of fluoride in drinking water. Am. Dent. A. J., 71:1121-3, Nov. 1965.
55. Gish, C. W., and Muhler, J. C. Effectiveness of a SnF_2-$Ca_2P_2O_7$ dentifrice on dental caries in children whose teeth calcified in a natural fluoride area. II. Results at the end of 24 months. Am. Dent. A. J., 73:853-5, Oct. 1966.
56. Gish, C. W., Muhler, J. C., and Howell, C. L. A new approach to the topical application of fluorides for the reduction of dental caries in children: results at the end of five years. J. Dent. Child., 24:65-71, 2nd Quar. 1962.
57. Goulding, P. C. Why doctors vote yes to fluoridation. Today's Health, 43:8, 76-7, Oct. 1965.
58. Gounelle, Hugues, and Billette, Jacqueline. La carie dentaire dans ses rapports avec l'alimentation et la nutrition. Annales de la Nutrition et de l'Alimentation, 6:211-42, 1952.
59. Grainger, R. M., and Coburn, C. I. Dental caries of the first molars and the age of children when first consuming naturally fluoridated water. Canad. J. Pub. Health, 46:347-54, Sept. 1955.
60. Green, G. E. Inherent defense mechanisms in saliva. J. Dent. Res., 45:624-9, May-June 1966.
61. Grøn, Poul, and Brudevold, Finn. The effectiveness of NaF dentifrices. J. Dent. Child., 34:122-7, Mar. 1967.
62. Gustafsson, B. E. Sugar and dental caries. p. 5-18. (In Volker, J. F., chairman. Conference on diet and oral health. Birmingham, University Alabama, 1956. 77 p.)
63. Gustafsson, B. E., et al. The Vipeholm dental caries study. The effect of different levels of carbohydrate intake on caries activity in 436 individuals observed for five years. Acta Odont. Scandinav., 11:232-364, 1954.
64. Hagan, T. L. Effects of fluoridation on general health as reflected in mortality data. p. 157-65. (In Muhler, J. C., and Hine, M. K., eds. Fluorine and dental health; the pharmacology and toxicology of fluorine. Bloomington, Indiana University Press, c1959. 216 p.)

65. Heyroth, F. F. Toxicological evidence for the safety of the fluoridation of public water supplies. Am. J. Pub. Health, 42:1568-75, Dec. 1952.
66. Hodge, H. C., and Smith, F. A. Some public health aspects of water fluoridation. p. 79-109. (In Shaw, J. H., ed. Fluoridation as a public health measure. Washington, American Association Advancement Science, 1954. V + 232 p.)
67. Horowitz, H. S. Stannous fluoride solutions for the control of dental caries. p. 5-20. (In Young, W. O., and Shannon, Jean H., eds. The utilization of fluorides applied topically for the prevention of dental caries. Lexington, Department Community Dentistry, College Dentistry, University Kentucky, 1966. VII + 272 p.)
68. Horowitz, H. S., et al. Evaluation of a stannous fluoride dentifrice for use in dental public health programs. I. Basic findings. Am. Dent. A. J., 72:408-22, Feb. 1966.
69. Horowitz, H. S., and Heifetz, S. B. Effects of prenatal exposure to fluoridation on dental caries. Pub. Health Rep., 82:297-304, Apr. 1967.
70. Horowitz, H. S., et al. School fluoridation studies in Elk Lake, Pennsylvania, and Pike county, Kentucky—results after eight years. Am. J. Pub. Health, 58:2240-50, Dec. 1968.
71. Horowitz, H. S., Law, F. E., and Pritzker, Theodore. Effect of school fluoridation on dental caries. St. Thomas, V. I. Pub. Health Rep., 80:381-8, May 1965.
72. Hurtarte E., Augusto, and Scrimshaw, N. S. Dental findings in a nutritional study of school children in five Guatemalan highland villages. J. Dent. Res., 34:390-6, June 1955.
73. Interdepartmental Committee on Nutrition for National Defense. Ecuador nutrition survey. Washington, Government Printing Office, 1960. X + 230 p.
74. Jackson, D., James, P. M. C., and Slack, G. L. Stannous fluoride-calcium pyrophosphate dentifrice trials; a review. Brit. Dent. J., 123:14-5, July 4, 1967.
75. Jackson, D., and Sutcliffe, P. Clinical testing of a stannous fluoride-calcium pyrophosphate dentifrice in Yorkshire school children. Brit. Dent. J., 123:40-8, July, 4, 1967.
76. James, P. M. C., and Anderson, R. J. Clinical testing of a stannous fluoride-calcium pyrophosphate dentifrice in Buckinghamshire school children. Brit. Dent. J., 123:33-9, July 4, 1967.
77. Jay, Philip, Beeuwkes, Adelia M., and Husbands, Julia. Dietary program for the control of dental caries. Ann Arbor, Overbeck, c1965. 30 p.
78. Jiraskova, M. An epidemiologic study of the caries incidence in localities with an optimal content of fluorine in drinking water. Arch. Oral Biol., 6:209-13, July 1961.
79. Jordan, W. A., and Peterson, J. K. Caries-inhibiting value of a dentifrice containing stannous fluoride: final report of a two-year study. Am. Dent. A. J., 58:42-4, Jan. 1959.
80. Katz, Simon, and Muhler, J. C. Prenatal and postnatal fluoride and dental caries experience in deciduous teeth. Am. Dent. A. J., 76:305-11, Feb. 1968.
81. Klatsky, Meyer. Studies in the dietaries of contemporary primitive people. Am. Dent. A. J., 36:385-91, Apr.-May 1948.
82. Klein, Henry, and Palmer, Carroll E. Medical evaluation of nutritional status. X. Susceptibility to dental caries and family income. Milbank Mem. Fund Quar., 20:169-77, Apr. 1942.
83. Knutson, J. W., and Scholz, Grace C. The effect of topically applied fluorides on dental caries experience. VII. Consolidated report of findings for four study groups, showing reduction in new decay by individual tooth and by tooth surface, and frequency distribution of newly decayed teeth in treated and untreated mouth halves. Pub. Health Rep., 64:1403-10, Nov. 11, 1949.
84. Korrodi, H., et al. Fluor und Schilddruse. Beitrag zum Problem der Kariesprophylaxe mit Fluor. Zeitschrift für Praventivmedizin 1, 7:285-96, 1956.
85. Law, F. E., Wallace, D. R., and Spitz, Grace S. Use of a bacitracin mouthwash in dental caries control. Pub. Health Rep., 76:1094-6, Dec. 1961.
86. Leone, N. C., et al. A roentgenologic study of a human population exposed to a high-fluoride domestic water. Am. J. Roentgen., 74:874-85, Nov. 1955.
87. Littleton, N. W. Dental caries and periodontal diseases among Ethiopian civilians. Pub. Health Rep., 78:631-40, July 1963.
88. Littleton, N. W., and White, C. L. Dental findings from a preliminary study of

children receiving extended antibiotic therapy. Am. Dent. A. J., 68:520-5, Apr. 1964.
89. Manly, R. S., and Harrington, Dorothy P. Release of fluoride to enamel by an adhesive bandage. Am. Col. Dent. J., 35:34-44, Jan. 1968.
90. Mann, A. W., et al. A comparison of dental caries activity in malnourished and well-nourished patients. Am. Dent. A. J., 34:244-52, Feb. 15, 1947.
91. Marthaler, T. M. The value in caries prevention of other methods of increasing fluoride ingestion, apart from fluoridated water. Internat. Dent. J., 17: 606-18, Sept. 1967.
92. Marthaler, T. M., and König, K. G. Der Einfluss von Fluortablettengaben in der Schule auf den Kariesbefall 6- bis 15 jähriger Kinder. Schweiz Mschr. Zahnheilk, 77:539-54, June 1967.
93. McCann, H. G. The effect of fluoride complexes on the uptake of F by enamel from topical solutions. Abstr. Internat. A. Dent. Res., 46:159, Mar. 1968.
94. McCauley, H. B., and McClure, F. J. Effect of fluoride in drinking water on the osseous development of the hand and wrist in childhood. Pub. Health Rep., 69:671-83, July 1954.
95. McClure, F. J. Fluoride domestic waters and systemic effects. I. Relation to bone-fracture experience, height, and weight of high school boys and young selectees of the armed forces of the United States. Pub. Health Rep., 59: 1543-58, Dec. 1, 1944.
96. ———. Fluoride in food and drinking water. Dental health benefits and physiologic effects. Am. Dietetic A. J., 29:560-4, June 1953.
97. ———. Fluorine and other trace elements in nutrition. Am. Med. A. J., 139:711-6, Mar. 12, 1949.
98. ———. Nondental physiological effects of trace quantities of fluorine. p. 74-92. (In Moulton, F. R., ed. Dental caries and fluorine. Washington, American Association Advancement Science, 1946. 111 p.)
99. McClure, F. J., and Kinser, C. A. Fluoride domestic waters and systemic effects. II. Fluorine content of urine in relation to fluorine in drinking water. Pub. Health Rep., 59:1575-91, Dec. 8, 1944.
100. McClure, F. J., et al. Balances of fluorine ingested from various sources in food and water by five young men. Excretion of fluorine through the skin. J. Ind. Hygiene and Toxicol., 27:159-70, June 1945.
101. Ministry of Health, Department of Health for Scotland, and the Ministry of Housing and Local Government. The fluoridation of domestic water supplies in North America as a means of controlling dental caries. Report of the United Kingdom mission. London, H. M. Stationery Office, 1953. 101 p.
102. Ministry of Health, Scottish Office, and the Ministry of Housing and Local Government. The conduct of the fluoridation studies in the United Kingdom and the results achieved after five years. London, H. M. Stationery Office, 1962. III + 50 p.
103. Mühlemann, H. R. Fluoridated domestic salt. A discussion of dosage. Internat. Dent. J., 17:10-7, Mar. 1967.
104. Muhler, J. C. Mass treatment of children with a stannous fluoride-zirconium silicate self-administered prophylactic paste for partial control of dental caries. Am. Col. Dent. J., 35:45-57, Jan. 1968.
105. Muhler, J. C., Bixler, David, and Stookey, G. K. The clinical effectiveness of stannous hexafluorozirconate as an anticariogenic agent. Am. Dent. A. J., 76:558-63, Mar. 1968.
106. Naylor, M. N., and Emslie, R. D. Clinical testing of stannous fluoride and sodium monofluorophosphate dentifrices in London school children. Brit. Dent. J., 123:17-23, July 4, 1967.
107. Oakley, K. Fluorine and the relative dating of bones. Advance. Science, 4:336-7, 1948.
108. Paul, B. D., Gamson, W. A., and Kegeles, S. S., eds. Trigger for community conflict: the case of fluoridation. J. Soc. Issues, 17, Dec. 1961.
109. Peterson, J. K., and Williamson, Lois. Three year caries inhibition of a sodium fluoride acid orthophosphate dentifrice compared with a stannous fluoride dentifrice and a non-fluoride dentifrice. Abstr. Internat. A. Dent. Res. Abstr., 46:101, Mar. 1968.

110. Policy statement on alternatives on water fluoridation. (In Chronicle of the 55th Annual Session and XIVth World Dental Congress.) Internat. Dent. J., 17:782-3, Dec. 1967.
111. Posner, A. S., et al. X-ray diffraction analysis of the effect of fluoride on human bone apatite. Arch. Oral Biol., 8:549-70, July 1963.
112. Restrepo, Dario. Salt fluoridation: an alternate measure to water fluoridation. Internat. Dent. J., 17:4-9, Mar. 1967.
113. Richards, L. F., et al. Determining optimum fluoride levels for community water supplies in relation to temperature. Am. Dent. A. J., 74:389-97, Feb. 1967.
114. Robinson, H. B. G. The metabolism of minerals and vitamins and the effect of systemic conditions on dental caries. Am. Dent. A. J., 39:51-8, July 1949.
115. Robinson, W. O., and Edgington, G. Minor elements in plants, and some accumulator plants. Soil Science, 60:15-28, 1945.
116. Roholm, Kaj. Fluorine intoxication. A clinical-hygienic study with a review of the literature and some experimental investigations. London, Lewis, 1937. 364 p.
117. Rovelstad, G. H. What about a vaccine for the prevention of dental caries? Am. Col. Dent. J., 35:74-81, Jan. 1968.
118. Russell, A. L. Dental fluorosis in Grand Rapids during the seventeenth year of fluoridation. Am. Dent. A. J., 65:608-12, Nov. 1962.
119. ———. The inhibition of approximal caries in adults with lifelong fluoride exposure. J. Dent. Res., 32:138-43, Feb. 1953.
120. ———. International nutrition surveys: a summary of preliminary dental findings. J. Dent. Res., 42:233-44, Jan.-Feb. 1963.
121. Russell, A. L., Consolazio, C. F., and White, C. L. Dental caries and nutrition in Eskimo scouts of the Alaska National Guard. J. Dent. Res., 40:594-603, May-June 1961.
122. Russell, A. L., and Elvove, Elias. Domestic water and dental caries. VII. A study of the fluoride-dental caries relationship in an adult population. Pub. Health Rep., 66:1389-401, Oct. 26, 1951.
123. Russell, A. L., and Hamilton, Peggy M. Dental caries in permanent first molars after eight years of fluoridation. Arch. Oral Biol., 6:50-7, July 1961.
124. Russell, A. L., et al. Dental caries and nutrition in South Vietnam. J. Dent. Res., 44:102-11, Jan.-Feb. 1965.
125. Schlesinger, E. R., Overton, D. E., and Chase, Helen C. Study of children drinking fluoridated and nonfluoridated water. Quantitative urinary excretion of albumin and formed elements. Am. Med. A. J., 160:21-4, Jan. 7, 1956.
126. Schlesinger, E. R., et al. Newburgh-Kingston caries-fluorine study. XIII. Pediatric findings after ten years. Am. Dent. A. J., 52:296-306, Mar. 1956.
127. Schulerud, T. A. Dental caries and nutrition during wartime in Norway. Oslo, Fabritius & Sønners Trykkeri, 1950. 77 p.
128. Scola, F. P., and Ostrom, C. A. Clinical evaluation of stannous fluoride when used as a constituent of a compatible prophylactic paste, as a topical solution, and in a dentifrice in Naval personnel. I. Report of findings after first year. Am. Dent. A. J., 73:1306-11, Dec. 1966.
129. Scott, E. M. Nutrition of Alaskan Eskimos. Nutrition Rev., 14:1-3, Jan. 1956.
130. Ship, I. I., and Mickelsen, Olaf. The effects of calcium acid phosphate on caries in children: a controlled clinical trial. J. Dent. Res., 43:1144-9, Nov.-Dec. 1964.
131. Siegel, E. H., Waugh, L. M., and Karshan, Maxwell. Dietary and metabolic studies of Eskimo children with and without dental caries. Am. J. Dis. Child., 59:19-38, Jan. 1940.
132. Singer, L., and Armstrong, W. D. Regulation of human plasma fluoride concentration. J. App. Physiol., 15:508-10, May 1960.
133. Slack, G. L., et al. Clinical testing of a stannous fluoride-calcium pyrophosphate dentifrice in Essex school girls. Brit. Dent. J., 123:26-33, July 4, 1967.
134. Slack, G. L., et al. Clinical testing of a stannous fluoride-insoluble metaphosphate dentifrice in Kent school girls. Brit. Dent. J., 123:9-16, July 4, 1967.
135. Slack, G. L., and Martin, W. J. The use of a dentifrice containing stannous fluoride in the control of dental caries. Report of an unsupervised clinical trial. Brit. Dent. J., 117:275-80, Oct. 6, 1964.

136. Smith, A. J., and Striffler, D. F. The reported frequency of toothbrushing as related to the prevalence of dental caries in New Mexico. Pub. Health Dent., 23:159-75, Fall 1963.
137. Smith, F. A. Safety of water fluoridation. Am. Dent. A. J., 65:598-602, Nov. 1962.
138. Smith, F. A., et al. The effects of the absorption of fluoride. V. The chemical determination of fluoride in human soft tissues following prolonged ingestion of fluoride at various levels. Am. Med. A. Arch. Indust. Health, 21:330-2, Apr. 1960.
139. Sognnaes, R. F. Analysis of wartime reduction of dental caries in European children. Am. J. Dis. Child., 75:792-821, June 1948.
140. Spinelli, M. A., and Amdur, B. H. Time studies on the mechanism of fluoride action on hydroxyapatite: solution equilibria. Abstr. Internat. A. Dent. Res. Abstr., 46:106, Mar. 1968.
141. Stookey, G. K., Carroll, R. A., and Muhler, J. C. The clinical effectiveness of phosphate-enriched breakfast cereals on the incidence of dental caries in children: results after two years. Am. Dent. A. J., 74:752-8, Mar. 1967.
142. Stralfors, Alan. The effect of calcium phosphate on dental caries in school children. J. Dent. Res., 43:1137-43, Nov.-Dec. 1964.
143. Sweeney, E. A., Shaw, J. H., and Childs, E. L. Effect of passive immunization on the dental caries incidence of caries-susceptible rats. J. Dent. Res., 45:993-7, July-Aug. 1966.
144. Syrrist, Arvid. A seven-year report on the effect of topical applications of sodium fluoride on dental caries. Odont. Revy, 7:386-96, 1956.
145. Szwejda, L. F., Tossy, C. V., and Below, Dorothy M. Fluorides in community programs; results from a fluoride gel applied topically. J. Pub. Health Dent., 27:192-4, Fall 1967.
146. The ten year Askov Dental Demonstration has come to a close; what did it prove? Edit. Am. Dent. A. J., 61:112-3, July 1960.
147. Thompson, T. G., and Taylor, H. J. Determination and occurrence of fluorides in sea water. Ind. Eng. Chem., Anal. Ed., 5:87-9, 1933.
148. Torell, P., and Ericsson, Y. The value in caries prevention of methods for applying fluorides topically to the teeth. Internat. Dent. J., 17:564-81, Sept. 1967.
149. Toverud, Guttorm. The influence of general health supervision on the frequency of dental caries in groups of Norwegian children. Brit. Dent. J., 86:191-7, Apr. 14, 1949.
150. Toverud, Guttorm, Rubal, Louis, and Wiehl, Dorothy G. The influence of war and postwar conditions on the teeth of Norwegian school children. IV. Caries in specific surfaces of the permanent teeth. Milbank Mem. Fund Quar., 39:489-539, July 1961.
151. U.S. Public Health Service. Public Health Service drinking water standards 1962. Washington, Government Printing Office, 1962 (P. H. S. Publication No. 956). VIII + 61 p.
152. Wagner, M. J., and Weil, T. M. Reduction of enamel acid solubility with electrophoretic fluoride applications. J. Dent. Res., 45:1563, Sept.-Oct. 1966.
153. Wallace, D. A. Therapeutic dentifrices; a review of the literature on clinical investigations. Dent. Progress, 2:242-8, July 1962.
154. Water cure. Edit. Washington Post, Feb. 14, 1963.
155. Zacherl, W. A. A clinical evaluation of sodium fluoride and stannous fluoride dentifrices. Abstr. Internat. A. Dent. Res. Abstr., 46:101, Mar. 1968.
156. Zander, H. A. Effect of a penicillin dentifrice on caries incidence in school children. Am. Dent. A. J., 40:569-74, May 1950.

CHAPTER 8

MEASURES AVAILABLE FOR THE PREVENTION AND CONTROL OF PERIODONTAL AND OTHER ORAL DISEASES

By A. L. RUSSELL, D.D.S., M.P.H.

As the dental caries problem is reduced, both the private and the public health dentist will be able, and will be required, to turn more attention to those other oral conditions which have, until now, been overshadowed by dental decay. Chief among these are diseases of the soft tissues.

ACUTE GINGIVITIS

Outbreaks of acute gingivitis sometimes occur in schools, dormitories, or barracks. Isolation or quarantine measures have shown little value in controlling these outbreaks, and sterilization of dishes or other fomites has proved equally ineffective. As a general rule, such epidemics in young children are due to acute viral infections, with incubation periods ranging up to nine days. These infections are highly communicable, and the virus is usually well disseminated through a group before the first case is detected. The child ordinarily goes through a period of malaise before the onset of oral symptoms, and may actually feel better when the lesions appear. The typical lesion is a shallow ulcer, usually on, but not confined to, the buccal mucosa. Treatment is largely supportive; a bland mouthwash may help to control secondary infection. Local treatment with caustics is contraindicated.

Ulcerative gingivostomatitis (Vincent's infection) is probably not a communicable disease. It tends to occur in people older than 14 or 15 years who may be living under similar conditions in dormitories or barracks, though individual cases are not unusual. In the typical case the onset is rapid. Pain may be the only prodromal symptom. As the process advances:

> ... the interdental papillae become acutely inflamed, stand away from the teeth, bleed easily on the slightest touch, and are exquisitely painful. Necrosis occurs, beginning with the tip of the interdental papillae, with subsequent development of a characteristic greyish-white pseudomembrane which is easily removed, leaving a raw, profusely bleeding surface. The characteristic odor is a diagnostic point of significance.[12]

The patient is sometimes acutely ill, with an oral temperature rising to 103 or 104°F. In such cases the symptoms are quickly relieved by antibiotic therapy. Recurrence is the usual experience, however, unless antibiotic therapy is supplemented by more comprehensive treatment, including irrigation with a bland mouthwash, the meticulous removal of calculus, and the elimination of periodontal pockets.

With the increasing diversification of industry, more and more chemical and physical agents with deleterious oral effects have come into general use. Workers are usually well protected by safety devices. Failure of one of these devices may lead to an outbreak simulating the clinical and epidemiological picture of an infectious gingivostomatitis, such as trench mouth. This possibility should be considered when an outbreak is confined to men in a single plant whose duties are closely associated.

CHRONIC DESTRUCTIVE PERIODONTAL DISEASE

If maintenance of an efficient natural dentition throughout the life of the individual is a principal objective of dental public health practice, then periodontal disease ranks close behind dental caries as a matter for concern. After surveying the needs of 15,672 white male and 22,239 white female dental patients in 1952, the Bureau of Economic Research and Statistics of the American Dental Association reported:

> More teeth required extraction because of decay than for any other reason, through age 39 in women and through age 34 in men. For patients over these ages, periodontal disease was the reason for between two and three times as many extractions as dental decay. The average need for extractions because of decay did not decline

greatly with age, but the number of extractions owing to periodontal disease increased markedly. The average need for extractions because of periodontal disease was over 50 per cent higher in men than in women.... Decay was the reason given for 41.4 per cent of the extractions required; periodontal disease, 38.3 per cent.[1]

About the same conclusion was reached at the end of a second survey, carried out in December of 1965 with 5,379 male and 6,048 female patients:[2]

> ... More teeth required extraction because of decay than for any other single reason through age 39 in both men and women. For patients over this age, periodontal disease was the reason for far more extractions being needed than was dental caries. The average need for extractions because of decay did not decline greatly with age, but the number of extractions because of periodontal disease ... was one third higher in men than in women.... Among males, decay was given as the reason for 39.0 percent of the extractions required; periodontal disease, 33.7 percent.... Among females, decay was given as the reason for 41.7 percent of extractions needed; periodontal disease, 28.6 percent. . . .[3]

Data from the two surveys are not strictly comparable, because they employed slightly different methods; the 1952 data are based upon the needs of all eligible patients seen on a given day,[1] while the 1965 data are based upon the needs of all *eligible patients* seen *for the first time* on a given day.[2] This difference in approach seems inadequate to account for the differences in needs reported for the two survey years. In 1952 the average male required the extraction of about 1.3 teeth for causes other than dental caries (most of which were attributed to periodontal disease); the average female, 1.0 teeth. For 1965 these needs were reported as about 0.6 teeth in males and about 0.4 teeth in females.[4] Substantially fewer patients of both sexes were indicated as needing periodontal treatment in 1965 as compared with 1952, and the average number of teeth involved was appreciably lower.[3] The findings in general are consistent with the hypothesis that persons who want dental care today are in better dental health than patients of a decade ago. If this is a true change for the better, it might be due to

> ... increasing fluoridation, steadily improving dental technics, greater utilization of dental services by an increasingly aware public, the relatively improved economic situation, and other socioeconomic causal phenomena.[4]

As noted in Chapter Six, periodontal disease in most populations studied epidemiologically has been associated with oral plaque, debris, or calculus to the virtual exclusion of other concurrent factors. This finding seems to be inconsistent, on superficial analysis, with the fact that certain therapeutic measures other than hygiene seem to have value in periodontal practice. Occlusal equilibration is regularly practiced when trauma seems to be aggravating existing conditions of disease.[14] There are well-documented, if relatively rare, instances in which bone destruction progresses rapidly in the absence of overt

PREVENTION AND CONTROL

local irritants, and there are many problem cases which fail to respond to ordinary scaling or curettage.[19] Many of the epidemiological studies have been carried out with primitive populations, without available dental care and without effective practices of oral hygiene. In such populations, inflammatory disease is so prevalent and so destructive that other factors might be overridden and masked. The studies do not negate the possibility that such factors as trauma might be of importance in a population with a lesser degree of inflammatory disease. Nevertheless, the present consensus seems to be that the principal etiologic agent in periodontal disease is bacterial plaque at the point of opposition to the gingival crest. As Stahl has said:

> A review of the literature demonstrates quite clearly that specific and universal agents for the initiation of periodontal disease are unknown at present. There is, however, overwhelming evidence that these initiating agents are local and affect the gingival attachment at the crevicular level. There is high probability that, in most instances, these agents are bacterial products acting on the underlying tissue integrity. There is further evidence that other physical or chemical agents may also break the attachment seal.
> The resultant lesion in all probability depends, both in extent and severity, on the host resistance and more specifically on the ability of the local tissues to resist the irritant or repair the injury that has taken place. . . .[56]

This typical picture is one of chronic inflammation in the gingiva which

> . . . progresses, following the course of the blood vessels, into the bone marrow spaces and on the periosteal side of the alveolar bone; only in exceptional instances does it penetrate into the periodontal membrane. Resorption of the alveolar crest from the gingival side leads to destruction, first, of the supporting alveolar bone and then to the lamina dura. The fatty marrow is replaced by fibrous marrow.[61]

There is destruction of the crevicular epithelium with an increased round-cell infiltration. A pocket is formed which becomes progressively deeper as the result of apical proliferation of the epithelial attachment alongside the cementum, with subsequent separation at the crevicular margin. The pocket is, typically, one with a lateral wall consisting solely of soft tissue. Annular deposits of calculus seem invariably to be associated with the process.[57] It does not follow that calculus is necessarily the causative or even the triggering factor in disease; it may simply serve as a protective shelf under which bacterial plaque can proliferate. Removal of deposits and elimination of the pocket is the first objective of any method of periodontal treatment.

Control Methods

If the relative lack of severity of inflammatory periodontal disease in American populations, as contrasted with peoples in other areas, is the result of some difference in their several ways of life, and if this difference is something which can be managed, then control of this form of disease, at least, becomes a practicable possibility. A brief review of evidence to this point is in order here.

Evidence that periodontal disease is less prevalent and less severe in people of the more favored social status has been adduced from such diverse populations as rural children in Indiana,[46] workers in a manufacturing plant in Oslo,[33] and school children in Bombay.[36] These differences in the prevalence of active disease are reflected in higher rates for tooth loss from periodontal destruction in persons from the less favored status groups. Table 19 shows relative tooth loss from dental caries, periodontal disease, and all other reasons in two closely comparable studies in Washington, D.C. Krogh recorded reasons for extractions for one year in his oral surgery practice, with a group of patients who were predominantly white and from a middle- to high-socioeconomic group.[31] Andrews, with Krogh, repeated the observation over one year with a group of patients classified by the social service of the Episcopal Eye, Ear, and Throat Hospital as being of low economic status. More than 80 percent of these patients were Negroes.[5] Low-income patients lost more teeth to periodontal disease than to dental caries, by a factor of two or three to one, in the age span from 40 through 69 years. Losses from the two causes were approxi-

TABLE 19. RELATIVE CAUSES OF TOOTH LOSS, BY AGE, IN MIDDLE- TO HIGH-INCOME AND IN LOW-INCOME GROUPS, WASHINGTON, D.C.

AGE GROUP	PERCENTAGE OF TEETH EXTRACTED FOR		
	DENTAL CARIES	PERIODONTAL DISEASE	ALL OTHER CAUSES
2,337 persons with middle to high income*			
10-19	34	0	66
20-29	49	2	49
30-39	43	16	41
40-49	34	35	31
50-59	35	37	28
60-69	32	32	36
70 and over	48	24	28
805 persons with low income†			
10-19	75	0	25
20-29	63	10	27
30-39	53	28	19
40-49	19	55	26
50-59	17	52	31
60-69	8	62	30
70 and over	4	69	27

*Krogh.[31]
†Andrews and Krogh.[5]

mately equal in the middle- to high-income group of the same ages. At all ages over 30 years the high-income group lost about five teeth to dental caries for each four lost to periodontal disease; the low-income group lost about twice as many to periodontal disease as to caries. The comparison shown in Table 19 is not corrected for the fact that the high-income group included a higher proportion of females. At ages 30 and over, both males and females in the high-income population lost more teeth to dental caries than to loss of supporting tissues. Low-income group males of the same ages lost about two and one-third times as many teeth to periodontal diseases, and females about one and one-third times as many.

This finding might be ascribed to the fact that most of the latter group were Negroes. Negroes have consistently scored higher than whites in the same localities when examined for active periodontitis.[45] The hypothesis that periodontitis might be associated with ethnic background, however, seems to be unfounded. A study in Birmingham demonstrated that differences in scores between white and Negro groups were equalized when comparisons were restricted to persons with the same degree of mouth cleanliness, even when it was assessed by such a weak population measure as the presence or absence of materia alba on the incisal third of two or more incisor teeth.[48] Bone loss in the group of Oslo workers was found, on radiographic examination, to be significantly related to the efficiency of oral hygiene in the individual.[52] Data from the series of international nutrition surveys already summarized[47] indicated that age and poor oral hygiene were the significant factors in periodontal disease in those populations, leaving little variation to be accounted for by such other factors as nutritional status. Similar correlations between clinical disease and calculus or hygiene were found by Greene, in a study of young males in Bombay and Atlanta, and in studies in Ecuador and Montana, and by Ramfjord in a survey of boys in Bombay.[21, 22, 44] On the basis of these studies mouth cleanliness and periodontal disease seemed to be as intimately associated as dental caries experience and fluoride ingestion in children of the 21 cities.

Evidence that this relation is one of cause and effect is provided in a study by Lövdal, Arno, Schei, and Waerhaug which merits something more than superficial mention.[34]

Their study with workers in an Oslo manufacturing plant has already been cited as indicating that there were differences in periodontal status between workers which corresponded with their socioeconomic status,[33] but that these differences could be explained on the basis of their more or less effective oral hygiene.[52] Having established these points, the Oslo group set out to "evaluate the combined effect of subgingival scaling and controlled oral hygiene, i.e., measures which are focused on removal of local irritants in the form of calculus, bacterial plaque, food debris and overhanging margins of restorations."[34] All of the 1,150 male and 278 female workers in the plant were invited to participate. Of this number 808 were actually followed throughout a five-year period of study. Patients were scored according to the percentage of gingival areas in the mouth showing evidence of gingivitis.

After instruction in home care, including proper toothbrushing and the use of toothpicks, each patient received a thorough scaling for the removal of supragingival and subgingival deposits. This scaling was repeated every six months for most patients; for some others, every three months. The objective was to keep each mouth essentially free of local irritants throughout the period of the trial. In order to simplify evaluation of this simple regime, no other treatment (such as gingivectomy or occlusal adjustment) was given.

This is another of the key reports which should be read in its entirety by everyone interested in the control of oral disease. A summary of the findings after five years is shown in Figure 10. Patients had been classified as "good," "fairly good," or "not good" in oral hygiene practice without reference to their examination scores. Comparisons are shown for the buccal, lingual, and interproximal gingivae for each of the three hygiene groups.

Each of the groups was markedly better at the end of the five-year term than in the beginning, in each of the three anatomical areas. Adequate scaling reduced gingival disease in all of the groups; in fact,

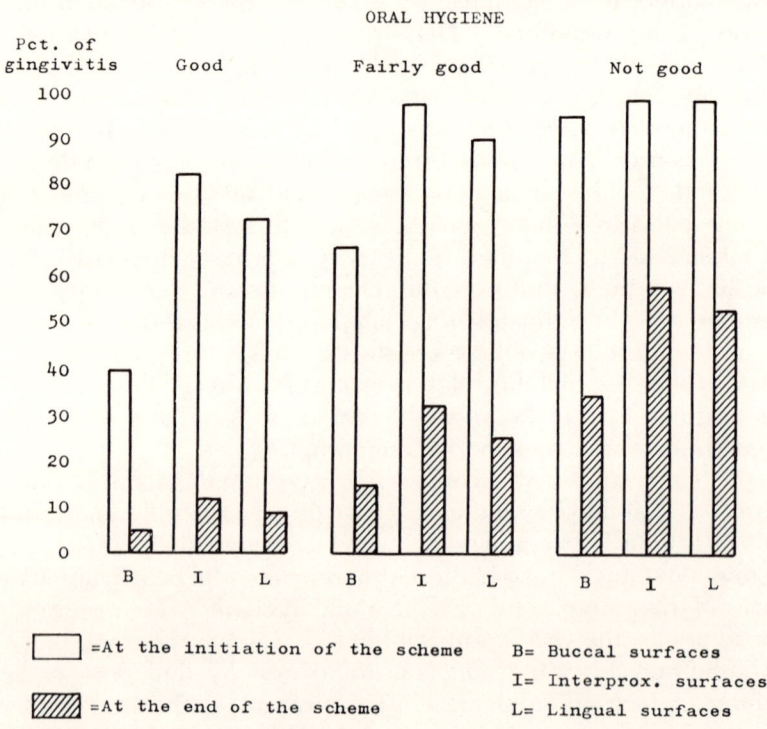

FIGURE 10. Percentage of gingival units (buccal, lingual, mesial and distal) showing signs of gingivitis at the initiation and at the end of the five-year period. (Lövdal, et al.[34])

those persons whose oral hygiene practices were faulty had less gingivitis at the end of the term than persons with good oral hygiene showed at the beginning. Conversely, scaling was most effective in persons with the more efficient toothbrushing and interdental cleansing with wooden picks.[34]

These conclusions are supported by the results of independent studies with such groups as Norwegian army recruits,[9] United States Air Force cadets,[32] and children.[30]

There is little epidemiological evidence on which to base an estimate of the relative importance of traumatism as a factor in population prevalences of periodontal disease. A committee assigned to study traumatism in the 1966 World Workshop in Periodontics concluded that there is a periodontal lesion attributable to trauma from occlusion, but that "there is no scientific evidence to show that a periodontal pocket or apical migration of the epithelial attachment is initiated by occlusal forces."[38] With the indices and procedures used in the population studies previously cited, disease possibly attributable to traumatism would ordinarily be overridden, and masked, by the concomitant presence of inflammation associated with plaque, debris, or calculus. Traumatic occlusion and malocclusion are not necessarily the same. Nevertheless, it might be argued that traumatism should occur more frequently in the maloccluded than in the normal dentition. The evidence in this regard is also inconclusive. Geiger observed a relation between crossbite and localized severity of periodontal disease in a series of 188 patients with periodontal disease, but could find no relation between disease and such factors as the occlusal plane, overbite and overjet, open bites, procumbency of the lower incisors, or crowding and rotation of teeth.[18] Poulton and Aaronson found a positive correlation between gingivitis and occlusion scores in 908 young males, and more Eskimo males with advanced periodontal disease showed marked crowding of the dental arches, at all ages, than men with simple gingivitis or with normal gingival tissues.[40, 49] These findings for Eskimos are shown in Table 1, page 47. The committee on traumatism in the 1966 World Workshop concluded that "there is a great need for controlled longitudinal studies after clinical measurements and criteria have been established for the various aspects of occlusion."[38]

The findings of Lövdal and his group in Oslo, however, supported as they are by independent observers, indicate that a considerable fraction of the total of periodontal disease can be intercepted and prevented by frequent and thorough supra- and subgingival scaling, accompanied by adequate personal oral hygiene.[15, 60] Both personal oral hygiene and professional prophylaxis must be carried out faithfully and completely; plaque tends to recur within a few days or weeks following conventional prophylaxis.[17] As Hard has put it:

> ... when mouths are kept clean enough, especially the subgingival areas, the periodontal tissues usually will be maintained in health

indefinitely.... Dentists have been too much concerned with the rehabilitation of mouths wrecked by periodontal disease and have not given enough attention to the prevention of such destruction.[24]

The teaching and practice of oral hygiene must begin early; the scaling program not later than puberty, as that is the point of onset of many cases of destructive disease. Greene has proposed that much more emphasis should be given in dental public health programs to the improvement of oral hygiene as a major step in the prevention of periodontal diseases.[21] On the basis of the available evidence it seems that such a program could be as effective in the control of periodontal diseases as fluoridation of community waters has proved to be in the control of dental caries.[29]

Some efforts have been made to control bacterial plaque through the use of enzymes,[13,15] urea in a dentifrice,[6] or antibiotics,[37] with some success. Coating the teeth with a thin film of an ion exchange resin seems to have failed.[27] Vaccine therapy has been given consideration;[8] studies with hamsters have shown that periodontal disease can be induced by a specific filament-forming organism,[28] and studies with humans have indicated that the return of plaque following a prophylaxis is correlated with the occurrences of filamentous organisms.[35] As with measures for the control of dental caries, the practitioner is well advised to follow the recommendations of the Council on Dental Therapeutics of the American Dental Association on the efficacy of newly developed measures for the control of periodontal disease.

There is little indication in data from the international studies, summarized earlier, that periodontal disease can be prevented to any important degree by the improvement of nutrition.

ORAL CANCER

It is fortunate that oral cancer is a relatively rare disease because, once contracted, its effects for the individual and his family are catastrophic. Age-adjusted death rates for cancer of the buccal cavity and pharynx have remained essentially the same—about 3.4 deaths per 100,000—since the year 1950.[43] Crude death rates from this cause have risen over the same span of time, due to aging of the population.[42] Rates adjusted to the age-composition of the United States as it was in 1940 indicate that the death rate in whites is in a slight downward trend, while death rates for nonwhites are sharply higher, increasing by about 35 percent between 1940 and 1963.[59]

It has been estimated that, in a typical year, less than three percent of deaths from this cause will occur in persons 34 years of age or younger, and more than three quarters in persons 55 years of age or older. Much the same association with age appeared in a series of 1,594 cases of cancer of the lip or buccal cavity reported by 29 general hospitals in Connecticut from 1935 to 1946. About 85 percent of these deaths occurred in persons 50 years of age or older. About 85 percent of the deaths occurred in males.[11] Approximately seven percent of all new cancers occur in the mouth or on the lip in males as against about two percent in females. Buccal cancer accounts for about four percent of all cancer deaths in males and for about one percent in females.[41] Oral cancer, then, is predominantly a disease of the male in middle and later life.

But it is a significant cause of death in females and in younger persons as well, and no person can be considered to be immune; the dentist should be alert for suspicious tissue changes in every patient he sees. Oral cancer caused about nine times as many deaths as poliomyelitis in the United States in 1959, and "nearly as many people die from oral cancer as die from being hit by a car."[26] In the United States, in those areas in which the best medical care is available, the cure rate for cancer of the oral cavity does not exceed 30 percent. It is probably even less for the country as a whole.[10] This seems to be due principally to the fact that most mouth cancers are detected, and brought to treatment, at a relatively late stage. Hayes has estimated that the cure rate in cancer of the tongue could be doubled or tripled by early detection.[26]

Recognition

The first visible sign of the lesion of oral cancer may appear to be innocuous. It may be characterized by nothing more than a slight change in tonus or color, compared with tonus and color in the adjacent soft tissues. Some lesions, such as leukoplakia, have been considered to be precursors of cancer.[55] Not all lesions diagnosed as leukoplakia progress to oral cancer, but when cancer does ensue the outcome may be disastrous for the patient. Pindborg and his associates have reported on a follow-up study of 248 patients with the following conclusion:

> ... All patients with oral leukoplakic lesions referred to the dental department, University Hospital, and the department of surgery, Royal Dental College, Copenhagen, were registered for the follow-up study. ... Among 248 patients with oral leukoplakic lesions, 214 were reexamined with a median observation period of 3.7 years. Eight showed malignant transformation. Among 26 patients with oral leukoplakia who died before reexamination, cancer had developed in 3. Eight patients did not come for reexamination but had not, according to the Cancer Registry, been registered with a diagnosis of oral cancer. Thus, a period prevalance of malignant transformation of 4.4% was found under the conditions of the present study.[39]

Histologically, most malignant tumors of the oral cavity are squamous cell carcinomas. These are sudden, chaotic new growths originating in the squamous epithelium that lines the oral cavity.

Squamous cell carcinomas in and about the lip tend to be of lower grades of malignancy than those in the floor of the mouth or the tonsillar area. These usually begin as a superficial surface ulcer or area of thickening. Less common are the adenocarcinomas, which arise from the submucous glands. These first appear, clinically, as a lump or bulge under overlying normal mucosa. A third category is made up of malignant tumors arising in the jaws. It includes bone sarcomas or locally invasive epithelial tumors, such as ameloblastomas. Excellent descriptions and photographs of these conditions are included in the monograph by Cahn and Slaughter.[10] This handbook or its equivalent should be within ready reach of every dentist in practice.

Most clinical photographs show the lesions at stages so advanced that treatment is futile. Recognition at these late stages has little value. In cancer, time is of the essence; the earlier the treatment, the better the patient's chances to survive without disfiguring mutilation. A primary aim in every routine dental examination should be the discovery of any abnormal tissue change in or near the oral cavity. A standard procedure should be followed to ensure inspection of all soft tissues in the mouth, with due attention to the lips, buccal mucosa, tongue, floor of the mouth, hard and soft palates, and uvula. Palpation is an important part of the physical examination for the detection and appraisal of lumps, swellings, or irregularities. Asymmetry of the head, face, and neck and lesions of the skin should be looked for and noted. Most persistent lumps in the lateral neck triangles of the adult are malignant tumors.[10]

Both the symptoms and clinical course are mild at the outset. The initial lesion is rarely if ever markedly painful or disabling. Squamous carcinoma begins as a small indurated plaque or ulcer that infiltrates the tissue in which it arises. If untreated, the tumor grows by infiltration into deeper tissues and by extension around its borders. As it progresses, the possibility of successful treatment diminishes. In the final stages of its course the lesion spreads to new sites in the adjacent lymph glands, and ultimately (unless death intervenes) to distant organs, such as the lungs or liver. In uncontrolled mouth cancer, death usually results from sepsis, malnutrition, dehydration, pain, hemorrhage, respiratory obstruction, metastasis, or a combination of several of these conditions.

Within recent years exfoliative cytology has evolved as an aid in early detection of the squamous cell lesion. There is one compelling finding in the series of studies on the practicability of oral exfoliative cytology: the large numbers of lesions considered to be innocuous which proved to be malignant on cytological study, even though the initial appraisals were made by clinicans with exceptional skill in diagnosis plus a high index of suspicion about abnormalities of oral tissue. A three-year study in 13 participating dental services of the Veterans Administration elicited a total of 315 confirmed mouth cancers. Of these, 62 cases (about one case in five) "... were completely unsuspected at the time of examination, and were not recommended for biopsy.... It was only because the protocol of this study required that *all* lesions be scraped for cytological examination, whether or not cancer was suspected, that these cancers were discovered."[50] In one of Silverman's series, "... 100 patients with clinically innocuous keratotic or ulcerous lesions, where in our judgement biopsy was not immediately indicated, were examined cytologically. Smears on 7 of these patients surprisingly revealed malignant cells."[54] In the series reported by Tiecke, Kendrick, and Calandra, four of 25 small ulcers or white patches "that were only suspicious in appearance and did not warrant immediate biopsy were actually already malignant."[58]

Preparation of slides for cytological examination is simple. Squamous cells are shed constantly and may be gathered from any mucous surface by scraping with a spatula, tongue blade, or cotton swab. The scrapings are transferred to and distributed over a clean microscope slide. Slides are then placed in a solution of one-half ether and one-half ethyl alcohol and allowed to fix for at least 30 minutes. Immersion may continue until the slides are stained; this period may be maintained indefinitely. Accurate interpretation requires staining and examination by a qualified pathologist. Such services are available to the practitioner through state and local health departments, professional schools, and teaching hospitals.

The smear procedure is painless and can be undertaken without arousing unnecessary fears in the patient. Routine application of the measure would undoubtedly result in an improved cure rate. Cahn has said:

> It is a paradoxical fact that, although squamous carcinoma is more prevalent in the uterus than in the tongue, the cure rate is much higher for uterine cancer than for lingual cancer. This would seem strange, since the upper vaginal vault is certainly less accessible than the oral cavity. Uterine cancer has a higher cure rate because it is discovered early mainly during routine cytologic examination.[51]

The unique value of cytological examination lies in the ease with which it may be applied to the early and innocent-looking lesion. However, specific diagnosis must be made on the basis of microscopic examination of tissue obtained by biopsy. A negative cytology report does not preclude the existence of cancer. A suspicious or positive report makes biopsy mandatory. This should be skillfully done, and done without delay. In most instances it should be performed by the person who will be responsible for the ultimate plan of treatment. Treatment requires eradication of the primary and all metastatic lesions by surgery, radiation therapy, or a combination of both. If the patient survives, extensive maxillofacial prosthesis may be required.

Most authorities believe that the removal of local irritants, or the avoidance of irritating agents, may have some value in the prevention of oral cancer. Bernier lists sunlight, extreme cold, wind, dust, tobacco, and mechanical, thermal, and chemical injuries as predisposing factors which have been implicated in the etiology of carcinoma of the lip.[7]

The most effective control measure for oral cancer remains early detection and prompt and adequate treatment. The opportunity for early detection is most apt to occur in the dental office. The responsibility to be alert for soft tissue changes is not the responsibility of the dentist alone; it is shared by the dental hygienist and by the dental assistant as well. Given any small persistent abnormality in or about the mouth, cancer should be considered first because it is more serious than any other condition with which it may be confused. If the lesion is actually malignant, speculative extraction of teeth will, at best, delay definitive treatment and may, at worst, accelerate the growth and invasion of the tumor. Application of medicaments to the lesion may speed invasion and metastasis. With cancer, the conservative policy of "wait and see" is literally fatal.

FLUOROSIS AND OTHER ENAMEL DEFECTS

Dental fluorosis is sometimes cited as the sole oral disease which can be prevented with complete certainty. This is done by restricting the intake of fluorides by children to optimum levels during the period of enamel formation. Removal of excess fluoride from a community water supply is, in general, more difficult and more costly than methods for adding fluoride to a fluoride-deficient water. The problem can sometimes be solved, as previously described in Oakley, Idaho, by a change to an alternate source of water. Where these solutions are impractical, mottled enamel can be prevented if the fluoride intake of children through the age of eight years is held to one milligram per day or less. This can be accomplished by utilizing a fluoride-free water, or milk, for all or part of the child's requirements for fluids. After crowns of the teeth have become calcified, they cannot be mottled by subsequent use of a fluoride-bearing water.

It should be noted that fluoride ingestion is not the only or even the most frequent cause of opacities in dental enamel. Enamel opacities are found as frequently in the low- as in the optimum-fluoride areas, and those unassociated with fluoride are frequently the most disfiguring.[16] Many of these conditions are hereditary. Witkop has indicated that the group of genetically controlled conditions called hereditary amelogenesis imperfecta includes diverse types characterized by general or localized hypoplasia, by hypocalcification, and by hypomaturation (which may be pigmented). Pigment is deposited in enamel in congenital erythropoietic porphyria. Teeth may be small and malformed in the individual exhibiting the Marshall syndrome. Enamel hypoplasia may involve the entire dentition in pseudohypoparathyroidism. Intrinsic staining of the enamel and enamel hypoplasia are common findings in erythroblastosis fetalis (due to Rh or other blood-group incompatability). All of these conditions are heritable.[62] None can be prevented by alteration of the physical environment.

Hypoplastic enamel stained yellow to brown often results from administration of tetracycline during the period of tooth formation.[23, 63]

A wide variety of other opacities of unknown etiology is found in enamel developed in fluoride and nonfluoride areas alike. These conditions, as well as those known to be hereditary, are frequently found in the deciduous dentition. True fluorosis of deciduous tooth enamel is extremely rare.

OTHER PROBLEMS

Greene has estimated that about 6,000 children are born alive in the United States each year with cleft lip or palate or both.[20] There is no known method for prevention of the condition. Prevention, or at least management, is not an impossible dream; clefts can be induced in laboratory animals by many factors, including deficiencies in specific nutrients, cortisone injection, and radiation. Identification of factors harmful to human mothers would lead, logically, to their proscription during pregnancy.

Control requires the close cooperation of a skilled team including, among others, physicians, surgeons, dentists, orthodontists, speech therapists, and psychologists. Clefts of the lip are usually repaired surgically when the infant is three to four months of age. The palate is closed later by surgical or prosthetic means. Speech therapy is highly important to the patient's rehabilitation.

Similarly, there is no mass measure, or present prospect of a mass measure, for the prevention of malocclusion. Preventive or interceptive orthodontics is an individual affair, consequent upon recognition of the opportunity in the specific patient by an alert practitioner.

SUMMARY

The end result is the same whether disease is controlled by preventive measures or by treatment. Every minute in dental practice is a minute applied toward improvement of the public health. Hence every measure which makes for more effective practice — earlier diagnosis, more efficient procedures at the chair and in the laboratory, better materials, more economic utilization of auxiliary personnel — is a public health measure. This efficiency in practice is an obligation of every dentist, and few would argue to the contrary.

But treatment facilities now, and in the immediate future, appear quite inadequate to cope with demands for dental care in the United States, much less the total dental needs. This mountain of need could be brought down to more nearly manageable size by the widespread application of three simple measures: fluoridation of the community water (or, where there is no common water supply, the application of fluorides by other means); the teaching of oral hygiene to all children at the youngest receptive age, so that they will be motivated to care for their mouths properly and assiduously; and complete and adequate scaling for every person as often as he needs it.

These matters are the responsibility of the dental office team, but they should not mark the boundary of the team's interests. The dental team should be something more than an integrated machine for the restoration of carious lesions and the replacement of missing teeth. It should be a prime source for community information on matters of biological fact. This cannot occur unless the dentist, his assistant, and the dental hygienist have fulfilled the obligation to be informed, not only on matters relating to the oral cavity, but also on matters relating to the welfare of the patient as a whole person.

BIBLIOGRAPHY

1. American Dental Association, Bureau of Economic Research and Statistics. Survey of needs for dental care. II. Dental needs according to age and sex of patients. Am. Dent. A. J., 46:200-11, Feb. 1953.
2. ―――. Survey of needs for dental care, 1965. I. Methodology and composition of sample. Am. Dent. A. J., 73:1128-32, Nov. 1966.
3. ―――. Survey of needs for dental care, 1965. II. Dental needs according to age and sex of patients. Am. Dent. A. J., 73:1355-65, Dec. 1966.
4. ―――. Survey of needs for dental care, 1965. VIII. Summary and comparison with previous surveys. Am. Dent. A. J., 74:1561-2, June 1967.
5. Andrews, George, and Krogh, H. W. Permanent tooth mortality. Dent. Progress, 1:130-4, Jan. 1961.
6. Belting, C. M., and Gordon, Dorothy L. In vivo effect of a urea containing dentifrice on dental calculus formation. J. Periodont., 37:26-33, Jan.-Feb. 1966.
7. Bernier, J. L. Carcinoma of the lip: preliminary statistical analysis of eight hundred twenty-seven cases. Am. Dent. A. J., 36:262-70, Mar. 1948.
8. Bibby, B. G. A consideration of vaccine therapy in periodontal disease. J. Periodont., 28:300-3, Oct. 1957.
9. Brandtzaeg, Per, and Jamison, H. C. The effect of controlled cleansing of the teeth on periodontal health and oral hygiene in Norwegian army recruits. J. Periodont., 35:308-12, July-Aug. 1964.
10. Cahn, L. R., and Slaughter, D. P. Oral cancer; a monograph for the dentist. New York, American Cancer Society, c1962. VI + 42 p.
11. Connecticut State Dental Society, Tumor Committee. Cancer, a handbook for dentists. Hartford, Connecticut State Dental Society, 1948. VI + 52 p.
12. Dean, H. T., and Singleton, D. E. Vincent's infection—a wartime disease. Am. J. Pub. Health, 35:433-40, May 1945.
13. Demmers, Dorothy G., and Belting, C. M. Effect of surfactants and proteolytic enzymes on artificial calculus formation. J. Periodont., 38:294-301, July-Aug. 1967.

14. Dummett, C. O. Traumatism and atrophy: etiology, pathology and symptomatology. Am. Dent. A. J., 44:715-25, June 1952.
15. Emslie, R. D. Prevention in periodontal disease. Internat. Dent. J., 17:320-8, June 1967.
16. Forrest, Jean R. Caries incidence and enamel defects in areas with different levels of fluoride in the drinking water. Brit. Dent. J., 100:195-200, Apr. 17, 1956.
17. Gardner, Joan I., and Ash, M. M., Jr. Effect of oral hygiene instruction on plaque recurrence following a prophylaxis. Abstr. Internat. A. Dent. Res., 46:74, Mar. 1968.
18. Geiger, Arnold. Occlusion in periodontal disease. J. Periodont., 36:387-93, Sept.-Oct. 1965.
19. Glickman, Irving. Periodontosis: a critical evaluation. Am. Dent. A. J., 44:706-14, June 1952.
20. Greene, J. C. Epidemiology of congenital clefts of the lip and palate. Pub. Health Rep., 78:589-602, July 1963.
21. _____. Oral hygiene and periodontal disease. Am. J. Pub. Health, 53:913-22, June 1963.
22. _____. Periodontal disease in India: report of an epidemiological study. J. Dent. Res., 39:302-12, Mar.-Apr. 1960.
23. Harcourt, J. K., Johnson, N. W., and Storey, E. *In vivo* incorporation of tetracycline in the teeth of man. Arch. Oral Biol., 7:431-7, July-Aug. 1962.
24. Hard, Dorothy G. The conservative treatment of periodontal disease. Am. Dent. A. J., 44:725-33, June 1952.
25. Harrisson, J. W. E., et al. Effect of enzyme-toothpastes upon oral hygiene. J. Periodont., 34:334-7, July 1963.
26. Hayes, R. L. Oral cancer and occupational health. J. Occup. Med., 5:342-7, July 1963.
27. Hoffman, D. L., Stallard, R. E., and Schaffer, E. M. An *in vitro* attempt to inhibit calculus formation using an ion exchange resin. J. Periodont., 34:344-7, July 1963.
28. Jordan, H. V., and Keyes, P. H. Studies on the bacteriology of hamster periodontal disease. Am. J. Path., 46:843-57, May 1965.
29. Knutson, J. W. Recent developments in the prevention and treatment of periodontal disease. South. Calif. State Dent. A. J., 32:140-6, Apr. 1964.
30. Koch, Goran, and Lindhe, Jan. The effect of supervised oral hygiene on the gingiva of children: the effect of toothbrushing. Odont. Revy, 16:326-35, Oct.-Dec. 1965.
31. Krogh, H. W. Permanent tooth mortality: a clinical study of causes of loss. Am. Dent. A. J., 57:670-5, Nov. 1958.
32. Lightner, L. M., et al. Preventive periodontic treatment procedures: results after one year. Am. Dent. A. J., 76:1043-6, May 1968.
33. Lövdal, Arne, Arno, Arnulf, and Waerhaug, Jens. Incidence of clinical manifestations of periodontal disease in light of oral hygiene and calculus formation. Am. Dent. A. J., 56:21-33, Jan. 1958.
34. Lövdal, Arne, et al. Combined effect of subgingival scaling and controlled oral hygiene on the incidence of gingivitis. Acta Odont. Scandinav., 19:537-55, Dec. 1961.
35. Lynch, Maryjane, Crowley, Mary, and Ash, M. M., Jr. Correlation between the return of dental plaque and bacterial flora following a prophylaxis. Abstr. Internat. A. Dent. Res., 46:154, Mar. 1968.
36. Mehta, F. S., et al. Prevalence of periodontal (paradontal) disease. 5. Epidemiology in Indian child population in relation to their socioeconomic status. Internat. Dent. J., 6:31-40, Mar. 1956.
37. Mitchell, D. F., and Holmes, L. A. Topical antibiotic control of dentogingival plaque. J. Periodont., 36:202-8, May-June 1965.
38. Occlusion related to periodontics. Committee report. p. 265-70. (In Ramfjord, S. P., Kerr, D. A., and Ash, M. M., eds. World workshop in periodontics. Ann Arbor, American Academy Periodontology and University Michigan, 1966. XX + 454 p.)
39. Pindborg, J. J., et al. Studies in oral leukoplakia: a preliminary report on the period prevalence of malignant transformation in leukoplakia based on a follow-up study of 248 patients. Am. Dent. A. J., 76:767-71, Apr. 1968.

40. Poulton, D. R., and Aaronson, S. A. The relationship between occlusion and periodontal status. Am. J. Orthodont., 47:690-9, Sept. 1961.
41. Public Health Service, National Cancer Institute, and the New York State Department of Health. Cancer control: a manual for public health officers. Albany, New York State Department Health, 1952. 90 p.
42. Public Health Service, National Vital Statistics Division. Monthly vital statistics report. Annual summary for the United States, 1962. vol. 11, Aug. 9, 1963. 39 p.
43. Public Health Service, National Center for Health Statistics. Facts of life and death. Washington, Government Printing Office, 1967. 33 p.
44. Ramfjord, S. P. The periodontal status of boys 11 to 17 years old in Bombay, India. J. Periodont., 32:237-48, July 1961.
45. Russell, A. L. Some epidemiological characteristics of periodontal disease in a series of urban populations. J. Periodont., 28:286-93, Oct. 1957.
46. ———. A social factor associated with the severity of periodontal disease. J. Dent. Res., 36:922-6, Dec. 1957.
47. ———. International nutrition surveys: a summary of preliminary dental findings. J. Dent. Res., 42:233-44, Jan.-Feb. 1963.
48. Russell, A. L., and Ayers, Polly. Periodontal disease and socioeconomic status in Birmingham, Ala. Am. J. Pub. Health, 50:206-14, Feb. 1960.
49. Russell, A. L., Consolazio, C. F., and White, C. L. Periodontal disease and nutrition in Eskimo scouts of the Alaska National Guard. J. Dent. Res., 40:604-13, May-June 1961.
50. Sandler, H. C. V.A. cooperative study of oral exfoliative cytology. Paper delivered at third annual conference on exfoliative cytology, Miami, Oct. 29, 1962.
51. Sandler, H. C., et al. Exfoliative cytology for detection of early mouth cancer. Oral Surg., Oral Med. and Oral Path., 13:994-1009, Aug. 1960.
52. Schei, Olav, et al. Alveolar bone loss as related to oral hygiene and age. J. Periodont., 30:7-16, Jan. 1959.
53. Silness, John, and Löe, Harald. Periodontal disease in pregnancy. II. Correlation between oral hygiene and periodontal condition. Acta Odont. Scandinav., 22:121-35, Feb. 1964.
54. Silverman, Sol, Jr. Early detection of oral cancer. Chicago, Year Book, 1959. 31 p.
55. Silverman, Sol, Jr., and Rozen, R. D. Observations on the clinical characteristics and natural history of oral leukoplakia. Am. Dent. A. J., 76:772-7, Apr. 1968.
56. Stahl, S. S. The etiology of periodontal disease—review of the literature. p. 129-66. (In Ramfjord, S. P., Kerr, D. A., and Ash, M. M., eds. World workshop in periodontics. Ann Arbor, American Academy Periodontology and University Michigan, 1966. XX + 454 p.)
57. Stanley, H. R. The cyclic phenomenon of periodontitis. Oral Surg., Oral Med. and Oral Path., 8:598-610, June 1955.
58. Tiecke, R. W., Kendrick, F. J., and Calandra, J. C. Smear techniques in the diagnosis of intra-oral carcinoma. Dent. Progress, 1:192-8, Apr. 1961.
59. U.S. Department of Health, Education and Welfare. White-nonwhite differentials in health, education, and welfare. Health, Ed. and Welfare Indicators, Feb.-Oct. 1965. 77 p.
60. Waerhaug, Jens. Current basis for prevention of periodontal disease. Internat. Dent. J., 17:267-81, June 1967.
61. Weinmann, J. P. Progress of gingival inflammation into the supporting structures of the teeth. J. Periodont., 12:71, July 1941.
62. Witkop, C. J., Jr. Genetic disease of the oral cavity. (In Tiecke, R. W., ed. Textbook of oral pathology. New York, McGraw-Hill, 1965. XII + 873 p.)
63. Witkop, C. J., Jr., and Wolf, R. O. Hypoplasia and intrinsic staining of enamel associated with tetracycline therapy. Am. Med. A. J., 185:1008-11, Sept. 28, 1963.

CHAPTER 9

THE APPLICATION OF PREVENTIVE AND CONTROL MEASURES

Previous chapters have delineated what is known about the extent and prevalence of dental diseases and disorders and what is known of how to prevent and control them. Of necessity, professional dental education emphasizes technical procedures such as cavity preparation, the manipulation of dental materials, and the fabrication of prosthetic appliances. Each of these procedures is of importance primarily as it contributes to the ultimate objective of practice—the maintenance of optimum oral health for every patient. The attainment of this objective requires the utilization of a wide variety of procedures to *prevent* the occurrence of dental diseases and measures to *control* those diseases that do occur. A total view of dental practice, therefore, requires consideration of these measures. The transition of dentistry from a mechanical vocation to a health profession has been marked by a steadily increasing emphasis on the prevention of disease and concern for the total health of the individual.

IN THE DENTAL OFFICE

Characteristics of Preventive Practice

A committee of the American College of Dentists has defined preventive dentistry as follows:

> Preventive Dentistry consists of the various educational procedures, used by dentists, dental hygienists, physicians, nurses,

teachers, and others, which will develop scientific oral health knowledges and habits, and will prevent the development of improper oral health knowledges and habits; it consists of those technics which will prevent the initiation of oral diseases or conditions such as dental caries, diseases of the supporting structures of teeth, and nonhereditary malocclusion; and it includes the prevention of such sequelae of the neglect of these conditions as oral and systemic infection, interference with normal growth and development of the arches, loss of masticatory function and impairment of the personal appearance or the social adjustment of the individual. The procedures utilized may be effective, scientifically correct, health educational measures or specific preventive technics, such as the topical application of sodium fluoride to teeth, the addition of fluoride to public water supplies, proper toothbrushing, proper diet, the interference with oral habits and the prevention of accidents to teeth. A measure may be considered a control technic if it is corrective in nature at the time it is utilized and if it prevents the development of sequelae. Such control technics are the early detection and correction of carious lesions, timely and proper orthodontic interference, the early detection and treatment of diseases of the supporting structures of teeth, and the early detection and treatment of oral cancer and the developmental anomalies of the oral cavity.[56]

It is significant that this definition lists patient and public educational procedures as the first characteristic of preventive practice. Although not specifically stated, it is presumed that high standards of technical competence and professional ethics will ensure that dental treatment procedures themselves will not harm nor damage the patient. It is assumed, for example, that radiographic examinations are made using accepted procedures to reduce radiation exposure to the minimum. Meticulous cleanliness, use of proper sterilization technics, and methods of reducing trauma to the dental pulp and periodontal tissues during operative procedures also are assumed.

At the 1965 U.S. Army Workshop on "Actualizing the Potential of Preventive Dentistry," one discussion group defined preventive dentistry as "... the employment of all measures necessary to attain and maintain optimum oral health."[16] Perhaps this one statement sums up the foregoing two paragraphs.

Generally, clinical dental practice, whether private or public, should include the following routine preventive and control measures:

    1. Thorough examination and assessment of the patient including: general observation of the overall physical status; health history of the patient; careful inspection of the hard and soft tissues of the mouth, face, and neck; radiographic survey; biopsy and pathological examination of any suspected soft tissue lesions; and caries-activity tests.
    2. Thorough oral prophylaxis at regular intervals.
    3. Topical applications of fluoride when indicated.
    4. Recommendations for the use of dietary fluoride supplements for selected patients not served by a water supply with optimum fluorides.

PREVENTIVE AND CONTROL MEASURES

5. Instruction in proper personal oral hygiene and in an appropriate dietary regime.

6. Provision of or referral for interceptive orthodontic procedures when indicated.

7. Referral to dental and medical specialists where necessary for a more definitive evaluation or for specialized treatment.

8. Premedication of patients with histories of rheumatic fever.

9. Utilization of practical measures for the control of radiation.

10. Adequate methods of sterilization of dental instruments, particularly for all instruments which break the integument.

11. Provision of mouthguards for those patients engaged in hazardous activities such as contact athletics.

12. Treatment of oral and dental lesions, including replacement of missing teeth.

13. Provision for routine recall of the patient to ensure regular prophylaxis, examination, and treatment of dental diseases as they occur.

Building a Preventive Practice

The dentist will find that initially, at least, the characteristics of the community in which he chooses to locate may influence the type of dental practice in which he can engage. Both in rural counties and in local neighborhoods in metropolitan areas, the attitudes of the residents toward a new dentist and their expectations of the type of treatment they will receive have been determined by their past experience. A dentist may find, for example, that he has moved into a community that has never experienced preventive dental care, and where the residents have come to expect the loss of their natural teeth as a normal hazard of adulthood. Thus the failure of previous dentists to live up to the ideals of their profession may become a critical factor in determining the kind of practice that the new dentist can establish initially.

The new graduate can follow one of two courses in such a situation. First, he can work with the people in the community firmly but sympathetically to teach them modern concepts of dental health, to help them to understand that it is possible in most circumstances to maintain teeth throughout life, and to instill in them a desire for good dental health. This change will not happen overnight, cannot be done by force, and will not occur automatically just because the dentist bears the title of "doctor." The alternative is for the dentist to give up, either by leaving the community in disgust and disillusionment, or by slipping into the pattern of mediocrity established by his predecessors—if such had been the case.

The happier choice, of course, is to work toward the development of a preventive practice. It is a better choice for several reasons. Once the objective has been attained and the majority of patients are returning regularly for examination, prophylaxis and routine maintenance service, practice is less taxing for the dentist. Rarely is it necessary to perform major reconstructive procedures which are both difficult and demanding for the dentist and difficult for patients to accept.

The dentist can provide nearly ideal dental care and is called upon less often to "patch up" mouths and compromise with the ravages of neglect. A preventive practice is not only more comfortable but also more personally and professionally rewarding. The dentist has the satisfaction of knowing that he is providing a true health service for the patients who come to him, that he is living up to the ideals of his profession, and that he is contributing to the well-being of his community. From a strictly selfish standpoint there is some evidence that the dentist who strives to build a preventive practice will be remunerated more adequately than the dentist who does not.[7, 25, 40]

Sometimes the viewpoint of a layman to dentistry can be most refreshing. Galton, a free-lance science writer and visiting professor of journalism at Purdue, spent two-and-one-half months visiting some 10 dentists around the country who were supposedly conducting preventively oriented dental practices.[25] He did not pretend that he was examining a representative cross-section of the dental profession, but he was looking for a man who believed himself to be or whom others believed to be in the vanguard of the profession from a preventive standpoint. He came away "pleasantly impressed." He was convinced that they were successful in their preventive practices because they "exuded enthusiasm." They were not necessarily "supersalesmen," but they were sincere and earnest. Another characteristic of these practitioners was that they all made and took the time to educate their patients. One of his concluding paragraphs speaks for him:

> I simply found a group of men who are trying hard to put more and more emphasis on prevention. Who are getting patients to believe in and work at it. Who are getting more patients in the process. Who are being financially well rewarded. Who are getting a great deal of satisfaction out of their work. And whose activities, although certainly not the ultimate, may well serve as guidelines for many other dentists.

In addition to the important factors of enthusiasm, sincerity, and the willingness to try, there are other factors which are important in developing and maintaining a preventive dental practice which incorporates modern concepts of dental treatment and patient management. These are careful planning, effective management, continuous patient education, and professional development.

Planning. The dentist needs first to determine the objectives he wishes to attain in his professional career and then to decide how these objectives are to be reached. Usually this type of planning can be done most effectively by setting down on paper the goals to be attained and the steps required to reach them. A study of the community in which the dentist practices, the characteristics of the residents and their past experience with dentists, for example, will suggest the type of approach that the dentist will need to use in building his practice. For instance, dentists practicing in communities near Atomic Energy Commission installations (where significant proportions of patients, because of their educational background and employment, are acutely aware of radiation hazards) have found it necessary to emphasize the safety of dental radiographic procedures in patient educational efforts and to make more drastic modifications in their procedures than ordinarily would be indicated. In these communities, high levels of education actually have made it more difficult to utilize this important diagnostic tool. At the other extreme are communities where income and educational levels are low and routine dental care for children has been the exception—not the rule. In these communities a dentist cannot expect to provide good dental care for children unless he makes a special effort to educate parents about the important functions of primary teeth, the necessity for regular maintenance care, and the value of preventive procedures.

Dental fees should not be established on a "hit or miss" basis, nor should they be established in slavish obedience to established tradition. Initially, of course, the dentist must consider current practice in the area in which he locates. It may be necessary for him to make some modifications in the type of schedule he would like to institute. Nevertheless, he should have a clear idea in his own mind of the relative value of the services that he provides, the amount of time that it takes to perform them, and the costs of operating his practice. There seems little justification for the common practices of not charging for clinical examinations, of expecting a lower remuneration for caring for children than for adults, or establishing a relatively low fee for such important preventive procedures as topical applications of fluoride and oral prophylaxes. It is sometimes said that what a person does is more influential than what he says. In this case, the establishment of a relatively low fee for services such as prophylaxes or operative procedures for children suggests to the patient that these services are less important to their welfare than are other types of service. To change a tradition of long standing requires conviction on the part of the dentist, willingness to devote time and energy to educate patients to the importance of preventive procedures, and the organization of the practice in order to achieve these objectives. Pedodontists have found, for example, that parents are willing to pay a reasonable fee for preventive services when they are combined in a regular recall system which includes a clinical examination, a radiographic survey, a prophylaxis, and topical applications of fluoride. The parents, then, are billed for the total service in one fee. In this way several important preventive services are introduced into the practice as an integral unit of service on a periodic continuing basis.

The dentist should assume the responsibility of establishing the policies of the office, be sure that those working with him clearly understand these policies, and provide the tools to carry them out. The dental assistant, for example, should have clear instructions about how to answer questions by patients. She should have available health educational materials which will answer the questions raised most frequently by patients, and she herself should understand the reason why certain procedures are followed and appreciate the importance of preventive services.

In many instances the well-trained dental assistant can communicate more effectively with the patient than can the dentist himself, since she may find it easier to put technical information into language that is readily understood. This role is possible, however, only if the dentist has taken the time to prepare her.

One of the most important factors in building a dental practice—and a preventive one—is the establishment and maintenance of a system for recalling patients periodically. A variety of recall systems is in use, and each method has certain advantages and disadvantages.[9, 35, 59, 66] Probably the most common methods are the written reminder, the telephone recall, and the advance appointment procedure. In selecting a particular recall system, it is important to consider the philosophy and character of the practice, the number of auxiliaries employed, and the mobility of the practice's patient population. Regardless of the method or methods selected, one person in the office should be delegated the responsibility for maintaining the system. In many offices, the dental hygienist is responsible; in other practices, it is the responsibility of the dental assistant, secretary, or receptionist. The basic objective is the same regardless of the system used—to help patients receive regular maintenance care by relieving them of the necessity of determining on their own how frequently they should visit the dentist and remembering when it is time to return for an examination. Periodic care usually eliminates the necessity for emergency treatment, reduces the total amount of dental treatment to be provided at any one time, and for many patients, brings dental care within the reach of their financial resources.

Routine recall is an important factor in successful health education of the patient since it permits a frequent reiteration of dental health principles and an opportunity to check on oral hygiene practices. Furthermore, it permits patient education to be done in gradual steps, reinforcing and building on concepts previously introduced. For example, a patient who presents himself to the dentist for the first time after a long period of neglect is hardly in a position to understand or to accept all that he should know. During the first series of visits it may be appropriate to discuss only the necessity for regular examination and treatment and the basic essentials of oral hygiene. At subsequent recall visits the patient may be prepared to accept the necessity for replacing a lost posterior tooth with a fixed bridge.

Management. It is not sufficient to identify the objectives of a practice and to develop reasonable plans. A practice develops only if the dentist keeps these objectives in mind continuously and exercises reasonable and consistent management of the practice. The selection and training of the auxiliary personnel who work in the office (termed "personnel relations" by the businessman) are important factors in the dentist's success. The majority of dentists find it necessary to employ dental assistants without prior training or experience. The dentist must communicate to these individuals his fervor and sincere conviction about the importance of good oral health and practicing preventively. He must provide them also with the technical knowledge they need to deal intelligently with patients and to understand the necessity for the procedures followed in the office.

The dental hygienist has the professional education to function effectively in the dental office. She, too, deserves a clear understanding of the objectives of the dentist, the reasons why he has organized his practice in the way in which he has, and the types of procedures he follows in treating patients. Only in this way can she intelligently educate patients, make suggestions to the dentist, and interpret the dental practice to the patients that she sees.

To provide the dental assistant with the training she needs to function or the dental hygienist with an orientation to the office only once is not enough. Effective practice management requires a continuous effort to maintain communication among those who are working together for the patient's welfare. It is hazardous to depend upon casual opportunities to do this job. Instead, a definite procedure should be established for "staff meetings" to (1) review office practices and procedures; (2) provide the personnel with an opportunity to make suggestions, raise questions, or voice criticism; and (3) evaluate the way in which the office is functioning. Communication among the personnel in the office and periodic evaluation of performance is enhanced if written descriptions of the responsibilities of each person are available and if there are written copies of policies to be followed. The dental hygienist, for example, should have a clear understanding of the circumstances under which the dentist will recommend topical applications of fluoride or replacement of a missing tooth — preferably in writing. If these instructions are available to her, she can perform an effective job of patient education on her own and the recommendations of the office (whether by dentist or hygienist) will be consistent. Written descriptions of the responsibilities of the staff will help to eliminate frictions that often arise when individuals work together on a joint effort in relatively close quarters.

Patient Education. Patient education is such a vitally important component of preventive dental practice and of the professional responsibilities of the dentist, the dental hygienist, and dental assistant that an entire chapter has been devoted to dental health education (Chapter 14). Effective patient education does not happen by chance—it has to be planned, not only for the total office but also for each day and each patient. The office must be organized to allow time for the dentist and the dental hygienist to communicate with patients, and there must be a clear understanding of the concepts that are important for patients to understand. The necessary educational materials and teaching aids should be available. All of the steps which must be taken to build a practice that can be called truly preventive are based upon the fundamental function of patient education. Unless patients can be taught to value oral health and to take the steps necessary to maintain it, the dentist's technical skill and scientific knowledge may go for naught.

Professional Development. The concepts of preventive practice considered ideal today may not necessarily be the optimum practice of tomorrow. Dental research is going forward at an unprecedented rate and will result in many developments, some of which probably are not even suspected today. Therefore, the dentist must be a continuous student. Only in this way can he keep abreast of scientific advances in a rapidly changing and dynamic profession. In fact, there is the strong possibility that the practitioner will have little choice about whether he will continue his education. There is a growing demand both within the profession and from the public for periodic relicensing of dentists.[49] Relicensure would be granted either upon certification of acceptable performance in continuing education programs or upon the basis of challenge examinations. Accordingly, the dentist should budget his time and finances to permit regular attendance at dental meetings and postgraduate refresher courses. He should subscribe to the important dental journals and learn to read them critically. Before the dentist has been in practice long, he may anticipate that new preventive and control technics will be advocated which were unknown while he was in dental school. The dentist must understand at least the basic principles of scientific investigation and exercise discrimination and critical judgment in evaluating new developments. The dental supply salesman, while fulfilling an important service in alerting dentists to new developments, should not unduly influence the dentist's judgment in selecting the procedures and materials which he will adopt for his practice.

Just as he belongs to the dental society and study clubs and attends and participates in scientific meetings, the dentist should encourage his hygienist to belong to the American Dental Hygienists' Association, to attend scientific meetings, and to take advantage of refresher courses offered to dental hygienists. Similarly, the dental assistant should be urged to belong to her dental assistants' association and to take advantage of educational opportunities such as courses for certification.

IN THE COMMUNITY

Although the clinical practice of dentistry is the major factor in maintaining the oral health of the public, community programs of prevention are of vital importance to supplement and reinforce the efforts of the dentist in his office. Since probably only 15 to 20 percent of the population seeks dental services regularly, there is little prospect at this time that the efforts of the dentist in private practice can reach a majority of his community.[39] The remainder of the population will be reached by community programs or not at all.

Dental diseases represent a major public health problem, and it is logical, therefore, that public health preventive measures for the entire community are indicated. Among others, three important conditions help determine that a disease is a public health problem: (1) a disease or other threat to health is widespread; (2) knowledge exists about how to prevent, alleviate, or cure this condition; and (3) the knowledge is not being applied—at least not effectively nor to all who could benefit from it.[58] Dental diseases, affecting at least 95 percent of the population and for which both preventive and control measures exist that are not being applied as effectively as they might be, are among the major public health problems of the day.

Dentists can work to solve dental public health problems in many instances most effectively through cooperative community action. Some dental preventive procedures are applied most appropriately in the community for the benefit of groups of people because they may be more efficient, less expensive, or easier to control—as in the case of fluoridation. Other procedures, such as topical applications of fluorides or the provision of mouthguards, can be applied either in private practice or on a group basis, sometimes simultaneously in the same community but to different recipients. A dentist practicing alone in a small town with a large consolidated high school would be hard pressed to provide mouthguards, through the usual way in his office, to all of the high school athletes engaged in contact sports. Yet by working with a school or community committee to develop an efficient system for using volunteers, he might accomplish the task with ease. In most communities the dentists probably would be swamped if called upon to provide topical applications of fluoride to large groups of children—as many as three quarters of whom never have been in a dental office. By working with organized community groups, however, a plan could be developed to have a dental hygienist employed by the local department of health or by the school system to provide the applications to groups of children.

These examples point up the importance to the dentist and the dental hygienist of participating in the development of community programs. By working with community groups, the professional person can save his own time—and frequently money as well—and he has the satisfaction of meeting dental needs in his community through the use of preventive measures applicable to the community.

The preventive procedures which are of particular value when applied in the community are (1) adjustment of the fluoride content of the drinking water (either by fluoridation or defluoridation); (2) topical applications of fluorides; (3) screening and referral programs to ensure early detection of disease (such as dental caries or oral cancer) and referral for treatment; and (4) the provision of mouthguards to athletes engaged in contact sports. Other methods available but less applicable to community use are the restriction of carbohydrates in the diet and the use of dietary supplements of fluoride.

Use of Dental Surveys in Preventive Programs

In a previous chapter, the use of surveys of population groups for epidemiological investigations was described. Dental surveys also play an important part in planning community dental health activities.[61] When used for this purpose, they frequently require less detailed clinical information about the oral health status of the individuals examined and are often supplemented by surveys of other facets of the community, such as the resources available and the population characteristics and distribution. Community dental surveys aid in identifying the dental problems of a community, in suggesting mechanisms and discovering resources and facilities for attacking these problems, and in evaluating the success of public health programs.

Before considering a community program to provide dental care for handicapped children, for example, it would be wise to survey

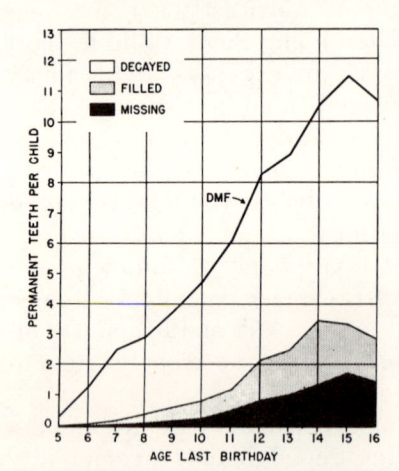

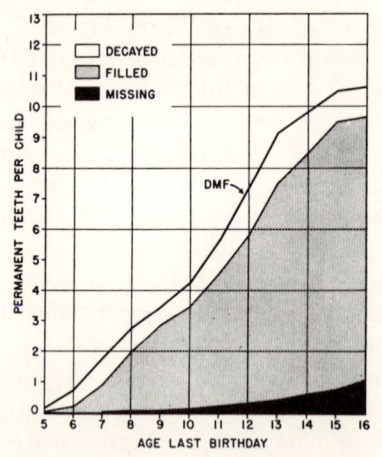

FIGURE 11. Prevalence of dental caries at the start of a community dental care study (left) and following the fourth treatment series (right). (Waterman, G. E., and Knutson, J. W. Studies on dental care services for school children; third and fourth treatment series, Richmond, Indiana. Pub. Health Rep., 69:247-54, Mar. 1954.)

both the dental status of the handicapped children in the community and the agencies available to provide care for them. Such a survey would serve both of the first two functions suggested—it would determine whether or not there was a problem and it would identify the resources that might be used to solve a problem if it did exist.

The third purpose of a dental survey in the community setting is to evaluate the success (or lack of it) of an operating program. Whenever any new program is instituted, it is wise to have a survey of the status of the community, often called a base-line study, since it will serve as a basis for future comparisons (Fig. 11). In the early days of fluoridation it was routine to conduct a base-line survey before the procedure was instituted so that the child population could be resurveyed several years later and the decrease in caries rates documented. Such surveys are no longer important to professional health workers because the benefits of water fluoridation occur consistently and have been demonstrated in a variety of independent studies. Community surveys of dental caries rates before and after water fluoridation, however, remain useful in demonstrating to community leaders the results of water fluoridation in their own community (Fig. 12). Community dental surveys for program planning and for periodic program evaluation are of value, of course, not only in preventive programs but

FIGURE 12. Data from community dental surveys demonstrating the caries attack rate (DMF teeth) in 12 to 16-year-old children in Grand Rapids, Michigan, before and 15 years after fluoridation. (From Englander, H. R., and Keyes, P. H. Dental caries: etiological factors, pathological characteristics, therapeutic measures. p. 221-74. [In Steele, Pauline F. Dimensions of dental hygiene. Philadelphia, Lea & Febiger, 1966. 520 p.] Adapted from data of Arnold, F. A., Jr., et al. Fifteenth year of the Grand Rapids fluoridation study. Am. Dent. A. J., 65:780-5, Dec. 1962.)

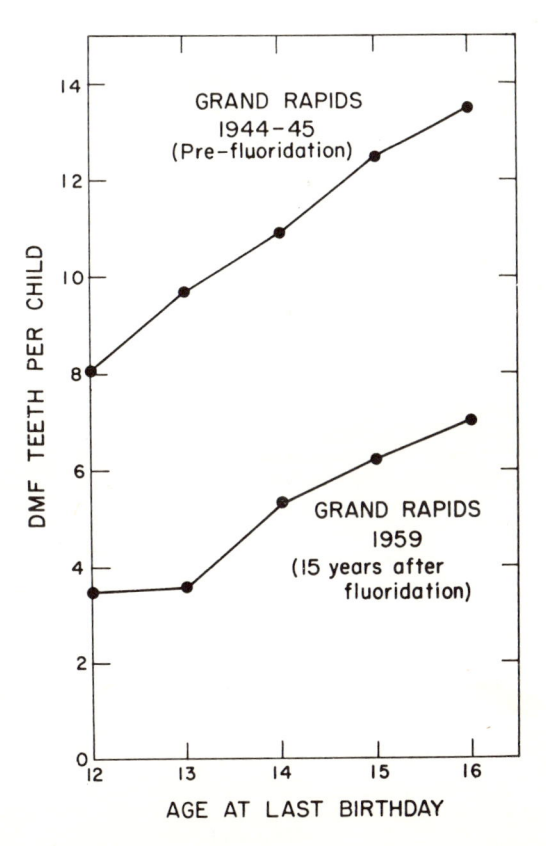

in community efforts to promote dental treatment and to provide dental health education. Just as the practicing dentist turns to dental specialists such as orthodontists or oral surgeons for consultation on certain clinical problems, so should he turn to dental public health specialists for assistance in surveying.

Fluoridation

An earlier chapter reviewed the abundance of scientific evidence that demonstrates the effectiveness of community water fluoridation. It is important to remember that fluoridation, unlike many other public health measures, is effective regardless of parental or patient cooperation, of the income or educational level of the community, or of the amount of dental treatment received. Because of the magnitude of the benefits, their lifelong character, and the fact that they are not dependent upon a change in health habits by the population, the value of this preventive procedure dwarfs all others now available to dentistry.

Despite almost a quarter century of effort, however, only about half of the people having access to public water supplies in the United States are being provided either natural or controlled fluoridation, and most of these people are in larger cities. As of January 1, 1968, 26 percent of the public water systems in the United States were providing natural or controlled fluoridation to about 82 million persons, or to about 53 percent of those people having access to public water supplies.[17] The great majority (approximately 80 percent) of the unfluoridated water systems were small ones serving fewer than 5,000 persons. Indeed, it has been estimated that, at the present rate of achieving fluoridation, the goal of 100 percent fluoridation will not be reached for over a century.[8, 22]

Paul has summarized the problem succinctly:

> The current controversy over fluoridation is the spectacular and unexpected by-product of a remarkable health measure introduced more than ten years ago. Seldom has there been a measure to protect the public's health which has been so effective, so certain, and so simple. And yet, curiously enough, seldom has a program for safeguarding health evoked an outcry so vehement, so sustained, and so successful in blocking action.[50]

The struggle to institute fluoridation has been so dramatic that it became the subject of an entire book by McNeil, titled *The Fight for Fluoridation*.[47]

The policy of the American Dental Association in regard to the role of the dental profession in the promotion of fluoridation is quite clear:

> Traditionally, the individual dentist and the dental society have made their scientific knowledge and resources available to the community. They have sought the acceptance of fluoridation by pro-

viding leadership in keeping with their professional competence. The tactics of those who oppose fluoridation, however, are of such nature as to warrant, and command, professional leadership beyond the usual point. The antisocial program of the antifluoridationists must be countered, and the individual dentist and the dental society must exercise aggressive leadership in all phases of activity which lead to the acceptance of fluoridation. The individual dentist and the dental society now have not only the obligation to support but also to initiate, when necessary, programs for the acceptance of fluoridation of the community water supply. This leadership should be amplified whenever possible by the enlistment of aid from other professions and individuals and agencies interested in public health.[13]

Despite the clear-cut policy of the American Dental Association, the recommendations of the Commission on the Survey of Dentistry, and the endorsement of fluoridation by countless official and voluntary health agencies and countless professional scientific organizations, many practicing dentists in the United States have not accepted their responsibility to promote fluoridation. The National Opinion Research Center study on preventive dental practice indicated, for example, that only two percent of the dentists questioned claimed to have participated in the organization of a fluoridation movement in their communities.[40]

FIGURE 13. United States: Total population in communities with controlled fluoridation, 1950-1967. The large increase in 1965 is attributed to New York City's fluoridating, and the increase in 1967 is attributed not only to Detroit's fluoridating but also to an audit of Public Health Service records for each state by the state dental director which apparently corrected under-reporting for previous years. (Data supplied by Community Programs Branch, Division of Dental Health, Public Health Service.)

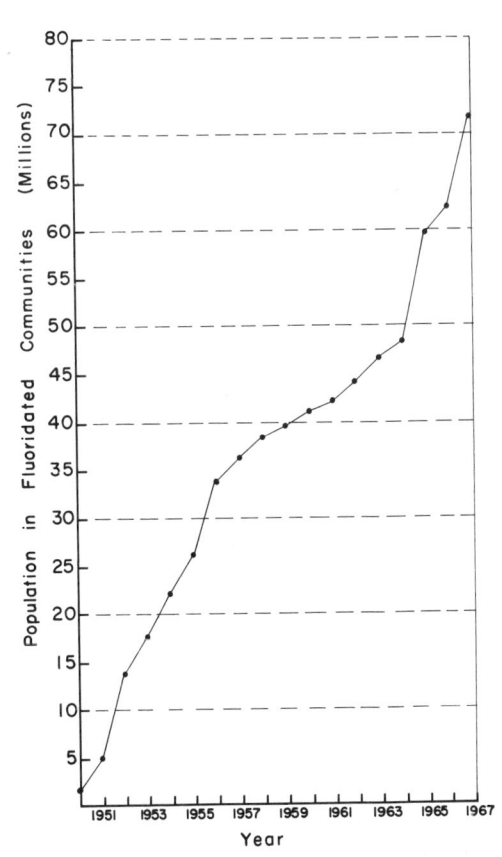

Despite the seeming apathy, the progress that has been made in fluoridation has been due largely to the dedicated efforts of a small but hardworking group of dentists whose enthusiastic support of this public health measure has done much to raise the prestige of dentistry in the eyes of the other health professions, as well as the public.

This same group of dentists working cooperatively with public health officials and dedicated legislators in the past year or two has been able to secure state-wide legislation requiring that all water supplies over a certain size be fluoridated in South Dakota, Connecticut, Illinois, Minnesota, Delaware, and Michigan. A number of other states have either introduced or are considering similar laws. Most of this legislation does not apply to the smallest communities and it usually allows a period of several years for the communities to comply. Each year, then, should show the graph (Fig. 13, page 155) increasing rather dramatically as state-wide fluoridation is implemented.

At a National Dental Health Conference, McNeil, in a paper titled "Time to Walk Boldly," outlined the challenge that fluoridation has presented to the dental profession:

> I maintain that as professional leaders and as spokesmen of science, the dentist, the physician, and the public health official cannot escape their public responsibility to fight with every resource at their command the vicious half-truths, outright lies, and devious tactics of the misguided, often dishonest, opponents. For those sincerely following their charlatan leaders, the professional man has a major educational campaign before him. There simply comes a time when the dentist, physician, public health worker, and community leader has to face scorn, ridicule, and threats to put across what he believes in. He has a vast amount of community prestige and on some issues he must be prepared to risk it.[45]

Unfortunately, there is a great deal still to be learned about how to work effectively in the community to ensure a favorable public reaction to fluoridation. The information that is available comes primarily from two sources. Social scientists—from fields such as sociology, psychology, political science, and cultural anthropology, which study various facets of the reactions of individuals singly and together in the community—have initiated some studies on fluoridation in recent years, and their findings have made available at least some tentative suggestions. Dentists, physicians, public health workers, and community leaders who have been engaged actively in fluoridation campaigns during the past decade can make suggestions based on experience and empirical judgments.

Social Science Studies. An entire issue of the *Journal of Social Issues*, titled "Trigger for Community Conflict: The Case of Fluoridation," was devoted to studies of fluoridation campaigns by behavioral and social scientists.[51] The initial paper includes a bibliography that contains virtually all known research papers dealing with the social science aspects of fluoridation—a bibliography that lists only 44 references.[50] The next few years saw only about another dozen papers published and only two or three serious studies.[15, 28, 32] This relatively small number of references, when compared with the thousands of published papers dealing with the engineering, medical, and dental aspects of fluoridation, makes it apparent that social sciences have made only a small contribution to this field. A few studies are under way and it is hoped that findings from them may provide more definite guidelines to successful fluoridation efforts. Some of the studies reported to date, while perhaps of not sufficient scope to warrant acceptance as a definite statement of fact, do present concepts which should be useful to those who must plan community efforts for fluoridation.

For example, Crain and Rosenthal conducted a survey by mail of the local public health officer, the city clerk, and the publisher of the largest newspaper in 1,186 cities. From the responses to their questionnaires, they concluded that fluoridation has the following political properties:

1. It has almost unanimous support among the elite.
2. Very few members of the elite have a strong interest in seeing it adopted.
3. The opposition comes from an organized minority, usually including chiropractors, Christian Scientists, natural food faddists, and, in a few cases, the radical right.
4. The public at large is uninformed, but is cautious because of the possible side effects of any medical innovation.
5. The medical profession is virtually unanimous in support of fluoridation.[15]

They found also that the mayor and city manager appear to play exceptionally important roles in the decision a city makes either administratively or by referendum. When the mayor favors fluoridation, it has a 60 percent chance of adoption, but when he opposes the measure, or takes no public stand, its chances of acceptance are minimal.[55]

PARTICIPATION IN FLUORIDATION CAMPAIGNS. Probably all professional health workers hope that a fluoridation effort can be conducted in a quiet, dignified manner, devoted primarily to the education of key leaders and groups in the community and avoiding the public controversy that may be expected if a referendum is held. Although it has been possible to secure adoption of fluoridation by action of the governing body of some communities following a relatively quiet and noncontroversial educational effort, a referendum has been unavoidable in many instances.

Raulet studied the efforts of professional health workers in fluoridation referendums and found that, because these workers were naive in the ways of power and propaganda, they tended to defeat their own purposes.[54] The health professionals were caught in the dilemma of conflicting "role expectations." In an issue concerning health, such as fluoridation, they are expected by their colleagues and by laymen to participate as professional experts. Furthermore, the "role" of expert was the type to which they were accustomed and in which they could operate most comfortably. But once the issue of fluoridation was to be decided by referendum, it became an open political question. In this instance the community expected that those who were supporting fluoridation would act as partisan lobbyists for an issue which had been defined by the community as controversial and political. In these campaigns the professional health workers, not surprisingly, chose to spurn the role of a political partisan and to assume a detached professional role. They refused to engage in public debate but held themselves aloof after having given their professional advice.

The efforts of the dentists and other members of the health professions met with unfavorable reaction from segments of the community for two different reasons. The community expected partisans in a political campaign to be motivated by their own self-interest and to conduct a propaganda campaign to further those interests. Since the health professionals supporting fluoridation were seen as political partisans, their endorsements of fluoridation and their attempts at health education (presented in their professional role) were not accepted as expert testimony. At the same time their efforts to maintain professional dignity and to avoid engaging in open controversy were interpreted as undemocratic arrogance. The decision to refuse to engage in public debates with the opponents, although appearing perfectly reasonable to the professional health workers, was interpreted as high-handedness and evasiveness both by those who were opposed to fluoridation and by those who were sympathetic to the cause but not actual members of the group promoting the procedure.

This study would seem to suggest that once the issue of fluoridation has become the subject of referendum, physicians, dentists, and public health workers cannot expect to maintain the detached role of a professional expert in the health field. They must expect that their actions will be interpreted by the public as those of a partisan participant in a political debate. McNeil has outlined what is then required: "When the 'antis' insist on making a political issue out of fluoridation, then it is time for those who believe in its effectiveness to get busy. They must meet the anti-fluoridationists on their own ground—on the political hustings, using political methods, and striving for a political victory."[46]

NATURE OF OPPONENTS. A number of attempts have been made to determine the type of individual most likely to oppose fluoridation, and to identify some of the factors influencing the decision to oppose fluoridation. Although the evidence to date does not provide a clear picture of these factors, it does give some insight into the nature of the opposition to fluoridation that should be useful to those who

PREVENTIVE AND CONTROL MEASURES

will experience the frustration of dealing with opponents who may appear irrational. Early findings demonstrated that young, highly educated, middle-class persons favored fluoridation and older, poorly educated, lower-class persons were against fluoridation.[43] It was found further that persons between 21 and 35 with college training and with children under 12 are most likely to favor fluoridation. This attractively simple classification has not been borne out in further studies. Analysis of the voting patterns in a New England community, in fact, indicated that many white-collar workers, persons between 41 and 50, and persons who had finished high school voted against fluoridation while many unskilled workers with little formal education voted for the measure.[27]

Kirscht and Knutson studied the attitudes of individuals toward science.[41] They found that the vast majority of people considers that the world is better off because of scientific endeavors. However, those who oppose fluoridation, while still generally favoring scientific advances, were more likely to have misgivings about some aspects of science. In particular, the opponents felt uneasy about some indirect effects of scientific efforts, such as the production of deadlier weapons and the weakening of moral values, which they saw as threatening their way of life. It has been suggested by Simmel that one of the common denominators among opponents to fluoridation is that they have received fewer advantages than others and that they are unable to influence political action in the world around them.[57] He tested four ways in which people could feel a sense of "deprivation," or feel that they were relatively less well-off than members of other groups. These four measures included: "economic deprivation" (awareness that a person is in a low-income bracket, or that his income has decreased); "prestige deprivation" (recognition that levels of living are below average and that the individual's occupation carries relatively little prestige); "political deprivation" (the feeling that the individual has very little influence on government action and is ignored by public officials); and "rank disequilibrium" (holding a status that is widely divergent from an individual's own social evaluation, such as a person who is highly educated but poor or a man in a high-ranking occupation belonging to an ethnic group with little social acceptance). In all four instances, individuals who showed the greatest measure of "deprivation" were more likely to oppose fluoridation than were those occupying more favorable positions. This study suggests that opposition to fluoridation is, at least for many individuals, a revolt against society by those who are frustrated by society's failure to satisfy their needs. A fluoridation campaign provides an opportunity to express this revolt politically. In attempting to answer why many fluoridation campaigns have aroused those with feelings of helplessness, Gamson and Green decided to turn their attention from the opponents of fluoridation to the proponents.[26, 30] Gamson suggests that it may be something in the "campaign posture" of fluoridation proponents which mobilizes the opposition, and Green feels it is the "authoritarian elements in the pro-fluoridationists' stance toward the public" that provokes the opponents of fluoridation.

The attitudes of those who had been active public opponents of fluoridation were studied in an attempt to determine why the argument that fluorides were a "poison" played such a prominent part in most fluoridation campaigns.[31] It is suggested that:

> ... opponents of fluoridation are troubled above all by what the measure means, and only secondarily by what, as a scientific or practical matter, fluoridation is. To them the issue is moral, a direct confrontation with threatening forces that illuminates and sharpens their sense that the society in which they live is radically out of shape.

Thus, this seemingly innocent issue triggers tensions which may have their source in industrialization, the growth of "big government and big unions," and the anxieties of the nuclear age. Green suggests that the plausibility of the "poison argument" is that it primarily serves as a symbol, or metaphor, of all that these individuals see as dangerous and threatening in society:

> ... poisoning involves an agent with malicious intent and a victim. The poisoner relies on deception: the success of the act depends entirely on how persuasively the poison is disguised as something harmless or even desirable. The effect of poison is to put the victim under the control of his assailant; with slow poisoning, as fluoridation is almost always characterized, the process is prolonged and, as the poison accumulates, the victim becomes increasingly weakened and helpless.[31]

The opponents of fluoridation interviewed by Green were opposed primarily on ideological and philosophical grounds. Surprisingly, although they frequently used the argument in public that fluorides are a poison, they themselves did not see that as the dominant objection. In fact, there is a suggestion that the conviction that fluorides are harmful was not strongly held but was found attractive by the opponents because of its obvious effectiveness when used in public debate.

These studies have several important implications for fluoridation campaigns. Although the opinions of some opponents of fluoridation can be changed, an individual whose opposition to fluoridation is triggered by hostility toward society is not likely to be influenced by factual arguments about the safety or effectiveness of water fluoridation. Furthermore, although opposition to this public health procedure may not be based on rational or scientific grounds, the bulk of the opposition is sincere and the convictions are held strongly. Their efforts to oppose what they conceive to be a real threat should be countered with sympathy and consideration. If the opponents are ridiculed or belittled, it usually only arouses public sympathy for them and antagonism against the supporters of the measure.

One of the difficult tasks in convincing laymen to support water fluoridation is to counter the frequently held opinion that "where there is smoke there must be fire." In other words, a considerable number of individuals, although basically sympathetic to fluoridation, find it difficult to believe that charges by the opposition (such as that fluoridation is poisonous or causes cancer) would be made at all unless there were some element of truth in them. The local opponents of fluoridation should be studied carefully to identify possible reasons and motives for their opposition to the procedure. Frequently it is possible to explain sympathetically some of the possible motivations of those in opposition and thus reassure those who favor fluoridation or are undecided.

Findings of Experience. If the dentist is to discharge his professional responsibilities in the community, he must recommend fluoridation if it is indicated and must be prepared to help the community secure its adoption. Although all of the answers to planning successful fluoridation campaigns may not be available, the dentist and the dental hygienist should profit from the knowledge that is available, try to apply the lessons of experience suggested by other fluoridation campaigns, and move forward. The self-employed, self-disciplined dentist who attempts to stimulate action in the community is now working with a group. He is no longer his own boss, seeing people one at a time, telling them what to do, making decisions, taking action, and seeing results rather quickly. He must reorient his thinking to what the groups around him want and must adjust his pace to the speed with which they are willing to move. He must learn patience and tolerance of his fellow citizens and try to understand their views and ways of making decisions and taking action.

BECOMING INFORMED. The first step is to become informed thoroughly about the technical aspects of fluoridation. The dentist or hygienist should first find out whether or not fluorides are now present in the drinking water.* The state or local health department can provide this information as well as a description of engineering characteristics of the water system. The dentist should have some general understanding of the sources of water and the present methods used for water treatment. In most instances, the state or local health department can provide at least tentative estimates of cost and identify any particular engineering problems that may complicate fluoridation, such as multiple sources of supply—each of which would require separate fluoridators.

At this point it would be wise for the dentist to refresh his

---

*Obvious as this step may seem, it has sometimes been ignored, and fluoridation efforts have been initiated in communities with optimum or near optimum amounts of fluoride in the water supply. The dentist practicing in a fluoride area may not recognize immediately the low caries prevalence because the patients coming to him are the very ones who need treatment—a self-selected, biased sample. Also, if he has never practiced in a nonfluoride area, he has no basis for comparison.

knowledge of the medical and dental studies which provide the scientific basis for fluoridation. In addition to the basic studies reviewed in Chapter Seven, it would be wise to contact the state and local health departments for the most recent information available and for more detailed answers to specific objections frequently raised by the opponents of fluoridation. Excellent references such as *Fluoridation Facts* are available from the American Dental Association[4] (and also from most state health departments) as well as Elwell and Easlick's *Classification and Appraisal of Objections to Fluoridation* published by The University of Michigan.[20]

It is important to find out whether or not any previous efforts have been made to institute fluoridation and, if so, the individuals who were involved and a history of what transpired. It is also wise to study the history of other controversial issues which may have arisen in the community in recent years. Those who oppose efforts such as the establishment of mental health clinics or the adoption of other public health procedures frequently are the ones who may be expected to form the hard core of opposition to fluoridation. It is also wise to determine the influence of "food faddists," "health food" stores, chiropractors, and naturopaths. Although not usually considered a significant part of the health services of a community, these persons often possess "expert" status with many laymen and sometimes become important members of the opposition.

One of the most important steps is to analyze the power structure in the community and locate the individuals who are most likely to assist in bringing about favorable action. Every community is unique, and there is no easy formula for identifying correctly all of the key persons and groups in any specific public issue. It is helpful, however, to try to determine the individuals who are influential because they occupy official positions in government, the various voluntary organizations that are a part of the life of the community, and those persons who, although perhaps not active in community groups, mold the opinion of a significant number of others.

Among those who occupy official positions of responsibility, it is natural to think first of those who can take official action to institute fluoridation, such as the mayor and members of the city council or village board. For example, the mayor, simply by remaining neutral, can successfully foil a fluoridation campaign.[55] The health officer and members of his department can play an important role, as can the school administration—particularly if a parent-teacher organization is expected to be an active group. The role of other public employees, such as the superintendent of the waterworks, or the town clerk, may not be apparent immediately. These individuals may not be in a position to initiate action or make major policy decisions, but they often can prevent action by subtle and covert efforts. (Dentists have found that fluoridation may be delayed for long periods of time, for example, by dilatory tactics in purchasing equipment or ordering chemicals.)

PREVENTIVE AND CONTROL MEASURES 163

Others, although not elected to official positions, have an important impact on community life because of what might be called "quasiofficial" positions. The attitude of the editor and staff of the local newspaper can be an important consideration. Similarly, the support or opposition of the management of a radio or television station (or of a key "personality" in their programming who has been given independent responsibility for the material he presents) can make the difference between success and failure.

It has been quite common in fluoridation campaigns to work through existing community organizations such as parent-teacher groups, service clubs, sororities, fraternal orders, and labor unions. Valuable as these organizations are, it is important to remember that they ordinarily reach only a small segment of the population. Characteristically, these groups often do not touch the lower economic groups in a community—the same groups that are not reached by communications through the newspapers, radio, and television. This segment of the community must be reached by face-to-face contact. To do so effectively requires the identification of individuals who are influential with certain groups but who may not be well known in the community. (These factors are discussed at more length in Chapter 14.)

GAINING CONSENT WITHOUT A REFERENDUM. Experience from many fluoridation efforts suggests several additional steps which a dentist or a dental hygienist might follow to promote fluoridation.

The first task is to gain the support of the local dentists and establish the fluoridation efforts as an activity of the entire dental society. From this point on, the dentist's efforts should be within the framework of the dental society. The dental hygienist would first solicit the support of her own professional society and urge the development of a joint project with the local dental society.*

It is important that members of the dental society sound out informally the opinions of members of the medical profession and other health-related groups that are of influence in their community. They should work with the water superintendent to ensure that he is disposed favorably toward fluoridation. Where professional education is indicated, it must be provided—preferably in a subtle manner. It is essential to develop a consistent and favorable opinion in the professional and technical groups in the community.

After taking steps to ensure the support of professional and technical personnel, members of the dental society might begin to meet informally and individually with those public and private indi-

---
*Dental hygienists generally have not taken an active part in fluoridation campaigns, to the writers' knowledge. Although the dental profession probably must take the initial leadership in a community effort, dental hygienists would appear to have an equal professional obligation to work for fluoridation. Furthermore, because of their special skills in health education, and their ability to relate to women's and parents' groups, they would seem to have a unique role to play. Hygienists who have "retired" to raise a family, as well as those in active practice, might be expected to assist.

viduals who have been identified as members of decision-making groups. They will preferably begin with those members with whom they already have established good working relations. By careful and indirect probing they should be able to determine what these people know and how they feel about community dental needs and about fluoridation. If this "scouting expedition" suggests that opinions are negative on the basis of incorrect or insufficient knowledge, it would be wise to slow down attempts to initiate fluoridation and change the emphasis to a low-pressure educational program with the community leaders. This program might be done partially through informal discussions and partly by indirect efforts to promote discussions of fluoridation at various group meetings at which representatives of the dental society or other experts would be invited to speak. As previously mentioned, responsible community leaders who oppose fluoridation frequently have no strong objections to the procedure itself but rather to the symbolism of fluoridation. Low-pressure campaigns of this kind may well succeed in providing needed information and thus modify initial negative opinions that were based on inadequate understanding. Those opponents whose initial negative reactions to fluoridation are based on strong emotional grounds are unlikely to be changed by any action.

At such time as the dental society has reason to believe that knowledge and opinions among leadership groups have become generally favorable to fluoridation, it should be possible (again through indirect and low-pressure technics) to prevail upon one or two such leaders to introduce the subject of fluoridation through the appropriate local government channels. If the educational campaign has been effective, the proposal to fluoridate well may come spontaneously from the leadership group without additional stimulation.

After the decision has been reached to place a fluoridation proposal before the governing body (but before it actually is discussed in an open meeting), the dentists have an additional educational task. It is important that they provide members of the governing body and other key individuals with knowledge of the existence of the opposition to fluoridation and the arguments that probably will be advanced against the procedure. To the extent possible, it is also desirable to predict the specific individuals and groups who probably will oppose fluoridation. Such a procedure not only may arm the "decision-makers" with facts in answer to the opposition, but it also may serve to make the arguments of the opposition seem anticlimactic. Throughout the campaign, the *public* "roles" of the dentists are those of professional resource persons to the governing body. In those roles, they provide requested information on need, effectiveness, safety, and finances involved in fluoridation.

It is important to solicit the aid of the mass media. Newspapers, radio, and television can turn a fluoridation issue into an unwholesome public spectacle in which the real issues may be forgotten.

PREVENTIVE AND CONTROL MEASURES

The combined experience of many workers suggests that widespread publicity of this type should not be encouraged at this point. The question now is how publicity can be kept in proportion. Experience shows that if full discussion is conducted with representatives of the mass communications media, many of them will agree not to magnify the fluoridation issue unnecessarily and to keep coverage on as scientific a plane as possible.

Since the meeting of the governing body that will decide the fluoridation issue probably will be well attended by the opposition, it also should be well attended by those favoring the proposal. On request, the dentists and other health professionals should provide "decision-makers" with information during such meetings, in the role of "expert witnesses."

Clearly it is not possible to spell out all the details of such a campaign, since improvisation will be needed to meet local conditions. However, it is important to note how the suggested procedure differs from many past attempts. The dentist and dental hygienist:

1. Begin by working with known official and nonofficial leaders in the health and welfare areas, including members of the professional groups concerned.
2. Assess the leaders' initial knowledge of and attitudes toward fluoridation.
3. Provide needed education subtly and at a slow pace.
4. Do not call attention initially to themselves as fervent fluoridation supporters; nor do they give evidence of any plan to promote fluoridation actively.
5. Do not identify themselves as the initiators or innovators of the change but leave it to another local group to take leadership.
6. Maintain a professional and nonpolitical role *on the public level*, avoiding the error of competing publicly with politicians in the political arena; they behave rather in a fashion that both lends dignity to and permits them to occupy professional roles in which they can be most secure. *On the private level*, they are most active, but their activities have been directed toward the decision-making group rather than toward the public in general.

WINNING A REFERENDUM. The plan that has been outlined presupposes the relatively ideal conditions under which it may be possible to avoid a referendum. Whenever possible, the adoption of fluoridation should be done without bringing the issue to a public vote. Fluoridation is a scientific and technical question which should be acted on by the elected representatives of the public, such as members of village boards or city councils. A referendum merely represents the abdication of decision-making responsibility by those who have been elected to perform this task. Furthermore, experience has shown that referendum campaigns are not debated on a basis which makes a rational decision by the electorate possible. If a common agreement has been reached on the facts—that fluoridation is safe, that it will produce a certain predictable reduction in dental caries, and that it will cost a certain amount of money—there might not be any great problem in asking the entire public to act on the question. During fluoridation referendums, however, the opposition is based generally either on the contention that fluorides do not reduce dental decay or that they are harmful in some way to the body. These two questions are resolved by scientific evidence, not by opinion, and are hardly an appropriate subject for public ballot. It would be as logical to expect the public to vote on whether the world was round, flat, or elliptical.

Under some circumstances, however, public balloting cannot be avoided; for example, in communities that previously have voted against fluoridation. Also, there are some states in which the opponents have been able to secure legislation which makes a referendum on fluoridation mandatory before it can be adopted. There are also instances in which the opponents of fluoridation themselves will force the issue to a public vote by petition.

In these instances, the task of gaining acceptance of fluoridation is much more difficult, and the dental society must be prepared to plan a different kind of campaign and to assume, in some cases, a different kind of "role." Much more intensive efforts now are necessary to enlist community leaders who are willing to engage in active political efforts to influence those who will vote on the issue.

A successful effort will require the planning of an educational and informational campaign to reach as large a segment of the population as possible. Every available method of health education should be utilized including advertisements and news releases. A speakers' bureau, to provide talks to civic groups, and mass mailings are among the procedures often indicated. Any respectable method to combat the efforts of the antifluoridationists must be considered. Leaflets and pamphlets should be printed in terminology and language understandable by the group to which they are directed. Experts in community organization and communication should be consulted to find out how to reach the large segment of the population that ordinarily does not participate in organizations such as service clubs and parent-teacher associations, and who are not influenced to a major extent by mass media.

As much as possible, in *public*, members of the dental society should attempt to stay in the background and to maintain their role as professional persons providing the scientific and technical information for those who are carrying out the campaign. One of the important roles is in organizing training sessions for the lay persons participating in the fluoridation campaign. In conducting educational efforts, dentists must attempt not only to be scientifically accurate but also to express the facts and concepts in simple, clear, positive terms. It will be necessary to discuss the nature of those who are opposing fluoridation and the reasons for their opposition. Extreme care should be taken that these comments are not derogatory nor of the "name-calling" variety. No matter how strongly dentists may feel personally about the opposition, their public statements should be confined to the fact that the opponents are sincere and conscientious individuals who are misinformed and whose efforts are misdirected. Impugning their intelligence or honesty is likely only to arouse sympathy for the opponents.

Although it is desirable for members of the dental society to remain in the background, it usually is not possible. They often will be asked to appear before public meetings and sometimes are challenged to public debates by members of the opposition. Whether or not to accept an invitation to debate a fluoridation opponent cannot be answered definitely. Findings from behavioral science research indicate that a refusal to debate may be interpreted by the public as professional arrogance, the lack of a sense of fair play, and evidence of a dictatorial attitude. On the other hand, it must be recognized that a debate with a skillful opponent of fluoridation cannot be "won." Experience has shown that false "objections" to fluoridation can be raised far faster than they can be answered by facts. The opponents charge that fluoridation causes cancer. Once this charge has been disproved at considerable length, the opponent merely changes ground and charges that it causes falling hair or ingrown toenails. This process can continue as long as the meeting.

Under most circumstances, local dentists and physicians can be more effective in public appearances in their own community than can those coming in from "the outside" no matter how expert the outsiders are in their field. Local practitioners do not experience the suspicion and resentment frequently encountered by outsiders, they are generally not the subject of the suspicion held toward "experts," and they usually have earned the respect and admiration of their fellow citizens. Often a positive and forceful endorsement of fluoridation with the assurance that it has been studied carefully, that it has been proved to be effective, and that it is absolutely safe is more apt to influence an audience than a long technical presentation.*

---

*An example of the effectiveness of local practitioners can be found in a fluoridation hearing that was held in a small community in the Northwest some years ago. The city council requested that both the proponents and the opponents of fluoridation present an hour and a half of testimony. Speaking for fluoridation were local dentists, a local physician, and an engineer and a dentist from the state health department. Speaking against fluoridation were a physician and a dentist from a city outside the state. The engineer and dentist from the state health department spoke briefly, confining their remarks to a discussion of local experience with fluoridation in communities in the state that were familiar to the audience. The bulk of the proponents' time was given to the local dentists and physician. The out-of-state physician and dentist spoke for the opposition for a full hour and a half. In the question and answer period that followed, the "experts" appearing for the opposition were strongly critical of the local physicians and dentists who were supporting the proposal. At the end of the question and answer period one of the citizens who been listening patiently during the discussion rose from the back of the room and emphatically stated, "We like our local dentists and doctors and we don't like people coming from ＿＿＿＿＿＿ criticizing them." At this point the audience broke into applause, and it was obvious that the sentiments strongly favored fluoridation and were opposed to the "big-city experts." Immediately after the meeting was adjourned the council met and voted to institute fluoridation.

It is pointless to attempt to suppress the opposition or to deny them an audience. First, they will find a way to express their views by one device or another. Second, efforts to suppress their presentations are likely to backfire and make the public sympathetic with their cause. On the contrary, every effort should be made to see that the opponents ventilate their strong feelings and gain their place in the spotlight (which may be all they wish to do in the first place). At the same time they often defeat themselves by their irrational, illogical, and unscientific statements.

Finally, it is important to persuade those in favor of fluoridation to go to the polls. As in any other political campaign, it is the opinion expressed in the ballot, not necessarily the total opinion of the community, that determines the decision. Free baby-sitting service, provision of transportation to the polls, and round-robin telephone efforts to persuade citizens to vote are among the devices that may be used.

Possibly the strong recommendations of the Commission on the Survey of Dentistry have spurred the American Dental Association, the Public Health Service, and various state and local dental societies and health departments to renewed, reinvigorated efforts to secure fluoridation.[67] The American Dental Association has devoted two entire issues of the *Journal* to fluoridation, as well as a special supplement which reported the findings from Evanston.[2, 3, 6] The Association's Council on Dental Health has begun publishing the *ADA Fluoridation Reporter*, devoted entirely to the promotion of fluoridation, and commissioned Donald McNeil to prepare a book titled *How to Get the Benefits of Fluoridation for Your Community*, a step-by-step guide to the successful conduct of a fluoridation campaign, also available from the Association.[44] State dental and public health societies and health departments are launching new campaigns for fluoridation.[53] These efforts appear to be effective since a definite trend toward mandatory state-wide fluoridation appears to have been established.

In addition, the problem of securing fluoridation for small communities and in rural areas has been attacked by state health departments and the Public Health Service. Two studies have shown that subsidies and technical assistance to extremely small communities can result in fluoridation of communities with extremely small populations.[62, 65] Another approach to providing fluoridated water to children in rural areas has been that of fluoridating the water supplies of public schools.[36, 37]

All of these efforts indicate a start in the right direction, but without the personal dedication of the majority of dentists and without the aggressive leadership of individual members of the American Dental Association, the children of the United States presently denied the benefits of fluoridation will continue to suffer the ravages of dental caries.

Other Preventive Measures Used in the Community

Topical Applications of Fluoride. While it is evident that fluoridation is the method of choice for the partial prevention of dental caries for children living on a communal water supply, there remains an increasing number of children who are not benefiting from drinking a water supply with optimum fluorides. Most of these millions of children live in rural or suburban areas and in small towns. Topical applications of fluoride to the teeth (fluoridization), despite some obvious disadvantages, are the most effective preventive measure available for community use in the absence of water fluoridation and should be used more widely. (See Chapter Seven.)

Topical applications of either sodium or stannous fluoride solutions are relatively expensive and require the use of valuable professional time. Tossy compared the costs of a community program of topical applications of sodium fluoride with the costs of fluoridation.[63] He calculated that topical applications would cost at least three times more per capita for a 40 percent reduction than fluoridation would for a 67 percent reduction.

The report of the Commission on the Survey of Dentistry indicated that one of the major barriers to the utilization of topical fluoride applications has been the shortage of personnel.[67] Dentists in private practice with full appointment schedules find it difficult to justify taking their own time at the chair to perform this time-consuming and relatively unremunerative task. Dental hygienists are in short supply and forbidden by law in some states to perform this service. Dental practice acts today, with a few exceptions, discourage and, in some instances, prohibit the dentist from exercising his professional judgment in delegating tasks to his auxiliaries. In most dental laws the dental hygienist, for example, is confined to performing prophylaxis type procedures and exposing radiographs. Only about 29 states, either informally or officially, permit dental hygienists to apply fluorides topically. Other states recently have revised their dental practice acts so that the dentist has considerable leeway, based on his professional judgment, in what services he may delegate to his auxiliary personnel to perform. A concise review of the current situation has been provided by Conway.[12]

The National Opinion Research Center study of dental practice indicated that only 23 percent of the dental practitioners provide topical applications of fluorides routinely when indicated.[40] It would seem that if dentists do not wish to perform this service for the patients in their offices they then have the responsibility to see that group programs are organized in their communities for the provision of this service. Many fine opportunities for concurrent dental health education can be capitalized upon when such programs are conducted

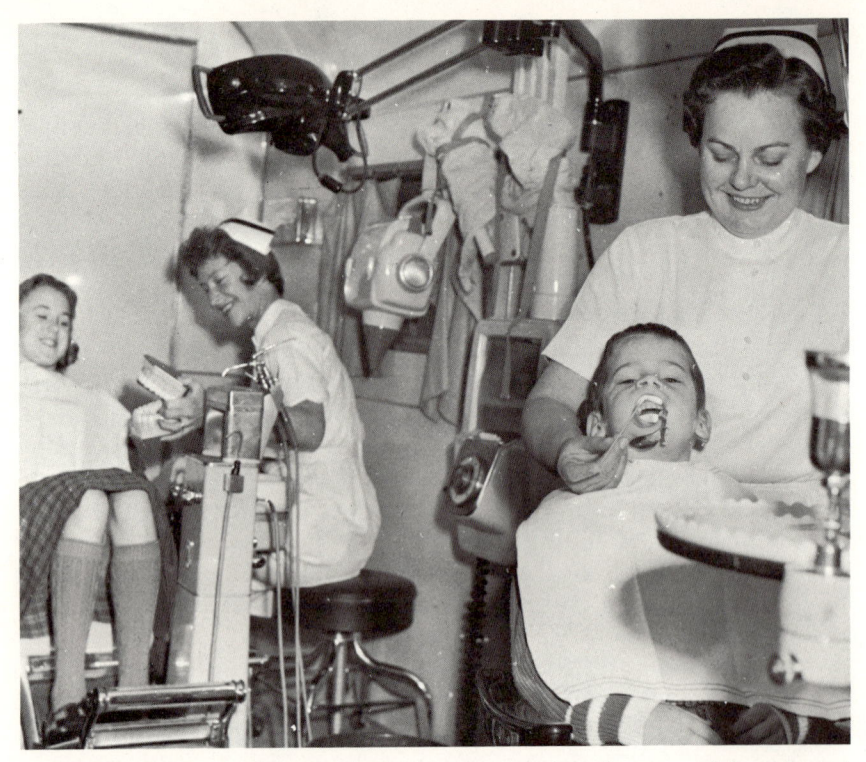

FIGURE 14. Dental hygienists applying topical applications of fluoride and giving instruction in toothbrushing technics on a mobile dental unit in a rural area. (Courtesy Idaho Department of Health.)

in cooperation with school systems and local health departments. Most state health departments stand ready to counsel with local dental societies in helping to organize these programs.

Community programs for the topical applications of fluorides have been developed in several states. The latest information indicates, however, that only 24 states conduct programs of topically applied fluoride at the state level, and nine more report activities by local health departments — a total of 33 states which have some type of public health program for the provision of topical applications of fluoride.[52] Only 10 percent of school administrators responding in a survey of school dental programs reported that fluoride applications were provided for any age group.[18]

Probably the most active promotion of the topical application of fluoride to groups of children has been the program sponsored by the Michigan Department of Health.[64] This program utilizes dental and dental hygiene students during vacation periods to provide topical applications of fluoride to groups of children on an organized community basis in various areas of the state where fluoridation is not feasible or has not been achieved. Teams of dental and dental hygiene

PREVENTIVE AND CONTROL MEASURES 171

students are sent out to the more remote areas of the state, usually summer vacation areas, where groups of children are provided topical applications at a nominal cost. The dental and dental hygiene students are able to earn a fairly good summer salary while gaining additional experience, particularly in the management of children in a dental situation. Further, it has been observed that when they return to school for their final year, those who have undergone this experience have a better understanding of public health. They also seem to be more active in the affairs of their communities once they have entered practice.

Galagan summarized the situation concerning topical applications of fluoride:

> ... there has been confusion and doubts about the place of topical fluoride treatments today, and they have not been used as extensively as they should have been.
> If topical fluoride treatments are to be used effectively to reach more of the 29,000,000 children not covered by water fluoridation (not even considering those who could benefit to some limited extent by topical fluoride treatments during the early years of community water fluoridation programs), we shall have to take action in the following ways:
> 1. Allow auxiliary personnel legally and actually to apply solutions, and provide for the necessary training of the additional personnel required for more extensive use.
> 2. Develop simpler and more effective techniques of application.
> 3. Develop more community programs to bring the benefits of topical fluoride therapy to large groups of children on an economical and practical group basis.[23]

Since Galagan's 1959 statement, several types of agents are being tested—which, if they work out, will perhaps be simpler to apply and even more effective.[21, 33] Final answers on these new measures will be determined by the American Dental Association's Council on Dental Therapeutics.

Other Community Fluoride Programs. In some communities experiments are being tried with dietary supplements of fluoride, usually in tablet form, on a group basis. When these procedures have been attempted, they usually are conceived as a partial substitute for community water fluoridation. There are many difficulties implicit in this type of administration of fluorides. It is particularly important to know the exact fluoride content of a child's drinking water supply and adjust the amount of fluoride being administered as the fluoride content of the water supply varies, as it will from time to time. Preliminary findings from studies going on in Switzerland and other European countries have encouraged the hope that the administration of fluoride tablets to school children would prove an effective community preventive procedure.[10, 48] Limited evidence from this country, however, suggests that relatively few parents will administer dietary fluorides to their children consistently during the years when the teeth are calcifying.[5] The possibilities of fluoridated salt are also being studied.

There also is the potential of establishing a program of fluoridating individual home water supplies in suburban and rural areas.[42] The movement of the American people from urban to suburban areas has removed many people from a community water supply and has necessitated the development of individual home water supplies. It is possible that soft water service companies, for example, could provide individual home fluoridation service to a group of customers on a regular route basis, servicing each home regularly and maintaining optimum fluoride in individual home water supplies. It is conceivable, too, that rural schools with their individual water supplies could be provided with individual fluoridators, perhaps serviced in the same way. It would seem that dentists have a responsibility to encourage such measures when the best source of fluorides, community water fluoridation, is not practical.

Screening and Referral Programs. Throughout the years emphasis has been given to the control of dental diseases through early detection and prompt treatment by the dentist. It is clear that the achievement of early detection and prompt treatment is far from being realized when only about 40 percent of the population even visits the dentist once in a given year. Therefore, the implementation of a comprehensive program of early detection and prompt treatment requires community action in the form of health education. Chapter 14, devoted to health education, discusses principles and methods of health education at length. In this section, however, specific programs of inspection or examination and referral will be discussed.

MASS INSPECTIONS OF SCHOOL CHILDREN. Probably the most prevalent type of program aimed at screening and referral to the dentist is that of mass dental inspections for school children. Well over half of the school administrators responding to a questionnaire indicated that "oral examinations" were provided to their students.[18] Of those schools that do provide this service, over half of the inspections are performed by a dentist, one quarter by a dental hygienist and the balance by school nurses, physicians, or the classroom teacher. In the vast majority of the schools providing the service, almost 90 percent of the examinations are performed within the school. Only seven percent of the reporting schools indicated that the examinations were conducted in the offices of private practitioners.

The benefits and limitations of dental examinations or inspections in the schools are subjects of controversy throughout the country. The foremost proponents, Stoll and Catherman, state:

> ... The continued use of these practices (school dental inspections) is advised for the purpose of stimulating parents to seek the professional services of the family dentist and family physician. The inspections in schools serve to motivate the child to better health atti-

PREVENTIVE AND CONTROL MEASURES 173

tudes and habits. The evaluation of a dental health program in terms of corrections and guidance depends largely on the data obtained during health appraisal inspections. Dental inspections help to determine the content of health instruction and serve as a medium of evaluation in health teaching.[60]

It should be noted that much of their thinking in regard to school dental inspections is predicated upon the situation prevalent in New York State and other eastern states where "dental hygiene teachers" are employed by school systems. These "dental hygiene teachers" are dental hygienists with bachelor's degrees and with teaching certificates. One of their chief duties is to inspect periodically the school children in the jurisdiction where they serve and to refer them for dental care. However, the supply of dental hygienists in most parts of the country is not such that this type of program could be carried out even if it were concluded that it was desirable.

The American Dental Association has listed the following benefits and limitations of school dental inspections:

> School dental inspections or surveys may afford certain benefits by:
> 1. Serving as a basis for school dental health instruction,
> 2. Building a positive attitude in the child toward the dentist and dental care,
> 3. Motivating the child to seek adequate professional care,
> 4. Serving as a fact-finding experience for students, teachers, dentists and others concerned with school dental health program,
> 5. Providing base line and cumulative data for evaluation of the school dental health program,
> 6. Providing information as to the status of dental needs so the advisability of supporting a sound dental health program may be recognized.
>
> School dental health inspections may have the following limitations and possible undesirable effects:
> 1. Even though the statement may be made that the school dental inspection is not intended to replace accurate and complete examination, parents and children frequently accept the inspection on this basis and depend on it rather than on a complete dental examination by the family dentist.
> 2. Unless it is possible to institute a definite follow-up program to assure that needed dental corrections are being made or to find out the reasons for lack of care, an annual dental inspection program primarily for the purpose of motivation is of questionable value.
> 3. It is desirable for parents to be present during a dental examination, particularly of children in the younger age groups. This procedure is not always feasible in school inspections.
> 4. It is desirable for a child to acquire early in life the habit of visiting his family dentist regularly for examination and care. Some school inspections may tend to discourage rather than to promote the development of this habit of personal initiative.[14]

In addition, the American Dental Association could have listed other limitations and detrimental effects of mass dental inspections in the schools. Mass inspections in the schools are a poor example, usually, of what a comprehensive, modern dental examination should be and, therefore, almost by definition are a poor teaching practice. Further, Study Group IV at the University of Michigan's Fifth Workshop on Dental Public Health concluded:

> Mass routine dental inspections should be discouraged because:
> a. At least 90 percent of all school-children need dental care routinely. The inspectors are looking for cavities they already know are there—cavities which they looked at last year, only this year they are bigger.
> b. The inspections are cursory at best, conducted under less than ideal conditions, and tend to lend a false security to the parents if nothing is found.
> c. The dental manpower spent on inspections could be better used in treatment.
> d. There is a possibility of inadvertent referral of a child whose dental needs recently have been completed.[19]

Any criticism of mass dental inspections does not apply to surveys conducted in the school for research purposes, to establish base lines for purposes of evaluation, or for purposes of estimating a group's dental needs. However, in such situations, inspections of all school children or of all children in certain grades usually need not be done. Rather, a scientifically selected sample of children can be examined to obtain the data needed.

If mass dental inspections are conducted in the schools, they should be planned so that concurrent dental health education, both at the time of the examination and in the classroom before and after the examination, can be provided. It is also important to arrange a mechanism for "follow-up" on the results of the inspection. School and public health nurses and the classroom teacher should attempt to see that, in some way, each child gets to a dentist or a community clinic for further examination and prompt treatment. However, in such a situation, while the follow-through is commendable, the system results in dual inspection and examinations (one inspection at the school and then a more thorough examination in the dental office) which would seem to be a waste of dental manpower.

REFERRAL PROGRAMS. Other community programs prefer to utilize a system of referral to private dentists or to community facilities without prior screening or mass inspection in the schools or elsewhere. Several different systems have been developed to meet the needs of different localities. The most usual system, however, is the development of a referral card which is distributed to selected children in the school system. Parents are asked to take the child to their family dentist or a community clinic for an examination. The dentist, at the private office or in the community clinic, indicates usually whether or not dental treatment is required and, if so, the present status of that treatment (that is, in progress or completed), and then the card is returned to the school. At a given time, all of the cards

PREVENTIVE AND CONTROL MEASURES

DENTAL HEALTH APPRAISAL CARD
New Mexico Department of Public Health
Division of Dental Health

Pupil's Name _____ School _____

Grade _____ Age _____ Date _____

A person's health, comfort, behavior, and personal appearance may be seriously affected by neglecting his teeth. It is advised that your (son) (daughter) see (his) (her) family dentist for an examination (including x-rays) and whatever care may be necessary. Early and frequent dental care protects and saves teeth and in the long run saves money.
Please check the appropriate boxes and complete the blanks:

☐ 1. My (son) (daughter) has a dental appointment with Doctor _____
   _____ on _____
                                    Date

☐ 2. My (son's) (daughter's) dental treatment was completed within the past six months by Doctor _____ on _____
                                                                    Date

☐ 3. I am financially unable to arrange for dental care for my (son) (daughter) at this time.

Signed _____
Address _____
Phone _____

Please detach and return the above card to the teacher within one week.   (over)

- -

DENTAL HEALTH APPRAISAL CARD
New Mexico Department of Public Health
Division of Dental Health

Please take this card to your family dentist.

Pupil's Name _____ School _____

Grade _____

Doctor: Please check the appropriate boxes and instruct the student to return the card to his or her teacher.

☐ 1. I have completed an oral examination for this student and find no dental attention necessary at this time.

☐ 2. This student is still under treatment at this time.

☐ 3. I have completed the necessary dental treatment for this student.

Remarks and Recommendations:

Date _____ Signed _____ D.D.S.

SH 2-57-5,000   *TO BE DISTRIBUTED WITH THE "SCHOOL HEALTH APPRAISAL FORM."

FIGURE 15. "Health Appraisal" card used to motivate parents to seek dental care for their children. The responses received also assist in the periodic evaluation of community dental health education efforts. (Courtesy New Mexico Department of Public Health.)

returned are tabulated and the referral program is evaluated. In Minnesota and Iowa, for example, there has been considerable emphasis on this type of referral program over many years, and considerable success has been achieved. In Minnesota, as high as 50 percent of all school children in the state actually have gone to their dentists through this method.

As with mass dental inspections, there are some dangers inherent in the referral systems. In some areas emphasis is placed on securing "100-percent-return classrooms." All children in each classroom are urged strongly, in some instances almost compelled, to see the dentist in order to achieve a 100 percent record for their classroom, for the school, and then finally for the school system. Many would agree that such a high degree of emphasis is not compatible with good health education practices. All too frequently, children from low-income families are pressured to "see their dentist" when most do not even have a dentist. Referral systems should not be established unless there are adequate dental facilities, including sufficient private dentists and community clinics, or a system for providing examinations for financially disadvantaged children so that all have a reasonably good chance of securing attention. Methods should be provided also for staggering the groups of children so that not all children are required to have a dental examination by the family dentist at the same time, thus overburdening the local facilities. A referral system should not be recommended unless someone is responsible for follow-up, such as the school nurse, public health nurse, or school dental hygienist.

Mouth Protectors. In 1962 the National Alliance Football Rules Committee made mandatory for all high school athletes engaged in interscholastic football the wearing of an intraoral mouth and tooth protector that includes an occlusal and labial portion. Several dentists over the years have been experimenting with mouth protectors for athletes, and in several programs considerable success was achieved in preventing or mitigating the effects of accidents to the oral structures. As a result of the 1962 ruling, dentists and dental societies all over the country suddenly were faced with the problem of providing mouth protectors for the members of the football teams of the high schools in their areas. A guidebook, the result of a joint effort of the American Dental Association and the American Association for Health, Physical Education and Recreation, gave considerable help to both high school coaches and local dental societies in their efforts to meet the requirements.[1] This guidebook recommended strongly that mouthguards be fitted individually to each player's mouth from individual impressions and favored the rubber-latex type of guard. However, as a result of the activity in the fabrication of mouthguards resulting from the 1962 ruling, several other types of individually fitted mouthguards are now being compared favorably with the rubber-latex types.[11, 29] There is some evidence that the use of mouth protectors not only provides protection against injuries to the oral structures but also affords additional protection against head and neck injuries.[34]

At its 1962 meeting, the House of Delegates of the American Dental Association resolved (1) that constituent and component dental societies, through their councils on dental health or similar agencies be urged to study all available information in order to be in a position to provide guidance to schools in the selection of mouth protectors as required by the National Alliance Football Rules Committee for students engaging in interscholastic football; and (2) that all members of the dental profession be urged to cooperate with schools in developing mouth protector programs that are mutually satisfactory to the schools and the dentists. The cooperation of the dental profession in following these resolutions has been outstanding. Dental society programs to provide mouth protectors have enhanced the public relations of the profession, since most societies have seen fit to carry the expense of the impression-taking themselves and, in many instances, the only cost to the schools has been for materials. In addition, dentists have instructed local committees of laymen in the methods of fabricating the mouthguards from casts, and excellent cooperative relations between local dental societies and various community groups have resulted.

Restriction of Fermentable Carbohydrates. Another avenue for the prevention and control of dental caries is through the restriction of fermentable carbohydrates in the diet.[38] It is questionable whether enough patients are willing to cooperate in modifying their diets to make the measure effective on a community basis. A few state and local health departments, however, have worked with groups of school children to establish such programs.

It would seem that dentists do have the obligation to inform their concerned patients and school and community groups that this method of control of dental caries does exist, that it is effective, and that it is considerably less expensive than prolonged sessions in the dental operatory. It would seem, too, that dentists have the obligation to recommend to schools, preferably through organized action with their dental society, that the sale of candy and sweetened beverages by and in the schools be abolished. Some school personnel oppose restricting the sale of these items in the schools because of their availability in stores and shops near the school premises. It is argued that, since the children will purchase sweets regardless, they might as well be sold by the school or school-related organizations and the profits devoted to a "worthy cause." However, the schools teach, or should teach, that these items are harmful to the teeth and result in poor dietary habits. Galagan points out: ". . . it would seem to be a measurable sign of progress . . . if a school becomes intellectually honest enough to practice what it teaches . . . even if carbohydrate consumption by the school-age child is not reduced by as much as a candy bar."[24] Merely recommending that the sale of sweets be abolished in the schools would not seem to be enough. Dentists and dental hygienists, and their professional societies, should make positive suggestions of acceptable substitutes to replace both the sweets and the money earned by their sale. The substitution of popcorn and nuts, for example, has worked well in some schools.

In summary, then, dentists and dental hygienists individually in their offices and in working with community groups through their professional societies have the ethical obligation to provide of their skill and knowledge and to contribute their time and energy to a reasonable degree to their communities. In these endeavors they should give high priority to the application of preventive measures.

Bibliography

1. American Association for Health, Physical Education and Recreation, and American Dental Association. Report of Joint Committee on Mouth Protectors. Chicago, American Dental Association, 1960. 21 p.
2. American Dental Association. Fluoridation. Am. Dent. A. J., 65:578-717, Nov. 1962.
3. _____. Fluoridation. Am. Dent. A. J., 71:1115-93, Nov. 1965.
4. _____. 1968 catalogue. Chicago, American Dental Association, 1968. 30 p. (p. 9)
5. Arnold, F. A., Jr., McClure, F. J., and White, C. L. Sodium fluoride tablets for children. Dent. Progress, 1:8-12, Oct. 1960.
6. Blayney, J. R., and Hill, I. N. Fluorine and dental caries. Am. Dent. A. J., 74: (special issue) 233-302, Jan. 1967.
7. Bureau of Economic Research and Statistics, American Dental Association. Survey of dentist opinion. II. Dental health education; dental fees. Am. Dent. A. J., 59:336-47, Aug. 1959.
8. Bureau of State Services, Public Health Service. Trends and developments in public health. Washington, Department Health Education Welfare, 1959. V + 127 p. (p. 72-81)
9. Campbell, R. H. The dental hygienist in private practice. Dubuque, Iowa, Brown, c1964. XIV + 130 p. (p. 55-65)
10. Cannell, W. A. Medical and dental aspects of fluoridation. London, Lewis, 1960. VII + 125 p. (p. 110)
11. Charendoff, M.D. The nature of oral injuries sustained in football and an evaluation of some protective devices. Ann Arbor, Rackham School Graduate Studies University Michigan, 1962. VII + 83 p. mimeog. thesis.
12. Conway, B. J. Modification of dental practice acts which will legalize expansion of auxiliary duties. Am. Dent. A. J., 76:1050-2, May 1968.
13. Council on Dental Health, American Dental Association. Statement of American Dental Association on role of dentists and dental societies in the promotion of fluoridation. Am. Dent. A. Tr., 103:44, 1962.
14. Council on Dental Health and Bureau of Dental Health Education, American Dental Association. A dental health program for schools. Chicago, American Dental Association, c1954. 24 p. (p. 14)
15. Crain, R. L., and Rosenthal, D. B. Structure and values in local political systems: the case of fluoridation decisions. J. Politics, 28:169-95, Feb. 1966.
16. Discussion Committee Report; Group A. p. 115-6. (In Workshop; Actualizing the potential of preventive dentistry. Columbia, Mo., University Missouri, 1966. XIV + 165 p.)
17. Division of Dental Health, Public Health Service. Fluoridation census 1967. Washington, Government Printing Office, 1968. V + 57 p.
18. Dollar, M. L., and Sandell, P. J. Dental programs in schools. J. School Health, 31:3-14, Jan. 1961.
19. Easlick, K. A., ed. The administration of local dental programs. Ann Arbor, Continued Education Service School Public Health University Michigan, c1963. VIII + 278 p. (p. 86-7)

20. Elwell, K. R., and Easlick, K. A. Classification and appraisal of objections to fluoridation. Ann Arbor, Continued Education Service School Public Health University Michigan, 1960. IX + 82 p.
21. Englander, H. R., et al. Clinical anticaries effect of repeated topical sodium fluoride applications by mouthpieces. Am. Dent. A. J., 75:638-44, Sept. 1967.
22. Flemming, A. S. Fluoridation I. Statement by Secretary Flemming. Pub. Health Rep., 74:511-3, June 1959.
23. Galagan, D. J. A public health dentist looks at topical fluorides today. J. Dent. Child., 26:164-72, 3rd Quar. 1959.
24. _____. Progress in school dental programs. Am. J. Pub. Health, 42:834-9, July 1952.
25. Galton, Lawrence. Preventive dentistry and a successful dental practice. p. 113-29. (In Hutchins, D. W., ed. Motivation and preventive dentistry; report of the proceedings of the fourth annual preventive dentistry workshop held in Washington, D.C., July 25 and 26, 1967, sponsored by the Army Medical Service Advisory Committee on Preventive Dentistry and the University of Missouri at Kansas City School of Dentistry. Columbia, Mo., University Missouri, c1968. XIII + 287 p.)
26. Gamson, W. A. How to lose a fluoridation referendum. Paper read to Panel on Social Science and Public Policy, Society for the Study of Social Problems, St. Louis, Aug. 1961. mimeog.
27. _____. Public information in a fluoridation referendum. Health Educ. J., 19:47-54, Mar. 1961.
28. _____. Social science aspects of fluoridation: a supplement. Health Educ. J., 24:135-43, Sept. 1965.
29. Godwin, W. C. A simplified mouth protector technic. Mich. S. Dent. A. J., 44:132-3, Apr.; 44:227-34, July-Aug. 1962.
30. Green, A. L. A critical look at pro-fluoridation campaigns. Paper read to Conference on Community Action for Fluoridation of Public Water Supplies, Albany, Mar. 1962. mimeog.
31. _____. The ideology of anti-fluoridation leaders. J. Soc. Issues, 17:13-25, Dec. 1961.
32. Hahn, H. D. Fluoridation and patterns in community politics. J. Pub. Health Dent., 25:152-7, Fall 1965.
33. Heifetz, S. B., Horowitz, H. S., and Driscoll, W. S. Evaluation of a self-administered procedure for the topical application of acidulated phosphate fluoride. Abstr. Internat. A. Dent. Res., 46:102, Mar. 1968.
34. Hickey, J. C., et al. The relation of mouth protectors to cranial pressure and deformation. Am. Dent. A. J., 74:735-40, Mar. 1967.
35. Hollander, L. N. Modern dental practice: concepts and procedures. Philadelphia, Saunders, 1967. XVII + 197 p. (p. 188-91)
36. Horowitz, H. S., et al. School fluoridation studies in Elk Lake, Pennsylvania, and Pike County, Kentucky—results after eight years. Am. J. Pub. Health, 58:2240-50, Dec. 1968.
37. Horowitz, H. S., Law, F. E., and Pritzker, Theodore. Effect of school fluoridation on dental caries. St. Thomas, V. I. Pub. Health Rep., 80:381-8, May 1965.
38. Jay, Philip, Beeuwkes, Adelia M., and Husbands, Julia. Dietary program for the control of dental caries. Ann Arbor, Overbeck, c1965. 30 p.
39. Kegeles, S. S. Why people seek dental care: a review of present knowledge. Am. J. Pub. Health, 51:1306-11, Sept. 1961.
40. Kesel, R. G. Dental practice. p. 95-238. (In Hollinshead, B. S., dir. The survey of dentistry; the final report. Washington, American Council Education, c1961. XXXIV + 603 p.)
41. Kirscht, J. P., and Knutson, A. L. Science and fluoridation: an attitude study. J. Soc. Issues, 17:37-44, Dec. 1961.
42. Maier, F. J. A system for fluoridating individual water supplies. Am. J. Pub. Health, 48:717-23, June 1958.
43. Mausner, Bernard, and Mausner, Judith. The anti-scientific attitude. Scient. Am., 192:35-9, Feb. 1955.
44. McNeil, D. R. How to get the benefits of fluoridation for your community. Chicago, American Dental Association, c1963. 40 p.
45. _____. Time to walk boldly. Am. Dent. A. J., 63:333-43, Sept. 1962.

46. McNeil, D. R. Political aspects of fluoridation. Am. Dent. A. J., 65:659-62, Nov. 1962.
47. ———. The fight for fluoridation. New York, Oxford, 1957. 241 p.
48. Montgomery, Adele T. Utilizing dietary fluorides; an appraisal of their effectiveness, practicality, and safety. Pub. Health Dent., 23:199-207, Winter 1964.
49. National Advisory Commission on Health Manpower. Report of the National Advisory Commission on Health Manpower. vol. I. Washington, Government Printing Office, 1967. VIII + 95 p. (p. 42)
50. Paul, B. D. Fluoridation and the social scientist: a review. p. 1-12. (In Paul, B. D., Gamson, W. A., and Kegeles, S. S., eds. Trigger for community conflict: the case of fluoridation. J. Soc. Issues, 17:1-84, Dec. 1961.)
51. Paul, B. D., Gamson, W. A., and Kegeles, S. S., eds. Trigger for community conflict: the case of fluoridation. J. Soc. Issues, 17:1-84, Dec. 1961.
52. Peterson, J. K. Use of topical fluorides in public health programs 1960; results of a mail survey. Pub. Health Dent., 20:106-7, Winter 1960.
53. Public Health Service. 1966 National Dental Health Assembly. Emphasis: fluoridation. Washington, Government Printing Office, 1966. VI + 22 p.
54. Raulet, H. M. The health professional and the fluoridation issue: a case of role conflict. J. Soc. Issues, 17:45-54, Dec. 1961.
55. Rosenthal, D. B., and Crain, R. L. Executive leadership and community innovation: the fluoridation experience. Urban Affairs Quar., 1:39-57, Mar. 1966.
56. Sebelius, C. L. Preventive service. Am. Col. Dent. J., 20:185-9, Sept. 1953.
57. Simmel, Arnold. A sign post for research on fluoridation conflicts: the concepts of relative deprivation. J. Soc. Issues, 17:26-36, Dec. 1961.
58. Sinai, Nathan. Quoted by Blackerby, P. E. Treatment in public health dentistry. p. 187-221. (In Pelton, W. J., and Wisan, J. M., eds. Dentistry in public health. Philadelphia, Saunders, 1949. XI + 363 p.)
59. Stinaff, R. K. Dental practice administration. 3rd ed. St. Louis, Mosby, 1968. XVI + 214 p. (p. 106-11)
60. Stoll, Frances A., and Catherman, Joan L. Dental health education. 3rd ed. Philadelphia, Lea and Febiger, 1967. 360 p. (p. 142)
61. Striffler, D. F. Surveying a community and developing a working policy. p. 69-81. (In Easlick, K. A., ed. The administration of local dental programs. Ann Arbor, University Michigan School Public Health Continued Education Service, c1963. VIII + 278 p.)
62. Striffler, D. F., et al. Fluoridation of water supplies in small rural communities. Pub. Health Rep., 80:25-32, Jan. 1965.
63. Tossy, C. V. A consideration of the cost of fluoridation in the control of dental caries. Am. A. Pub. Health Dent. Bul., 10:3-9, Nov. 1950.
64. ———. Organizing community programs utilizing topical fluorides: solutions. p. 173-89. (In Young, W. O., and Shannon, Jean H., eds. The utilization of fluorides applied topically for the prevention of dental caries. Lexington, Ky., University Kentucky, 1966. VII + 272 p.)
65. Trithart, A. H., and Collier, D. R. A program of financial assistance to small communities to fluoridate. Tenn. S. Dent. A. J., 46:325-8, Oct. 1966.
66. Ward, Margaret A. An effective recall system. Am. Dent. Hygienists' A. J., 40:24-6, 1st Quar. 1966.
67. Young, W. O. Dental health. p. 5-94. (In Hollinshead, B. S., dir. The survey of dentistry; the final report. Washington, American Council Education, c1961. XXXIV + 603 p.)

Additional Readings

Crain, R. L., Katz, Elihu, and Rosenthal, D. B. The politics of community conflict; the fluoridation decision. Indianapolis, Bobbs-Merrill, c1969. XX + 269 p.
Kimball, S. T., and Pearsall, Marion. The Talladega story; a study in community process. University, Ala., University Alabama Press, 1954. XXXIV + 259 p.
Maier, F. J. Manual of water fluoridation practice. New York, McGraw-Hill, c1963. V + 234 p.
Sapolsky, H. M. Science, voters, and the fluoridation controversy. Science, 162:427-33, Oct. 25, 1968.

Section Four

MEETING THE DEMAND FOR DENTAL CARE

CHAPTER 10
Dental Treatment Needs and the
Demand for Care

CHAPTER 11
The Purchase of Dental Care

CHAPTER 12
Public Dental Care Programs

CHAPTER 13
Dental Manpower Resources

    Ralph McCall has been active in his local dental society since he started to practice seven years ago. At the last monthly meeting it was reported that the largest labor union in the city had asked for help in establishing a dental care plan for its members to be financed from the union welfare fund. Ralph participated actively in the discussion that followed and by the end of the meeting had been named chairman of a special committee appointed to meet with union representatives.
    The members of the committee did not particularly welcome the assignment because there were many questions that they were not prepared to answer. First, the dentists wondered whether a union dental care plan was a legitimate attempt to improve dental health conditions or whether it was really a form of "socialized dentistry" that should be avoided at all cost. Even if it appeared wise for organized dentistry to cooperate, many other questions remained to be considered. What kind of plan would ensure good dental care at a reasonable cost yet would safeguard the interests of the dental profession? How could the administration of the plan be handled and

how much would it cost? If complete service could not be included, what age groups and what services should be assigned priority? And, finally, if a dental care plan resulted in an increased demand for service, were there enough dentists in the community to meet the demand?

A number of dentists have had to seek answers to the same questions that Ralph McCall and his committee are facing. There is every reason to believe that an ever increasing segment of the profession will be involved in various kinds of dental care plans. This Section will attempt to outline some of the more important factors that affect the provision of dental care, whether for individuals on a private basis or for groups of people through an organized program.

CHAPTER 10

DENTAL TREATMENT NEEDS AND THE DEMAND FOR CARE

The need for dental treatment may be measured and expressed in several ways. Russell, in the chapters on the epidemiology of dental diseases, demonstrated the need for treatment of the two most prevalent dental diseases on the basis of the disease *detectable* by dentists using standard methods of measurement. The precision of the method of measurement influences the extent to which disease will be detected, but no examination procedure can be expected to uncover all pathological conditions present. It must be recognized, therefore, that there will be a difference between *detectable* and *absolute* need.

Estimates of treatment needs based on the prevalence of dental disease assume that standards of care accepted by the dental profession are the norm for each individual seen. A realistic appraisal of treatment needs must include consideration of the influence of patient attitudes and the degree to which dental care will be sought or accepted. A clinical examination of the detectable disease in a patient may suggest to the dentist the need for extensive restorative procedures and periodontal therapy. The patient, however, may view his oral health status in a completely different light and perceive needs for treatment which include only extraction of the teeth and replacement by dentures. In this instance, there would be some difference between absolute and detectable need and a marked difference between "need" for treatment and *demand* for care.

In part, at least, the disparity between "need" and "demand" reflects differences between the dentist and the patient in their assessment of the severity of dental diseases and their concept of accept-

DENTAL TREATMENT NEEDS

The most striking characteristic of the dental treatment needs of the population is sheer magnitude.[33, 38] An excellent recent survey of an area probability sample of the adult population of the United States indicated that nearly 20 million men and women have no natural teeth.[29] Experience would suggest that the majority of these individuals need some type of prosthetic service. Among the 91 million others, there were an estimated 855.4 million missing teeth and 127.4 million teeth with unfilled carious lesions—although there were 637 million filled teeth. The "average" dentulous adult, 18 to 79 years of age, was estimated to have a total of 17.9 decayed, missing, or filled permanent teeth (1.4 decayed, 9.4 missing, and 7.0 filled). Figure 16 shows these estimates by age group and sex.

The treatment needs of an individual are determined both by

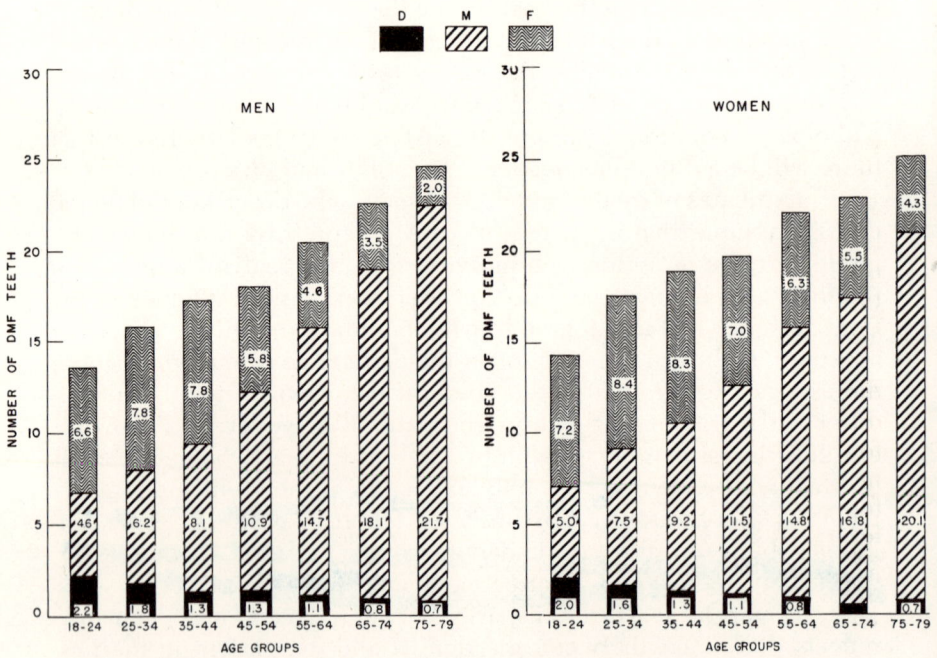

FIGURE 16. Mean number of decayed, missing, and filled teeth among dentulous men and women, by age, in the United States, 1960–62. (From National Center for Health Statistics, Public Health Service.[29])

the attack of dental diseases and by the amount of dental care received. The reduced incidence of dental caries resulting from the use of domestic water containing optimum fluorides, for example, cuts the need for restorative dentistry throughout life.[20] Yet, even if all known preventive procedures had maximum utilization—an ideal which is far from attainment—most persons would continue to be affected by dental diseases. The most important factor determining the amount of treatment needed by a group is its past utilization of dental services.

All of the influences that may determine the utilization of dental service, outlined later in the chapter, therefore, are related to the extent of accumulated treatment needs. Thus, males generally show greater unmet needs than do females; the poor, more than the well-to-do; Negroes, more than whites; the unlettered, more than the educated. Furthermore, because of the cumulative nature of dental diseases, unmet needs for service increase with age, at least until the final result of neglect, complete edentulousness, limits the need for care to prosthetic replacement.[7, 9]

Initial vs. Maintenance Needs

The occurrence of disease may be measured as *prevalence* (the total disease existing in the population at any one time) or as *incidence* (the number of new cases occurring in a given period of time). Because of the chronic nature of most dental diseases, prevalence rates, which reflect both recently occurring cases and the backlog due to neglect, are much higher than incidence rates. Prevalence data provide an estimate of the total treatment requirements at the time of study. If complete dental care is provided for a group, the services included in the first series of appointments, to care for "initial treatment needs," ordinarily are quite extensive. The need for service is lower once the accumulated defects have been corrected and the patient has been put on periodic recall for treatment of new disease as it occurs. In the latter instance, the incidence of new disease is being met on a "maintenance treatment" basis.

As would be expected, there is a close relation between the regularity with which care is sought and the extent of the backlog of needed services. A national study of patients who came to dental offices (in contrast to the total population and as reported by a systematic sample of dentists on mail survey) indicated that those who had seen a dentist within the previous 11 months required less than two restorations.[8] In contrast, about five fillings were needed by those who had not been seen for two or three years. (See Figure 17.)

The average dental practice includes patients receiving both initial and maintenance treatment. In the same morning a dentist will provide extensive restorative care for a patient who has not been seen for several years and only prophylaxis and minimal treatment for a regular patient who has been on periodic recall. Although the dif-

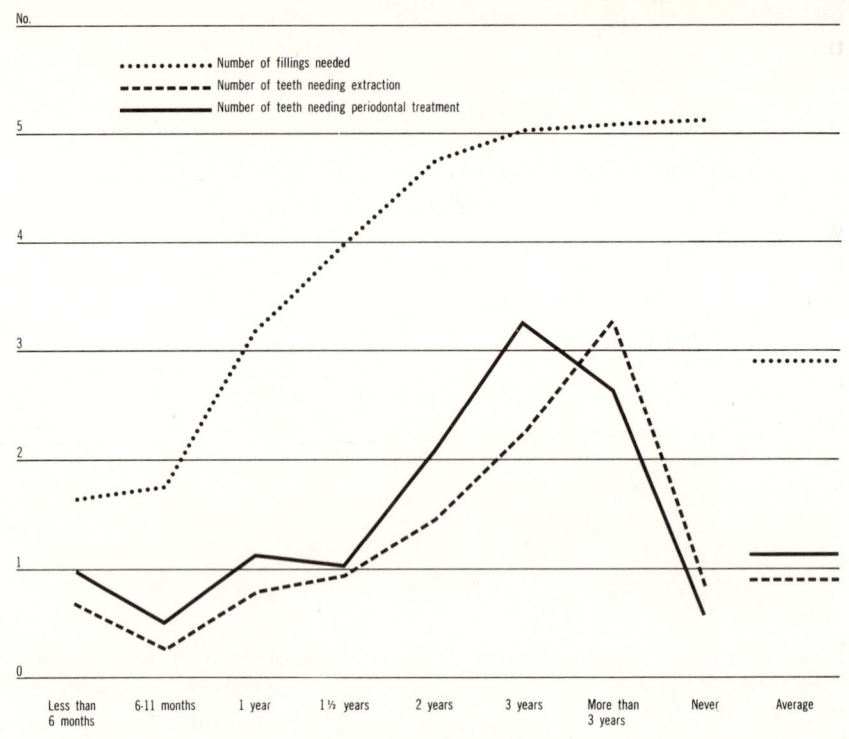

FIGURE 17. Average needs for fillings, extractions, and periodontal treatment, by length of time since last visit to a dentist. (From American Dental Association.[8])

ference in the magnitude and character of treatment needs of these two types of patients is evident, the concept of initial and maintenance service requirements is of only academic interest in private practice. When a dental care program is being planned, however, the determination of the need for care in the first stages of operation and the estimation of the level of need in subsequent periods (when most patients are on a maintenance basis) are of critical importance. For this reason, the consideration of dental treatment needs will be limited primarily to an analysis of programs in which relatively complete dental care has been provided to groups of individuals.

School Children — Services and Dentist-Time. In a study conducted by the Public Health Service in Richmond, Indiana, school children from kindergarten through the ninth grade were offered dental care without charge in order to gather data on initial and maintenance dental care.[40] The care was provided in school clinics. The children were given complete dental treatment in a series of four treatment periods extending over five years. The chief concern in the first series was caring for the accumulated defects in the permanent teeth; in the second and subsequent series, treating the incremental needs which occurred between treatment periods. Only limited care was provided for primary teeth in the first series. (The accumulated needs of children entering school after the first series were met.) Service provided the children under the program included the following: prophylaxes, permanent fillings, extractions, restorations of fractured anterior teeth with full and partial crowns, vital partial pulpectomies of permanent and primary teeth, root canal therapy of permanent anterior teeth, treatment for periodontal diseases, and topical applications of fluoride. Fillings and extractions constituted the principal treatments needed by the children. (See Figure 11, Chapter Nine, page 152.)

During the first series, in which accumulated needs were met, the number of teeth needing fillings was 4.28 per child and the number of teeth requiring extraction was 0.24 per child. In each treatment series thereafter, there was a reduction in needed services. In the final series, fillings were required in only 1.36 teeth per child involving 1.94 surfaces, and only 0.02 teeth per child required extraction. Because of the constant influx of children who had had little or no previous care, these average values tend to overstate somewhat the volume of service required to meet purely incremental needs.

A steady reduction in services required was observed at each age level. The most striking reduction took place, of course, among the older children, since they started the program with the greatest accumulation of unmet dental needs. The average number of teeth requiring fillings per 15-year-old child in the first treatment series was 7.20, and the average number of teeth requiring extraction was 0.45 per child. In the final series the average treatment requirements for a child at this age had been so reduced that the number of teeth requiring fillings was only 1.61 and the number of teeth requiring extractions was only 0.02 per child.

In the first treatment series each dentist was able to care for 530 children during the course of a year, providing 2.88 man-hours of treatment per child. Only 0.75 man-hours were required during the fourth treatment series, and each dentist was able to care for 1,343 children.

A program very similar to the Richmond study was conducted by the Public Health Service in Cambridge, Maryland.[15] The major difference was that the Cambridge water supply contained optimum levels of fluorides so that the data on treatment needs reflected the impact of reduced dental caries attack. In the first treatment series each dentist in Cambridge was able to care for 805 children, in contrast to 530 in Richmond. The man-hours required for initial treatment were reduced from 2.88 in Richmond to only 1.3 in Cambridge. Because fewer teeth were attacked by caries, there was less likelihood that neglect, in this young population, would result in accumulated unmet needs. For this reason the differential between initial and maintenance needs was less than in the Richmond population. The

TABLE 20. COMPARATIVE DATA FOR THREE SCHOOL DENTAL CARE PROGRAMS, GAINESVILLE, FLA., RICHMOND, IND., AND WOONSOCKET, R.I.*

LOCATION	TREATMENT SERIES			
	First	Second	Third	Fourth
Number of DMF permanent teeth per 8-year-old white child:				
Gainesville, Fla.	2.4	2.0	1.7	1.4
Richmond, Ind.	2.9	3.2	2.9	2.8
Woonsocket, R.I.	3.9	4.2	3.8	3.6
Percentage of new patients among total patients				
Gainesville, Fla.	100	38	39	26
Richmond, Ind.	100	35	22	17
Woonsocket, R.I.	100	48	23	19
Dentist man-hours, per child:				
Gainesville, Fla.	0.8	0.8	0.5	0.5
Richmond, Ind.	2.9	1.9	1.2	0.8
Woonsocket, R.I.	3.3	2.8	1.7	1.4
Children for whom treatment was completed, per dentist-year:				
Gainesville, Fla.	1,270	1,303	2,031	1,867
Richmond, Ind.	530	743	1,009	1,343
Woonsocket, R.I.	384	470	714	848

*Frank.[21]

man-hours required to complete a treatment series went from 1.3 initially to 0.4 in the fourth treatment series.

Another Public Health Service study similar to the Cambridge study was carried out in Gainesville, Florida (with fluoridation), and the data compared with the Richmond, Indiana, and Woonsocket, Rhode Island, data.[21] (See Table 20.) The findings are even more dramatic, but the communities are far from comparable.

School Children—Cost. Data have been reported for the first three years of a dental care program sponsored jointly by the International Longshoremen's and Warehousemen's Union and the Pacific Maritime Association (I.L.W.U.-P.M.A.)[14] About 10,000 children under the age of 15 received care under this program. The majority of them were eligible at no charge for complete care (exclusive of orthodontic treatment) without limitation. Only children who joined the program during the first year were studied, so these data do not reflect the impact of new children's enrolling in the plan during the study.

During the first year of operation the average cost per child receiving services was $71.73. In the second year the figure dropped to $42.24 but rose again to $50.82 in the third year. The "average" figures concealed a wide range of costs—from only a few dollars a year to over $800. In the average year, however, costs for the majority of children ranged from $10.00 to $50.00, and 10 percent fell below the $10.00 level. Considerably more than half the annual cost was for fillings, accounting for $41.62 of the total cost in the first year, for example. Diagnostic services, examinations, and radiographs represented the second largest expenditure, averaging just over $9.00 for the three-year period.

In assessing the impact of reduced incidence of disease, or of the relation between costs of initial and maintenance care, it must be recognized that certain fixed costs become proportionally greater when total treatment needs are reduced. The need for routine clinical examinations, radiographs, and oral prophylaxes, for example, does not drop in proportion to a decrease in total treatment requirements. Furthermore, in a group dental care plan, administrative costs will be relatively fixed since they are related primarily to the number of individuals receiving service rather than the amount of care provided for each person.

An indication of the magnitude of fixed costs was provided in a plan for a prepayment program for school children in two Idaho communities, based on the findings of an epidemiological survey.[42] In the community in which the water was deficient in fluorides, the first-year costs of $52.50 per child were expected to drop to $37.50 in subsequent years. Less than half this amount was for administration, topical applications of fluoride, prophylaxes, and diagnostic services. The cost in a community with optimum fluorides was estimated to be $17.50 per child the first year and $15.00 in succeeding years. Even without topical applications of fluoride and allowing for only one examination a year, fixed costs of $9.50 for administration, oral prophylaxis, and diagnostic services represented close to two thirds of the total maintenance costs.

Studies based on a total population of children include the treatment experience of children from families who can afford to purchase care. Differences between initial and maintenance needs may be expected to be even greater in programs which concentrate their efforts on the indigent segment of the population. Mumma studied this phenomenon recently in an analysis of the needs of children as expressed in estimated "15 minute time units" needed for extractions and restorations.[28] (Preventive and diagnostic procedures were not included.) The service requirements based on these time units for children classified as dentally indigent were 1.5 times greater (8.78 vs. 5.88) than those for the nonindigent.

As would be expected, differences in treatment time resulting from water fluoridation experience are reflected in differences in cost. Ast et al. reported a comparison of service time and costs from a program providing care for children from the "poorest socioeconomic areas" of a fluoride-deficient city and a city completing more than 20 years of water fluoridation.[1, 2] Relative initial care costs were 2.3 times as much in the fluoride-deficient area ($27.61 vs. $11.92). Relative maintenance costs were also about twice as high where fluorides were lacking ($11.51 vs. $6.17).

Adults. Among older persons, with a longer history of neglect, not only prevalent need but incremental need as well can be expected to vary according to the dental status of the individual at the beginning of his treatment. Thus, persons who enter a program with many teeth already missing (or indicated for extraction) will require fewer fillings and earlier prosthetic care, on the average, than will those of comparable age who enter a dental treatment program with a better preserved dentition. For this reason, considerably more experience will be needed with adults than with school children before sufficient data will be on hand to indicate with any precision what dental treatment will be required to maintain dental health, once prevalent needs are met.

An early experiment in which a group of dental patients received initial and regular maintenance care has provided valuable data about adults.[3] This study presented information about 485 adults who regularly received all "essential" care over a period of five consecutive years at a clinic operated by Dental Health Service, Inc., in New York City. They were predominantly a low-income, white-collar group who could not afford dental care in a private office but who were ineligible for treatment at free clinics.

This group presented a relatively large backlog of need. During the initial period the average patient required 7.5 fillings and 2.5 extractions, and seven in every 10 persons needed dentures. During maintenance care, an average of two fillings per person per year was required and only 0.15 extractions. Prosthetic needs also were reduced considerably, with only four complete or partial dentures placed per 100 patients. Initial need for fillings was greatest for those in their late teens and early twenties, with a steady decline in successive age groups. In general, annual maintenance needs for fillings showed this same general relation to age, but, at each age, were only about half the average accumulated needs at the same age. Maintenance needs for extractions and for prosthetic care, on the other hand, dropped to low levels for all age groups, although in initial care they had shown the characteristic pattern of increase with advancing age.

Information on initial and maintenance needs under a program of regular dental care is also available from a study conducted by the Public Health Service, in cooperation with the Group Health Association of Washington, D.C.[16] (Figure 18.) Participants in this study were persons of above-average income who agreed at the outset of the program to purchase all dental treatment recommended by the examining dentist in accordance with a standard of high quality, comprehensive dental care. Thus, they were persons who had an especially keen appreciation of the value of oral health and the financial means to attain it. Their accumulated needs were considerably less than those of the New York group. During initial care, they required only about five fillings, on the average, and about one half an extraction.

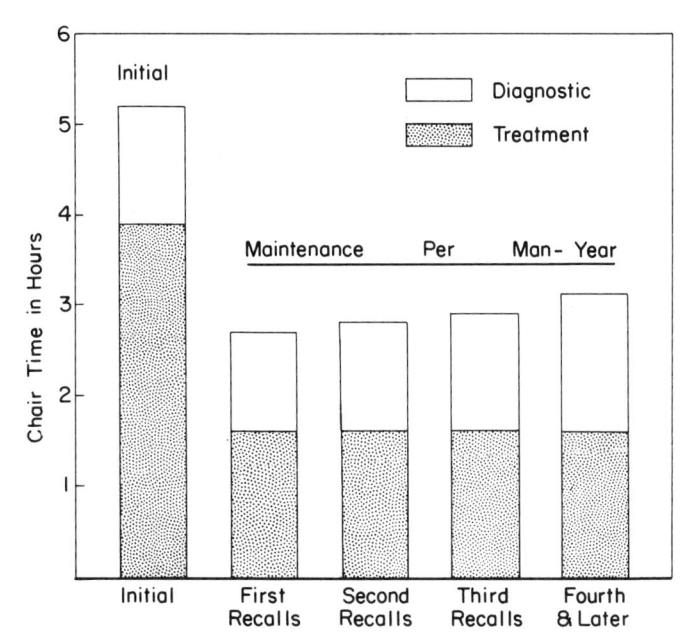

FIGURE 18. Average hours of chair time required per man-year for initial and maintenance treatment in the Group Health Association study. (Division of Dental Resources, Public Health Service.[16])

Only 13 dentures were placed per 100 persons. Initial needs for fillings among young adults were only about two thirds as great as those shown for the Dental Health Service group; for persons past 55 years, initial filling needs were 50 percent or more greater. Extractions, on the other hand, were about half as great among those in their late teens and early twenties, but only about one fourth as great in all other adult age groups.

Average maintenance needs for the two study groups were much closer. The Washington group required 2.5 fillings per year, on the average, during maintenance care, or only about one half a filling more than the New York group. However, about twice as many fillings were required for persons above 45 years. Similarly, the average needs for both extractions and dentures were alike in the two groups during maintenance care among older persons, but the Washington group showed the greater need for extractions. These differences in maintenance needs appear to stem from differences in the dental status at entrance of the individual participants in the two programs.

More recently, data have become available from a group practice which enrolled nearly 2,000 persons in a private prepayment program. Those who joined the plan were predominantly white-collar workers of above-average income who would be expected to have lower initial dental treatment needs than average. Among members 50 years of age and over who remained in the plan, the cost of service dropped by half in the second year, from $50.20 to $25.00. In the third year, the cost rose to $31.00. A similar pattern was observed in other adult age groups.[37]

Incremental Care

Incremental care, treating defects as they occur and thus avoiding a pyramiding of needs, is one of the basic objectives of dentistry. If patient cooperation can be obtained, incremental or maintenance treatment can be provided readily in private practice. In fact, the majority of patients in many well-managed dental practices may receive this kind of care. This objective is not always as easily attainable in public care programs or in plans for the group purchase of care. The high costs of providing initial care to meet accumulated needs may exceed the funds available for the program or require premiums or contributions large enough to discourage participation. Furthermore, the initiation of a program which offered services to a significant segment of the population in an area would probably overwhelm the available professional manpower.

Programs for the group purchase of care, whether public or private, can meet this problem by initiating services on an incre-

Year of Program	Age of Child											
	3	4	5	6	7	8	9	10	11	12	13	etc.
1 (1964)	A											
2 (1965)	B	A										
3 (1966)	C	B	A									
4 (1967)	D	C	B	A								
5 (1968)	E	D	C	B	A							
6 (1969)	F	E	D	C	B	A						
7 (1970)	G	F	E	D	C	B	A					
8 (1971)	H	G	F	E	D	C	B	A				
9 (1972)	I	H	G	F	E	D	C	B	A			
10 (1973)	J	I	H	G	F	E	D	C	B	A		
11 (1974)	K	J	I	H	G	F	E	D	C	B	A	etc.
etc.												

FIGURE 19. Pattern of incremental dental care. (Frankel.[22])

mental basis. A hypothetical example of such a plan, as applied to a school population, is illustrated in Figure 19.[22] In the first year, care is offered only to three year olds. The following year this group of children (A), now four years old, receives maintenance care and a new group of three year olds (B) is offered care. Each year an additional age bracket is added until, at the end of 11 years, children from three through 13 are receiving treatment.

This approach allows a program to start on a limited scale and expand gradually. At no time is there a large backlog of needs to be treated. During the developmental period, the financial and manpower requirements can be estimated relatively easily; once the desired age groups have been included, these requirements become stable.

[This concept is a basic part of the American Dental Association's national dental health program for children which will be reviewed in a later chapter.]

DEMAND FOR DENTAL CARE

As pointed out at the beginning of this chapter, the need for dental service often is confused with the demand for care. Obviously, one can be aware of a need and not demand care for it. Or one can be aware of a need, desire care for it, but not have the ability to obtain

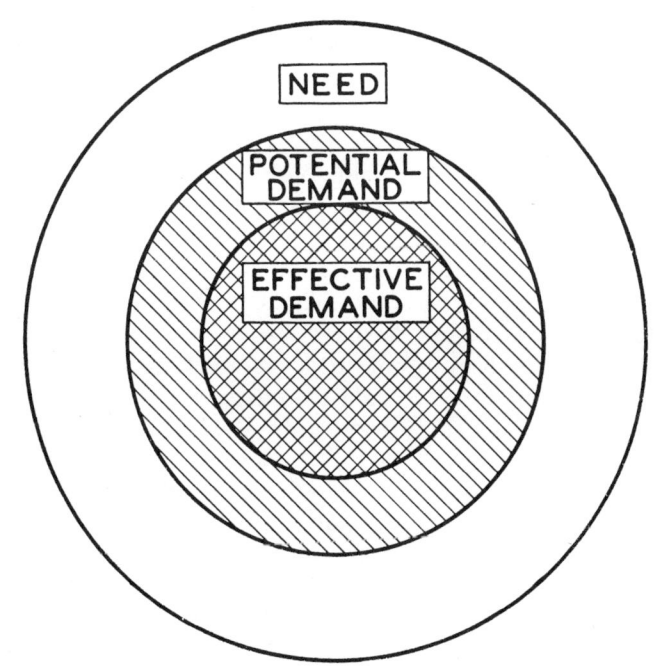

FIGURE 20. Dental treatment needs and the demand for care. (From Dollar and Kulstad.[19])

dental service to satisfy the need. The unqualified desire for dental care is defined as "potential demand," whereas the desire *plus* the ability to obtain dental service is defined as "effective demand."[19] The interrelation of the three factors, "need," "potential demand," and "effective demand," is depicted in Figure 20. (For purposes of discussion, "utilization" is equated with "effective demand" although economists probably would disagree.) Again, a person can be aware of a need, desire that something be done about it, and not know that something can be done. It should be realized, also, that even those who desire good oral health may not really wish to have to visit a dentist to maintain it. Thus, the needs, desires, wants, and demands — both potential and effective — are a complicated web of factors, all bearing in various degrees and interrelations on the utilization of dental services and the availability of those services.

Patterns of Utilization

Although almost everyone experiences dental diseases, only about 40 percent of the population visits a dentist during the course of a year; and it has been estimated that only about 15 to 20 percent of the population utilizes dental services on a routine periodic basis.[18, 24]

There are significant differences in the rate of utilization of dental services among various segments of the population. These differences provide clues about why individuals do, or do not, value optimum oral health and seek professional care to achieve it. An analysis of these factors suggests methods for improving the oral health of the public through private practice and through community efforts. Such a study also makes it possible to predict future changes in the demand for professional services.

Many studies have been made of the differences in *utilization* of dental services among people who visit a dentist.[13, 14, 16, 26] Only relatively recently, however, has information about representative cross sections of the entire population, including those who never visit a dentist, become available. The U.S. National Health Survey constitutes the most comprehensive survey of illness and disability ever attempted. The findings of this study indicate that only about 40 percent of the population even claimed to have visited a dentist in the year preceding the time they were interviewed, and only 23 percent within the preceding six months.[18]* One in three admitted not visiting a dentist in the preceding five years, including 18 percent who said they had never been in a dental office.

The utilization of dental services varied considerably with age.

---

*The survey measured utilization both by the interval between visits and the number of visits per year — different reflections of essentially the same phenomena. To illustrate both factors, the text will review data on the length of time since the last visit to a dental office, while Figures 21 and 22 will demonstrate variations in the number of visits per year.

Even among those from five to 44 years of age, less than 50 percent had received dental care within the previous year. Among older individuals the ratio was even lower. Moreover, 28 percent of the five to 14 year olds and nine percent of those from 15 to 24 years had never visited a dentist.

Substantial differences also existed between the white and nonwhite populations. Thirty-seven percent of the nonwhites had never visited a dentist, in contrast to 16 percent of the white population. Conversely, more than twice as many whites had visited a dentist during the preceding year. The same relation was found between race and the number of dental visits per year.

Urban residents were more likely to seek dental care than were residents of rural areas. Thirty-nine percent of the urban residents and 36 percent of those classified as "rural nonfarm" had seen a dentist within the preceding year. Only 27 percent of rural farm residents had sought care within the past 12 months. A larger proportion of females had visited a dentist recently than had males.

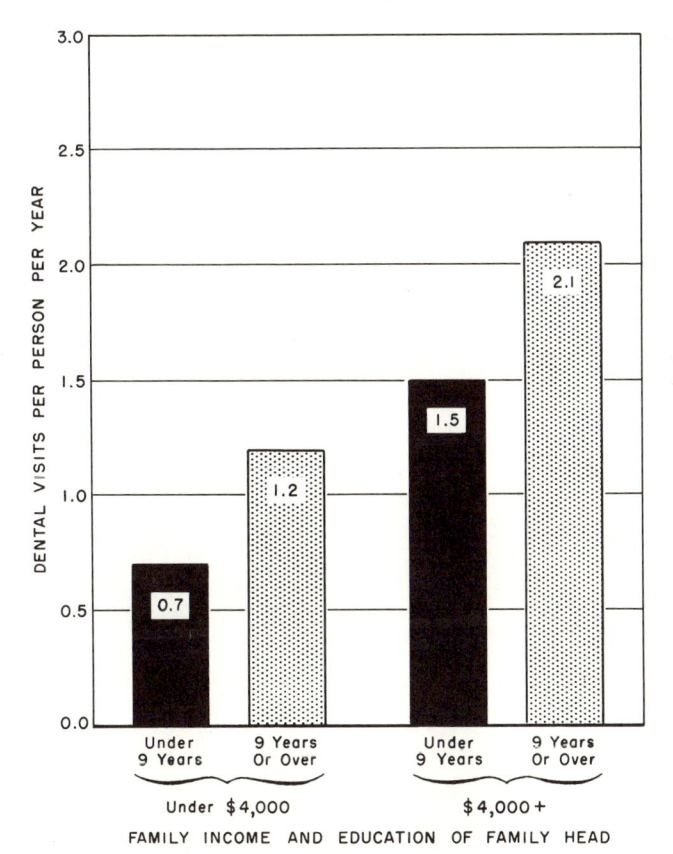

FIGURE 21. Number of dental visits per person per year by family income and education of family head. (Division of Public Health Methods, Public Health Service.[18] Graph courtesy Division of Dental Public Health and Resources, Public Health Service.)

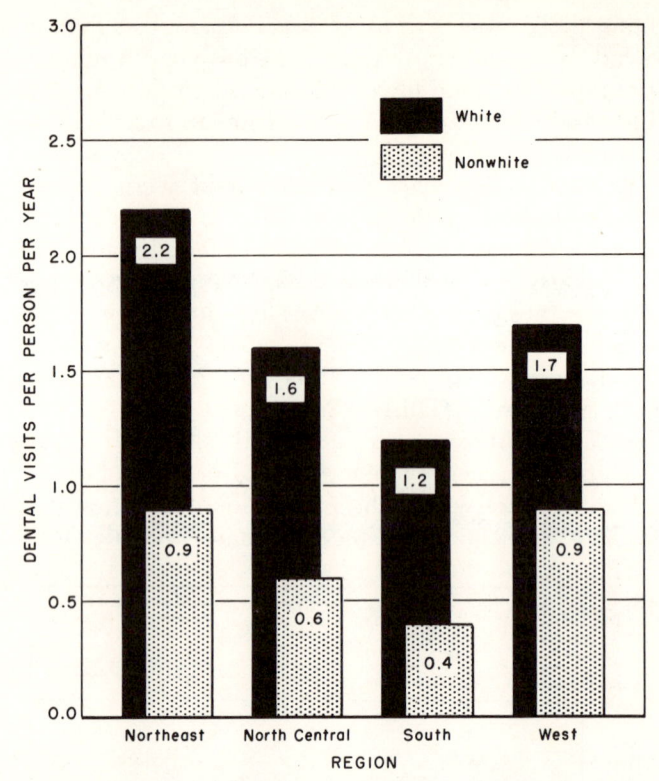

FIGURE 22. Number of dental visits per person per year by region and race. (Division of Public Health Methods, Public Health Service.[18] Graph courtesy Division of Dental Public Health and Resources, Public Health Service.)

The frequency with which dental service was sought bore a striking relation to family income. (Figure 21.) Almost one fourth of the individuals from families with an income of less than $2,000 had never visited a dentist, while only 10 percent of the members of families with an income of $7,500 or more were without dental experience. More than half of the individuals from the highest income group had visited a dental office within the previous year, in contrast to about 20 percent of those from the lowest income group. (The relation of dental utilization to income is not perfect; there is no level of income, no matter how low, at which some people are not receiving care.)

Very similar differences existed when the individuals were classified according to educational attainment. Only 17 percent of those persons in families headed by a person with less than five years of schooling had received dental care within the year prior to interview. Fifty-seven percent of those in families whose head had completed at least one year of college had visited a dentist within a year.

The study indicated that family income and the education of the family head were related independently to the frequency with which dental care was sought. In other words, when income was held constant, the utilization of dental service varied in proportion to the amount of education attained by the family head. When education of the family head was the constant, a correlation was still found between income and the frequency with which dental treatment was sought.

Utilization of dental services also varied between the four major geographic regions. In the group of states designated as southern, 25 percent of the individuals surveyed had never been to a dentist. The highest rate of utilization was found in the northeastern states where 43 percent of the respondents had visited a dentist within the previous year, and only 13 percent reported that they had never been to a dentist. The north central and western states were quite similar, with 38 and 39 percent of the population reporting a visit to a dentist within the preceding 12 months.

A similar study conducted five years later showed that, while overall patterns had not changed substantially, there were trends to increased utilization for all variables reported.[30]

Determinants of Demand

Knowledge. The action that an individual takes to maintain oral health is conditioned by his knowledge of proper hygienic procedures. It is pointed out in a later chapter that, in order to be motivated to take action to improve his health, an individual must believe (know) that there is something he can do which will be effective in improving health or preventing disease. Even if there is a desire to maintain optimum dental health and a belief that this can be attained, neglect can result from ignorance about the proper action to be taken. Unfortunately, ignorance about dentistry is widespread. Surveys conducted by the American Dental Association and the National Opinion Research Center of the University of Chicago illustrate some of the variables.

For example, there is agreement among scientific investigators that calcium cannot be withdrawn from the teeth once they have been formed. Yet 63 percent of the individuals surveyed by the American Dental Association believed that the unborn child absorbed calcium from the teeth of the mother.[5] The idea that eating foods with adequate vitamins and minerals will prevent tooth decay was held by almost seven out of 10. One fourth of the individuals felt that a toothache did not necessarily require the attention of a dentist "since it will often disappear by itself."

Less than 50 percent of the individuals stated that a child first should be taken to a dentist at two and a half or three years of age. Thirty-five percent said that the child did not need to go until five years of age, or just before he started school, and more than 14 percent would wait until the child had a toothache or a cavity could be seen.

The responses to this survey were tabulated according to the educational level of the respondent. The data showed that those individuals with the least education were most likely to give the "wrong" answers. However, even among the best educated, misinformation was common.

Respondents surveyed by the National Opinion Research Center were asked to state if they agreed with the statement, "Some people are just born with good teeth and others are not—and there is not much anyone can do about it."[26, 31] More than half of the individuals agreed with this fatalistic view. A smaller, but significant, number also expressed agreement with the statement, "No matter how well you take care of your teeth, eventually you will lose them."

A number of factors apparently influenced the responses to the questions. For example, 56 percent of those 65 years of age and older felt that the loss of teeth was inevitable regardless of the care taken, but this view was held by less than 30 percent of those from 20 to 34 years of age. Belief that tooth loss is inevitable was expressed by 57 percent of those with incomes under $2,000 but by less than 30 percent of those reporting an income of $7,500 or more. Those who had not visited a dentist in the previous five years were twice as likely to feel that they would lose their teeth regardless of what they did as were those who reported 10 or more visits to a dentist during the same period.

It is important to recognize, however, that information about the teeth and mouth is not the most important factor which determines whether or not an individual will seek dental care. In general, the respondents in the N.O.R.C. study who gave answers indicating correct knowledge about oral health were more likely to seek dental care on a routine preventive basis than those who gave incorrect answers. However, the positive correlation was not strong. For example, among those with an income of $5,000 or more, only 37 percent of those who felt that tooth loss was inevitable visited a dentist routinely; but 52 percent of those who did not view edentulousness as unavoidable utilized the services of a dentist on a regular basis. Apparently, the attitude of an individual toward oral health is a more important factor in determining his actions than is his knowledge.

Attitudes. The personal value system of an individual is established by many complex factors which are not easily explainable. Yet these factors have such a direct relation to the demand for dental services, and ultimately the level of oral health, that they deserve study. In *The Health of Regionville*, a sociological study of popular attitudes toward illness, Koos identified some of the factors which influence the attitude of individuals toward dental treatment.[25] Persons interviewed in this study were divided into three socioeconomic groups: business and professional (Class I); skilled and semiskilled workers (Class II); and unskilled workers (Class III).

Almost 95 percent of the Class I households reported that they had a family dentist, but only 12.5 percent of the Class III families had established such a relation. The striking differences in the attitude toward the utilization of a dentist were reflected in the reasons given for visiting a dentist. Fifty-seven percent of the individuals in Class III and nine percent of the individuals in Class II reported that they sought care only to have a tooth extracted. No members of the Class I families gave this reason for going to a dentist. In contrast, 52 percent of the individuals in Class I gave prophylaxis and examination as the reasons for seeking care. Only 14 percent of the individuals in Class III listed these preventive services as the purpose of a dental visit.

The attitude toward dental service that characterizes many in the lower socioeconomic brackets is illustrated by remarks made during the interviews. One Class III housewife summarized her view of dental service by saying:

> I wouldn't say we had a dentist, no. If one of us has to have a tooth pulled, we go—if it can't be pulled home. If a tooth's loose, there's no reason to fork over money to pay for pulling it. . . . Oh, you go to whatever one that can take you. It don't really make any difference—they're all alike, I think.[25]

A housewife in Class II illustrated the way in which dental care was neglected among families who could afford it but did not seek it because of the low value placed upon its importance:

> I'll be just right out and say that my back teeth are going to pieces. I had to put clove (oil) on one this morning. But I'm not going to spend a lot of money for a dentist every little while. . . . We've made up our minds that we're going to have a few things in this world, too, and I can get along just as well with a few teeth missing. There's this television coming before long, and I'd rather have that—and some other things—than all my teeth. . . . It isn't as though I didn't have some teeth to chew with, but when they all go it'll be cheaper to get a plate once than to have a lot of visits every year to the dentist.[25]

The answers to a hypothetical question asked in the study conducted by the National Opinion Research Center shed light on the variety of factors which influence demand for care.[31] The respondents were asked whether John Williams, a 31-year-old married man with two children, should spend $600 to have his natural teeth restored to good condition or whether he should spend only half that amount to have the remainder of his teeth extracted and dentures made. Sixty-three percent of those with an annual income of $7,500 or more thought that he should retain his natural teeth. Only 34 percent of those earning less than $2,000 indicated the same choice. There was an almost parallel correlation with age. Among those from 20 to 24 years of age, 61 percent indicated that he should spend the money to have his own teeth restored to normal. Only 32 percent of those 65 and older agreed. It can be surmised that the opinions of the older individuals reflected the cultural patterns prevalent during their adolescence and young adulthood 25 to 50 years ago. Their response also may have been conditioned by their experience with the loss of teeth and the wearing of dentures, or they may have reflected a situation in which they were living on a reduced income and hence viewed the expenditures within the framework of their personal budgets.

Those respondents who felt that they needed "little or no" dental care during a year were most likely to feel (62 percent) that the natural teeth should be retained. Only 44 percent of those reporting a "great deal" of need for treatment during a year favored the expenditure to restore the natural teeth. Those who had no natural teeth were least inclined (27 percent) to recommend treatment for the remaining teeth. Those who had sought dental care frequently in the past were most in favor of treatment. Sixty-five percent of those reporting 10 or more visits in the last five years said that the individual should try to preserve his own teeth; less than 30 percent of those who had not visited a dentist in that period of time recommended the same course of action.

A slightly larger number of females (53 percent) than of males (47 percent) felt that the expenditure for treatment was worthwhile.

The amount of education reported had an even more marked effect on the response than did income or age. Only 36 percent of those who had an elementary school education or less favored retention of the natural teeth. More than half the high school graduates and almost seven out of 10 college graduates recommended that treatment be obtained.

Other clues concerning the relative importance of various factors which influence desire for dental care were reported in a national survey conducted for the Health Information Foundation.[23] Respondents who did not see a dentist regularly were asked, "How is it that you don't see a dentist more often?" Sixty-seven percent of the answers related to the individual's knowledge of his own oral health and his need for treatment. These reasons (have false teeth, no natural teeth, teeth so bad it is not worthwhile to go, teeth cause no trouble) showed that the respondents had diagnosed their own state of oral health and found no necessity for professional services. The answers undoubtedly indicated a low valuation of the importance of oral health. More important, perhaps, was the indication of ignorance of the value of regular visits to the dentist to detect oral pathology early and institute treatment before extensive corrections are necessary. Negligence or laziness, cited in 16 percent of the answers, undoubtedly was a reflection of the same factors. What is designated as laziness, however, cannot be related completely to sheer inertia but must represent, at least in part, a judgment of the individual that the consequences of his neglect would not discommode seriously his future well-being.

TABLE 21. REASONS FOR NOT SEEING A DENTIST MORE OFTEN.*

REASON	PERCENT WHO DO NOT SEE DENTIST REGULARLY
Have false teeth, dentures, plates	29
Don't have any teeth (no mention of plates)	7
Teeth so bad it isn't worthwhile to go	4
Teeth are all right, cause no trouble; no need to go	27
Negligence, laziness; keep putting it off	16
Can't afford it; costs too much; don't like to spend the money	14
Don't like to go; afraid of dentists; it hurts	9
Too busy to go; don't have the time to spare	6
Don't know any good dentists; or dentist too far away	3
Miscellaneous reasons; too old, sick, etc.	3
Don't know; too vague to classify	1
TOTAL	119†

*Freidson and Feldman.[23]
†Some people gave more than one reason.

The cost of care was cited as a reason for neglect only 14 percent of the time by the group who reported that they did not see a dentist regularly, although some, at least, might hesitate to give this response to an interviewer.

Different responses were obtained from those who did not seek service regularly but reported that they, or a member of the family, should have received more care. In a large measure these responses eliminated the self-diagnostic factors. A third of these answers listed cost as a primary barrier to obtaining care. The answer was correlated sharply with family income. Cost was listed as a barrier by only eight percent of families making $7,500 a year or more, but by more than half of those making less than $2,000. One third of the answers cited

TABLE 22. REASONS WHY RESPONDENT, OR MEMBER OF FAMILY, DID NOT GET NEEDED DENTAL CARE*

REASON	PERCENT OF THOSE WHO FAILED TO GET NEEDED DENTAL CARE
Couldn't afford it; costs too much; hated to spend money	34
Negligence, laziness, just didn't get around to it	33
Spouse doesn't believe in going; can't get him to go	5
Didn't think condition was serious enough	6
Afraid to go; dread it; it hurts too much	21
Too busy; didn't have the time	12
Didn't know a good dentist; hard to get appointment; dentist too far away	7
Miscellaneous reasons	6
Don't know; just didn't do it, etc.	4
TOTAL	128†

*Freidson and Feldman.[23]
†Some people gave more than one reason.

negligence as the reason for not obtaining needed care. Twenty-one percent said that they were afraid to go. Socioeconomic factors did not appear to influence the responses listing either negligence or fear.

The study summarizes the factors influencing an individual's choices relating to dental care:

> All these factors can be joined into a whole, from the point of view of the patient, by considering the use of dental services to stem from an over-all assessment, or definition of the situation. The prospective patient assesses his dental condition and the seriousness of the consequences if he does not seek dental care. This self-diagnosis is weighed or balanced against the factors of cost, anticipated pain, and inconvenience, to see if going to the dentist "is worth it." The final result, the use or avoidance of dental services is thus a complex product of the education involved in self-diagnosis, of the income level involved in weighing costs, of the dental health and past dental experience involved in anticipating pain, and of the social experience involved in assessing inconvenience.

Past Dental Experience. A number of studies indicate that the attitude of patients toward dental care is influenced significantly by their experiences in the dental office. Among the important factors which influence patients' attitudes are whether or not they have experienced pain or discomfort; the amount of explanation and patient education provided; the degree to which the dentist utilizes accepted preventive procedures; and whether or not complete oral health care is recommended and provided. About one third of the respondents studied by the National Opinion Research Center were classified as seeking dental care "preventively."[31] Individuals included in this classification indicated that they ordinarily went to the dentist at least once a year and that they had visited the dentist within the last 12 months. Within each income level the likelihood that patients would go to the dentist "preventively" showed a strong correlation with the characteristics of the practice of the respondent's dentist. Among the practice characteristics which were related to the utilization of dental care on a routine basis were use of a recall system, regular use of dental x-rays, regular provision of oral prophylaxis, use of high-speed cutting instruments for cavity preparation, and the utilization of dental assistants.

Availability of Service. It is more difficult for certain segments of the population to obtain dental care than others. The consistent findings that those living in rural areas receive less dental care than do residents of cities, for example, reflects, in part at least, the barriers imposed by the lack of dentists and transportation problems. The supply of dentists is distributed unevenly and will not be equal among all geographic areas in the near future—nor should it be—since there are regional variations in the demand for care relating to economic conditions and educational levels. Nevertheless, the variation in the relative supply of dentists appears to be considerably greater than is desirable.

Difficulty in obtaining a dental appointment may become an increasingly important deterrent to the utilization of dental service in the future. A subsequent chapter will show that the relative supply of dentists has been declining in the United States since 1930. Due to increasing productivity of individual dentists, the dental profession so far apparently has been able to meet the increasing demands for dental services despite the relative decrease in supply of dentists. The coming explosive population growth, together with the steadily increasing per capita demand for dental services, threatens to overwhelm the ability of the profession to provide care for those who seek it.

Even if adequate numbers of dentists were available, a significant proportion of the population could not obtain treatment because it lacks the means to purchase care. Although cost is not the only factor which prevents people from seeking dental care, it is an important barrier for many. In today's complex modern society, the care of the needy has become primarily the responsibility of official and voluntary welfare agencies. In theory, these agencies have been assigned the responsibility of providing at least the minimum level of essential service for the disadvantaged segments of the population. Precise information on the number of needy individuals who receive a minimum level of dental service is not available. All available evidence indicates, however, that only a small proportion is receiving reasonably adequate dental care.

The special treatment needs of some make it difficult to obtain care, even if cost is not a barrier. Traditional methods of providing dental care were designed to provide service for those individuals who are in reasonably good health, ambulatory, and able to come to the dental office. Those who do not possess these qualifications—the institutionalized, the homebound, the chronically ill—frequently find it difficult to obtain the professional care necessary to maintain oral health.

Future Levels of Demand

The backlog of accumulated treatment needs in the population amply demonstrates that need far exceeds demand. It must be recognized, however, that this level of demand, inadequate as it may be, is higher than ever attained before in this country. There is also abundant evidence that the average American of the future will seek even more dental service than he does today.

Increases in per capita utilization of dental service can be predicted because of changes taking place in the characteristics of the population—characteristics that, in an earlier section, were shown to influence attitudes toward oral health and the extent to which professional care is sought. Because the better educated person is likely to appreciate dental health, for example, the steady advance in educational levels is creating new demands for care. And because the person with an income sufficient to permit a reasonably decent standard of living also is more likely to seek dental services, the steady rise in real income (purchasing power) also contributes to the increase in demands for care. Even though prices have risen along with income levels, income has risen relatively faster.

With the continuing improvement in both education and income levels during the past quarter of a century, the proportion of the population visiting the dentist each year has advanced strikingly. Prior to 1930 only 20 to 25 percent of the total population visited a dentist in the course of a year.[12] American Dental Association estimates, based on responses from dentists, have indicated that this percentage at least doubled in the following three decades.[10] An analysis of demand for care made by the Bureau of Economic Research and Statistics of the American Dental Association, based on annual per capita expenditures for dental care from 1935 to 1962 (corrected for price changes), showed a steady climb in the individual purchase of dental care.[4] During this period the per capita expenditure for dental care increased at the rate of 24 cents a year, rising from $4.58 to $11.03 (in 1957-1959 dollars). This expenditure represents an increase of 140.8 percent in the amount of dental care received per person in 27 years.

There is every reason to expect a continuation of these trends.[35] It has been estimated, for example, that between 1960 and 1970 there will be a 77 percent increase in the number of persons with baccalaureate and professional degrees. Moreover, per capita income (in 1955 dollars) is anticipated to increase from the $1,850 in 1955 to $2,550 in 1975. As Pelton and Bothwell have expressed it: "There can be no question but that the *automatic market* for dental services—the market consisting of those who recognize the value of dental services and are also fortunate enough to be able to pay for them—is going to expand, and expand substantially."[34] The factors which may be expected to increase the per capita demand for care have been documented in a number of studies.[17, 27, 32, 34-36, 39, 41]

The clearly predictable increases in per capita demand for service resulting from changes in the economic and educational characteristics of the population may be augmented by increases in demand created by new developments in the methods of financing dental care. Dentistry is just beginning to feel the impact of the third-party payment plans, both public and private, that have assumed an increasing share of the cost of other health services. There is no way of predicting the rate at which group dental payment plans will develop but, as Chapter 11 will show, it seems evident that growth will occur—possibly at a more rapid rate than expected.

A subsequent chapter will describe legislation currently being implemented nationally which may add as many as 40 million persons to the group eligible for dental care from public agencies. This group is in addition to the more than three million already eligible for care at the time the legislation was passed. It is impossible to predict with precision the extent to which governmental programs for the provision of dental care may grow, but in the light of current political trends it is safe to assume that they will expand.

Although the development of programs that eliminate the necessity for immediate payment for dental service does not mean that all individuals will seek care, it will result in a significant increase in the demand for dental service. Available evidence, therefore, points to greatly expanded levels of per capita demand for dental care because of increases in education and income, and the growth of private and governmental dental care payment programs. The last chapter in this section will show that the spectacular growth of the population—a rate of increase that may exceed the ability of the dental profession to increase its numbers or its productivity—compounded by the increase in demand will make it difficult to ensure adequate service for all who demand it.

Bibliography

1. Ast, D. B., et al. Time and cost factors to provide regular, periodic dental care for children in a fluoridated and nonfluoridated area. Am. J. Pub. Health, 55:811-20, June 1965.
2. _____. Time and cost factors to provide regular, periodic dental care for children in a fluoridated and nonfluoridated area: progress report II. Am. J. Pub. Health, 57:1635-42, Sept. 1967.
3. Beck, Dorothy F., and Jessup, M. F. Costs of dental care for adults under specific clinical conditions; an exploration of general issues on the basis of initial and maintenance care experience of 485 patients of Dental Health Service, New York City. (St. Louis), American College Dentists, 1943. 306 p.
4. Bureau of Economic Research and Statistics, American Dental Association. Expenditures and prices for dental and other health care, 1935-1962. Am. Dent. A. J., 68:125-31, Jan. 1964.
5. _____. Family dental survey. Am. Dent. A. J., 47:575-80, Nov. 1953.
6. _____. 1950 survey of the dental profession. IV. The dentist's work year. Am. Dent. A. J., 41:625-31, Nov. 1950.
7. _____. Survey of needs for dental care. II. Dental needs according to age and sex of patients. Am. Dent. A. J., 46:200-11, Feb. 1953.
8. _____. Survey of needs for dental care, 1965. III. Dental needs according to length of time since last visit to a dentist. Am. Dent. A. J., 74:145-50, Jan. 1967.
9. _____. Survey of needs for dental care. V. Dental needs according to income and occupation. Am. Dent. A. J., 47:340-8, Sept. 1953.
10. _____. The 1956 survey of dental practice. IX. Summary. Am. Dent. A. J., 55:126-33, July 1957.
11. _____. The 1962 survey of dental practice. X. Summary. Am. Dent. A. J., 68:132-5, Jan. 1964.
12. Committee on the Costs of Medical Care. Medical care for the American people. Chicago, University Chicago Press, 1932. XVI + 213 p. (p. 11)
13. Division of Dental Public Health and Resources, Public Health Service. Dental care in a group purchase plan; a survey of attitudes and utilization at the St. Louis Labor Health Institute. Washington, Government Printing Office, 1959. VI + 68 p.

14. Division of Dental Public Health and Resources, Public Health Service. Report on the dental program of the I.L.W.U.-P.M.A.: the first three years. Washington, Government Printing Office, 1962. VII + 43 p. (p. 4-11, 19-21)
15. ———. Unpublished data.
16. Division of Dental Resources, Public Health Service. Comprehensive dental care in a group practice. Washington, Government Printing Office, 1954. VI + 48 p.
17. ———. A study of dental manpower requirements in the West. Boulder, Colorado, Western Interstate Commission Higher Education, (1956). IX + 247 p.
18. Division of Public Health Methods, Public Health Service. Health statistics from the U.S. National Health Survey: dental care; interval and frequency of visits; United States, July 1957-June 1959. Washington, Government Printing Office, 1960. 42 p. (p. 1-8)
19. Dollar, M. L., and Kulstad, Hugo. The economic aspects of the dental health problem. p. 24-34. (In Pelton, W. J., and Wisan, J. M., eds. Dentistry in public health. Philadelphia, Saunders, 1949. XI + 363 p.)
20. Englander, H. R., and Wallace, D. A. Effects of naturally fluoridated water on dental caries in adults. Pub. Health Rep., 77:887-93, Oct. 1962.
21. Frank, J. E., et al. School dental care in a community with controlled fluoridation. Pub. Health Rep., 79:113-24, Feb. 1964.
22. Frankel, J.M. The child: an incremental program. Am. Col. Dent. J., 28:262-5, Dec. 1961.
23. Freidson, Eliot, and Feldman, J. J. The public looks at dental care. New York, Health Information Foundation, 1958. 16 p.
24. Kegeles, S. S. Why people seek dental care: a review of present knowledge. Am. J. Pub. Health, 51:1306-11, Sept. 1961.
25. Koos, E. L. The health of Regionville; what the people thought and did about it. New York, Columbia University Press, 1954. XIV + 177 p. (p. 118-25)
26. Kriesberg, Louis, and Treiman, Beatrice R. Socio-economic status and the utilization of dentists' services. Am. Col. Dent. J., 27:147-65, Sept. 1960.
27. Moen, B. D. Survey of present and future needs for dental manpower. p. 18-26. (In Proceedings of the workshop on the future requirements of dental manpower and the training and utilization of auxiliary personnel. Ann Arbor, University Michigan, 1962. 206 p.)
28. Mumma, R. D., Jr. The amount of dental care required by the dentally indigent elementary school child in Trenton, New Jersey. J. Pub. Health Dent., 27:140-54, Summer 1967.
29. National Center for Health Statistics, Public Health Service. Decayed, missing, and filled teeth in adults; United States—1960-1962. Washington, Government Printing Office, 1967. IV + 47 p.
30. ———. Dental visits; time interval since last visit; United States—July 1963-June 1964. Washington, Government Printing Office, 1966. 54 p. (p. 2-3)
31. National Opinion Research Center, University of Chicago. Marginal results and basic cross-tabulations: public attitudes and practices in the field of dental care. Chicago, University Chicago, 1960. 446 p. mimeog.
32. New England Board of Higher Education. Dental manpower needs in New England. Winchester, Mass., New England Board Higher Education, 1958. 79 p.
33. Pelton, W. J. Dental needs and resources. p. 61-92. (In Pelton, W. J., and Wisan, J. M., eds. Dentistry in public health. 2nd ed. Philadelphia, Saunders, 1955. X + 289 p.)
34. Pelton, W. J., and Bothwell, Ruth. The dental profession in the Great Lakes region. Am. Col. Dent. J., 26:3-27, Mar. 1959.
35. ———. The need and the demand for dental care. p. 12-7. (In Proceedings of the workshop on the future requirements of dental manpower and the training and utilization of auxiliary personnel. Ann Arbor, University Michigan, 1962. 206 p.)
36. Pelton, W. J., Bothwell, Ruth, and Vavra, Helen. The dental profession in the Midwest. Washington, Government Printing Office, 1960. 20 p.
37. Smith, Q. M., Mitchell, G. E., and Lucas, Gertrude. An experiment in dental prepayment: the Naismith dental plan. Washington, Government Printing Office, 1963. IV + 31 p.
38. Sognnaes, R. F. Dentistry at its centennial cross-roads. Science, 130:1681-8, Dec. 18, 1959.

39. Southern Regional Educational Board. Dental manpower needs in the South. Atlanta, Southern Regional Educational Board, 1957. IX + 60 p.
40. Waterman, G. E., and Knutson, J. W. Studies on dental care services for school children; third and fourth treatment series, Richmond, Ind. Pub. Health Rep., 69:247-54, Mar. 1954.
41. Young, W. O. Dental health. p. 5-94. (In Hollinshead, B. S., dir. The survey of dentistry; the final report. Washington, American Council Education, c1961. XXXIV + 603 p.)
42. Young, W. O., and Pelton, W. J. Planning a dental prepayment program for children in an area of low caries prevalence. Am. Dent. A. J., 53:38-46, July 1956.

Additional Readings

Andersen, Ronald, and Anderson, O. W. A decade of health services: social survey trends in use and expenditure. Chicago, University Chicago Press, 1967. XIX + 244 p.
Association of State and Territorial Dental Directors. Proceedings of 1959 biennial conference of state and territorial dental directors with Public Health Service and Children's Bureau. Washington, Government Printing Office, 1959. VII + 62 p.
Draker, H. L., and Allaway, N. C. Facets of motivation in dental care buyers (partial report from phase I, study of family expenditures for dental care in New York State). Pub. Health Dent., 23:208-21, Winter 1964.
Kegeles, S. S. Some motives for seeking preventive dental care. Am. Dent. A. J., 67:90-8, July 1963.

CHAPTER 11

THE PURCHASE OF DENTAL CARE*

Professional care is basic to the maintenance of oral health, whether for the individual or the community. Any exploration of methods of solving the dental health problem must include an analysis of improved methods for the purchase of dental services. The most important developments in financing dental care in recent years have been the growth in third-party payment by organizations such as labor unions and industry, the purchase of care on a group basis, and the use of prepayment plans. Even more dramatic changes will come about in the immediate future as the result of legislation which will bring about a major expansion in public care programs (see Chapter 12).

The changes that have taken place in the socioeconomic pattern in this country have resulted in a shift of emphasis from the individual to the group. In the rural culture of past decades, the provision of health care was almost entirely an individual arrangement between the patient and the physician or dentist. The increasing amount of collective action has created a new type of relation between patients as a group and dentists as a group. Although the professional responsibility of the dentist has not changed, he is now called upon to discharge this responsibility in a new context.

---

*The field of prepayment is in a state of rapid flux. The profession is in the midst of a period of change unparalleled in its history. For this reason an attempt has been made to emphasize broad principles and to minimize specific details. In order to be knowledgeable about current developments, the dental student is urged to read carefully the *Journal of the American Dental Association*, and the dental hygiene student to read the *Journal of the American Dental Hygienists' Association*. In the *Journal of the American Dental Association,* particular attention should be given to several regular features—"Dental Prepayment," "Washington Report," and "News of Dentistry"— in addition to the editorial page.

More than seven years ago the report of a commission studying prepayment and health care concluded:

> Health is considered a necessity ranking with food, clothing and shelter. There is no longer any question of whether people receive health services. It has become a matter of how only. A more affluent society well organized into groups, more sophisticated about health, and conditioned to time payments, gives indication of wanting to put more than acute hospital illnesses into prepayment or insurance. Over the next ten years an increasing percentage of the medical care dollar probably will be covered through prepayment, insurance or taxes. The consumer gives every evidence of wanting security and predictability.[1c]

The truth of this conclusion becomes more clearly evident every year.

Smith has stated clearly the challenge facing the dental profession as it relates specifically to one mechanism of financing:

> Dentistry, then, holds no veto over prepaid dental care. Whether prepayment grows and prospers will not be decided by the profession alone but by the public at large. Should the public become convinced that professional interest and public interest are conflicting and irreconcilable, we may discover that we are influencing no attitudes but our own. The veto we do have is over mediocrity and shortsightedness. Using that veto, we will be influential. We can see to it that prepayment plans, as they grow, grow in a healthy fashion, offering the highest quality of care to the consumer public and the greatest protection to our professional independence.[28]

A study by the National Opinion Research Center emphasizes the interest of the public in prepayment and its desire to obtain care under this mechanism.[16] In spite of a general lack of direct personal experience with dental insurance, some 42 percent of the persons interviewed thought it a "good idea." Those who had heard of dental insurance were more likely to approve than those who had not, and even a familiarity with group hospitalization insurance increased the number of approvals. Furthermore, over a third were interested enough in prepayment coverage to say that they would elect dental coverage as a fringe benefit in preference to a cash salary increase.

A significant finding of this study relates to the public attitude toward the use of the family dentist. In general, respondents felt that, given a choice, they would favor using a private dentist of their own selection. If, however, they had to decide between joining a prepaid plan and choosing their own dentist, they would prefer the dental coverage and were willing to give up the free choice of dentist. A similar finding about the public's attitude toward "free choice of dentist" was found in a study of recipients of care from the Labor Health Institute of St. Louis.[8] In this plan a great many members expressed preference for a private dentist, and many continued to use private dentists even though they were eligible for "free" care through the clinic. Yet interviews suggested that the preference for a private practitioner was in many cases not the expression of a general principle but of loyalty to a particular man.

The significance of these findings for the dental profession is that the public apparently values the right to choose its dentist only on the basis of an established satisfactory relation. The principle of free choice of a dentist, although strongly held by the dental profession, apparently is not of major consequence to the public. Only satisfactory performance by members of the profession creates support for this principle in the mind of the public. This performance should include both the satisfactory practice of dentistry and community leadership in developing improved methods of financing dental care through private practice.

POSTPAYMENT PLANS

Postpayment plans, sometimes termed budget-payment plans, are mechanisms for the individual purchase of service. Dentists have frequently arranged to allow payments for dental care to be made at intervals over a period of time. The first steps to offer this service through an organized dental society plan were taken in 1936 in Allegheny County, Pennsylvania, and in 1941 in Detroit, Michigan.[4] Today at least 100 such plans have been established by state, county, or city dental societies. Although postpayment plans represent a joint effort by members of the dental profession, they do not constitute, for the consumer, any major deviation from the traditional one-to-one relation with his dentist.

Under a budget-payment plan, the patient borrows money from a bank or finance company to pay the dentist's fee at the time that the contract for care is made. The bank processes and approves the application for the loan (which usually has been completed in the dentist's office). After approval by the bank, the dentist is paid his entire fee less a discount charge, which is placed in a special "loss reserve" fund to reimburse the bank for any uncollectible notes. The patient repays the loan, plus interest, to the bank in budgeted amounts. The "loss reserve" fund is the property of the dental society (or the participating dentists), and its use in reimbursing the bank for delinquencies permits greater numbers of patients to qualify for bank loans.[10]

Postpayment plans help patients pay for the restoration of accumulated defects by eliminating the necessity for a large immediate expenditure. Although it had been hoped that budget-payment plans would bring the benefits of routine dental care to a larger segment of the population, evidence to date has not indicated that they do so. Extensive study of two of these plans has shown that the budget-payment contracts were used primarily to finance prosthetic treatment.[7, 9] Only about a fourth of the loan recipients were from families with an income of less than $300 a month. The average size of the loans was large ($299.46 and $211.66), and only 10 percent of them covered services for more than one individual. Under present patterns of operation, budget-payment plans are a convenience for the public and are helpful to the dentist in reducing collection problems. However, these plans do not appear likely to create a significant increase in the utilization of dental services by minimizing the barrier of cost.

PREPAYMENT PLANS

A prepayment plan is an arrangement by which periodic, specified payments (premiums, dues, contributions) are made in advance and used to pay for health services when the need arises.[10] Although prepayment contracts may be written on an individual basis, the experience in dentistry has been almost exclusively with the group purchase of care. Prepayment for medical and hospital care was conceived as a mechanism for insuring against the cost of illness or injury which is unpredictable for the individual. Dental disease, on the other hand, may be expected to occur almost universally. The extent of future treatment needs will vary from individual to individual, however, and the frequency of occurrence and the extent of utilization may be predicted on a group basis with sufficient precision to allow reasonably accurate estimates of average costs. In this way prepayment plans can spread the individual risk of payment for dental care, eliminate unpredictability of costs, and provide a mechanism for regular budgeted payment.

Health Insurance Experience Applicable to Dentistry

Growth in Demand. Over the past 25 years the American public has made exceptional progress in providing itself with financial protection against the costs of medical and hospital care. The growth of health insurance has been spectacular—a growth directly related to the public's growing appreciation of the value of health care and the necessity of finding a mechanism to finance this care. From 1951 to 1961 the number of persons protected for hospitalization expense grew 60 percent; the number protected under surgical coverage increased 96 percent; those with regular medical insurance rose 240 percent; and those persons covered by major medical expense policies increased by more than three hundredfold. By 1965 over 156 million Americans, about four out of every five persons, had some form of health protection through voluntary insuring organizations.[30] Although most policies do not provide coverage adequate to the need, the continued rise in numbers demonstrates the viability of the prepayment concept (Figure 23).

Another significant aspect of the data on hospital and medical

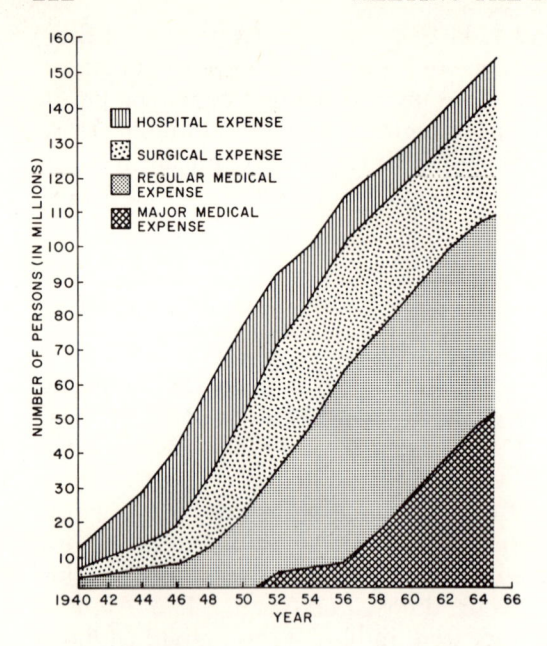

FIGURE 23. Number of people with health insurance protection in the United States by type of coverage. (Health Insurance Institute[30]).

care coverage is its near saturation level. The 156 million figure represented 81 percent of the civilian population. Such a large proportion of the population has been reached that the major gains in total numbers are coming from population growth rather than increases in the percentage who are covered. From 1940 to 1945, for example, the percentage of persons covered rose by 16 percent, but that increase represented only 20 million persons. However, from 1960 to 1965, the gain in coverage rose only by seven percent, but that gain represented 25 million persons.[30]

It will be some time before the additional impact of hospital and medical protection under Medicare or health services eligibility from public sources under Medicaid can be precisely measured. Precise estimates are not necessary to recognize the major increases in the number of persons who are protected against unpredictable costs of hospital and physician services — and who are now probably in a position to desire protection from the costs of other health services, including dental care.

In addition to demonstrating the increasing demand for prepaid health coverage, the experience in providing medical and hospital insurance has provided lessons which can be useful in planning dental prepayment plans.

Professional Leadership. From the beginning, hospital service plans made the greatest headway in areas in which strong, well-organized groups of hospitals existed to provide aggressive leadership in the development and establishment of community-wide hospitalization plans.[27] Similarly, although to a lesser extent, medical society leadership was an important factor in influencing the development of plans to provide coverage for medical and surgical benefits. In more recent years the efforts of unions and industrial management to extend "fringe benefits" have played a large role in the growth of health insurance. Nevertheless, the character of dental prepayment plans, and to a certain extent their rate of development, may be determined to a large measure by the leadership demonstrated by the profession.

The profession, if it is to be worthy of the name, must look at prepayment plans as meeting patients' needs as well as the profession's—for the general good. The dental service corporation, for example, should not be viewed negatively merely as a mechanism to stave off "socialized dentistry." Rather, positive values should be seen in a method by which more and better dental care can be brought to more people in the best interest of both the public and the profession. It is contended, also, that—in the long run—it would be to dentistry's best interests, if the profession developed more comprehensive plans and went more than halfway to meet with those most likely to be interested in purchasing dental care plans, such as labor leaders and industrial managers. In fact, representative leaders of consumers' groups might be appointed to the boards of dental service corporations and avoid the criticism which has fallen on Blue Shield boards of directors—that they do not have sufficient public representation.

Hillenbrand, the executive director of the American Dental Association, has branded as unfortunate the tendency to use the word "socialization" as a catch phrase to dismiss health proposals without giving them full and fair hearing. He has also warned that if the health professions fail to make available and support acceptable methods and devices for expanding health care, such as prepayment plans, the government may have no choice but to intervene.[15]

Selection of Risks. Successful development of health insurance plans requires enrollment procedures which will minimize an adverse selection of risks—the enrollment of persons whose health needs and utilization of health services are greater than normal. This task can be accomplished most easily by enrollment of employed persons (and usually their dependents) as a group. This mechanism results in economies in recruiting members and processing payment and eliminates the hazard that only those who anticipate high costs for care will enroll. Experience has shown that an adverse selection of risks in medical plans can be controlled even when offering independent membership through the use of community drives during which all promotional technics are used for a brief enrollment period. After this drive is completed, no additional policies are sold until they are again offered on a community-wide basis.

There has been only limited experience with individual enrollment in dental prepayment plans and, since none of these plans has been able to cover a major share of the community, several have experienced an unfavorable selection of risks. In the early 1940's, for example, McBride attempted to offer a prepayment contract to patients in his own practice but was forced to abandon the scheme because parents withdraw coverage from children with low treatment needs and retained it for those who required extensive attention.[19] In the late 1950's the Naismith Dental Group, a private group practice, offered prepaid dental care by individual contract for a monthly fee.[29] Families could enroll any or all of their members and could withdraw, on 10-days' notice, either the entire family or selected members. A sizeable number of subscribers received the dental care they needed and then withdrew, having paid dues only for the months of enrollment so that the value of the services received far exceeded payments to the plan. Recently, however, one of the nation's largest insurance companies announced that it would offer dental insurance to companies with as few as 10 to 49 persons on their payroll.[25]

Development in Urban Areas. Hospital and medical plans have shown the most progress in urban areas. In these areas, hospital and medical facilities are generally adequate, a high degree of industrialization permits widespread utilization of group enrollment and payroll deduction, and per capita income tends to be high so that a relatively large number of the population can meet hospital insurance charges. Experience to date with dental plans suggests that they will remain largely centered in the urban industrialized areas for at least the immediately foreseeable future.

Indemnity vs. Service Plans. Health insurance plans provide benefits either in the form of cash payment (indemnities), direct service, or a combination of both. Cash indemnity plans allow subscribers specific sums of money to be applied against the cost of hospital or medical services. Service plans, on the other hand, provide protection against the entire cost of specified services, usually by providing care through contractual arrangements with physicians, hospitals, and others. A few plans combine the two types of benefits by providing services to families with incomes of less than a stated amount and giving cash benefits to subscribers with incomes above this level. These plans provide complete coverage of the cost of care for individuals in lower-income brackets, while those with higher incomes must pay any differential between the indemnity and the fee established by the hospital or physician.

Indemnity plans apparently have been preferred by the medical profession because they seem to interfere least with the traditional practice of medicine, since the physician may make additional charges above the amount allowed by the indemnity schedule. They have not been, however, wholly satisfactory to the public since subscribers frequently resent having to pay additional fees when medical care is required. Some subscribers, and particularly administrators responsible for establishing plans on behalf of a corporation or labor union, have felt that indemnity programs are open to abuse by practitioners who can increase the fees charged to those eligible for benefits under the indemnity program.

THE PURCHASE OF DENTAL CARE

Fee Schedules. The establishment of fee schedules has presented particular problems in medical plans, since, while hospitals traditionally have operated on the basis of fixed charges, many physicians resented having any group, even members of their own profession, interfere with the establishment of fees. Where diverse areas are served by the same plan, a fee schedule which is appropriate for one area may not be suitable for another. Specialists often feel that they should receive a higher fee than should general practitioners for the same service, but such a dual schedule has proved neither satisfactory to the profession nor practical to administer. In an attempt to find a method of reimbursement more acceptable to the profession, insuring agencies developed a new approach to payment for service — a "usual-and-customary fee." This plan requires that each participating dentist submit periodically a listing of the fees he usually charges for each procedure. The fee listing is reviewed by the dental care plan administrators and, if accepted, becomes the basis for payments to that particular dentist until revised.

The "usual-and-customary" basis for reimbursement for professional services has proved to be the most acceptable mechanism to leaders of the profession, and the House of Delegates has urged that "priority consideration" be given to this method in future negotiations with public or private agencies. There has been some reluctance on the part of dental care plan administrators to put such a system into effect because of administrative complications and the fear of inappropriate increases in cost.

In addition, it has been difficult at times to obtain accurate and complete data necessary to plan and administer programs. The Council on Dental Care Plans of the American Dental Association has pointed out:

> A funding agency cannot be expected to accept the usual and customary fee concept without first being reassured that some responsible dental agency within the state has accurate, current data on usual and customary fees. Moreover, dental service corporations and private insurance carriers cannot calculate realistic premiums for dental care programs without reliable data on the normal charges of private practitioners. Constituent societies are at a disadvantage in objecting to fixed fee schedules or low tables of allowances when they do not possess data by which the validity of their challenges can be demonstrated. The Council, therefore, urges constituent societies and dental service corporations promptly to initiate a system of confidential prefiling of the fees usually charged by dentists within each state, subject to periodic up-dating, in order to have available a valid basis for insisting that prepayment programs provide reimbursement on the usual, customary and reasonable concept.[2]

The tradition that physicians' charges might be modified according to the financial ability of the patient to pay — the "Robin Hood" concept — also has created difficulty. The latter problem has sometimes been attacked by selling the combination of policies which provides either full coverage or indemnity according to the subscriber's income.

Controlling Costs. In order to keep the costs of health insurance protection within predicted ranges, administrative controls on the types of services offered have been necessary. A fee or indemnity schedule establishes the maximum obligation of the plan for each service sought by the subscriber. The types of services to be offered by the plan usually are specified carefully and limits are often established on the amount of service that may be received within a given period of time. One of the methods of limiting costs has been the use of coinsurance, an arrangement by which the beneficiaries pay part of the cost of service. This may be applied either as a deductible feature (such as the common $50.00 or $100.00 deductible automobile collision insurance), or on a proportional basis in which the subscriber pays a certain percentage of each claim and the plan pays the balance, or as a combination of both. Coinsurance reduces the total obligation of the plan for services sought and may, in some instances, also serve as a damper on utilization, which may or may not be good, depending on one's viewpoint.

The use of cost-control mechanisms is of particular importance in dental prepayment because of the unique nature of dental diseases. Because of the high incidence of disease, the cumulative nature, and the common failure to seek treatment, most people entering a plan will bring considerable accumulated treatment needs. In some instances, the funding of the plan may be sufficient to pay the high costs of initial treatment. If not, some method of reducing the obligation for "preexisting conditions" must be adopted. Other types of health plans often have met this problem by automatically excluding these conditions from coverage. Some dental prepayment plans do the same, in effect, by requiring that all accumulated dental needs be met at the patient's expense in the first year.

Management-Union Health Care Efforts

Sporadic efforts have been made to protect union members against the risks of accident and illness since the turn of the century. These plans were organized by private employers or labor unions, or were sponsored by consumer cooperatives. Labor-management health insurance plans did not grow rapidly at first. Benefits were generally low and limited in scope. Many of the plans failed because contributions were not adequate to meet the demand for benefits. During the 1930's a number of companies established—for their employees—group insurance plans financed either by management or through contributions from both management and labor. The plans were under the administration of management and had no obvious relation to collective bargaining.

The National Labor Relations Act, passed in 1935, provided

statutory authority for labor to bargain collectively on the issues of wages, hours, and working conditions.[5] The passage of this act was followed by a tremendous growth in labor organizations. During the early years of World War II, wages were frozen and many employers established health and welfare benefit plans as an inducement to maintain their labor force in the face of national shortages. Price-wage stabilization agencies approved the inclusion of these benefit plans in union contracts provided that they did not exceed a certain percent of the payroll. At the same time, employers were given the authority to include, as a business expense, the cost of providing group hospital and medical insurance for employees. An amendment (popularly known as the Taft-Hartley Act) to the National Labor Relations Act established the mechanism for carrying out health and welfare programs. Subsequent rulings of the National Labor Relations Board required employers to bargain concerning group health and accident insurance provisions.

In recent years, negotiations on health and welfare benefits for employees have provided a major area of activity in union-management bargaining. Programs which provide service benefits to union members have proved particularly attractive to many. Health and welfare programs provide a benefit to the employee which is not taxable—at least not to date. Furthermore, it is felt by some that union members are more likely to recognize the benefits gained when they come in the form of services provided through a union program rather than as a cash wage increase which, once spent, soon loses significance as a possible value of union membership.

Health and welfare programs may be administered by management, jointly by management and labor, or by the union. The first type of administration involves the provision of benefits directly by management on the basis of coverage which may or may not have been established directly through collective bargaining. Services may be purchased directly by management or through another agency such as a commercial insurance carrier or service corporation. Joint administration by labor and management involves the establishment of a welfare fund through management contributions stipulated in the contract with the union. This independent fund, usually governed by trustees equally representative of union and management, determines the manner in which the benefits are provided. If the health or welfare plan is administered directly by the union, the management usually provides the funds according to the collective bargaining agreement, but it is administered entirely by representatives of the union.

Development of Dental Care Plans

There appeared to be relatively little interest in solving the problems of financing dental care until after the majority of the population had achieved some protection against hospital and medical costs. The dental profession recognized early, however, that eventually the public would express interest in prepaid dental care. As early as 1943, a committee of the American Dental Association recommended a study of existing hospital prepayment programs and urged the establishment of experimental programs to provide experience with the utilization of the prepayment mechanism for the purchase of dental care. To provide guidance in the establishment of plans for the group purchase of dental care, the House of Delegates approved a statement of principles in 1953 and have subsequently revised it over the years. An abstract* of pertinent policies follows:

> The American Dental Association believes that dental prepayment programs provide a sound mechanism for making dental care more readily available. The development and growth of dental prepayment plans, therefore, are encouraged, provided that they meet the principles and standards established by the dental profession in the interest of providing the best possible level of dental care.
> 1. The areas of responsibility involved in the administration of dental prepayment plans should be clearly delineated:
>   a. The operation of the plan should be efficient and economical, and governing policies should provide freedom to experiment with methods of payment.
>   b. The administration of the professional phases of the plan should be entirely under the control of professional personnel. Professional standards and treatment should not be under the control of nondental administrators.
>   c. The method of authorization of dental care under a prepayment plan should prevent any interference with the dentist-patient relation or the professional judgment and decision of the dentist.
> 2. Provision should be made for public, consumer, and professional representation on the governing boards of dental prepayment and direct service organizations.
> 3. The development of dental prepayment plans in which dentists in private practice participate is preferred to the establishment of facilities staffed with salaried dentists (closed-panel systems).
> 4. High priority should be placed on comprehensive coverage for all patients, particularly children. Where funding limitations prevent consideration of a comprehensive prepayment program, deductibles and coinsurance should be considered but the minimization of such features should be given high priority in future developments of the plan or program.
> 5. The benefits available under the plan, and any limitations, should be clearly defined.
> 6. The patient must have freedom to choose, within the agreed limitations of the plan, the dentist to whom he may wish to apply for treatment. Similarly, the dentist, within the same limitations, must have the right to accept patients who apply for treatment.
> 7. All ethically and legally qualified dentists must be eligible to participate within the agreed limitations of the plan.
> 8. The plan should provide for the maximum use of existing facilities.

---

*Abstracted by Joan Keevil from *Policies on Dental Prepayment*.[3]

9. The promotional standards under which dental prepayment plans are developed should meet the requirements of the *Principles of Ethics* of the American Dental Association and the codes of ethics of the constituent and component societies involved.
10. The determination of policies relating to fees and methods of remuneration should be made at the state or local level by authorized representatives of the dental profession.
    a. The costs of dental care should be determined on the basis of accurate, current statistical data which reflect fees in the area in which the plan operates. Fee schedules and tables of allowances should be developed with the advice and assistance of the dental society in order that they may (1) ensure high standards of treatment in providing benefits under the plan and (2) be subject to adjustment at reasonable intervals in accordance with changes in the economic level.
    b. Priority consideration should be given for reimbursement for professional services on the basis of usual and customary fees.
11. The financial reserves of the plan should be adequate to ensure continuity of operation.
12. Constituent societies without dental service corporations are urged to establish dental service corporations so that this not-for-profit mechanism will be available when there is a group demand for dental services.
13. The active solicitation and promotion of dental prepayment plans by dental service corporations is encouraged within the policies established by the sponsoring constituent society and the individual dental service corporation.
14. Dental prepayment plans should include a sound program of dental health education for all beneficiaries.
15. The plan should make adequate provisions for the adjustment of any complaints arising from the dentist-patient relation.
16. Constituent societies have responsibility for evaluating dental prepayment plans which come within their jurisdiction, provided the societies' criteria are consistent with standards which have been established at the national level.

The dental profession's study of prepayment was timely, since it occurred at a time of rapid growth in plans for the group purchase of care. Although a dental care plan was organized as early as 1915 by the Metropolitan Life Insurance Company, and sporadic attempts were made to offer dental services through group plans in the years that followed, significant growth did not occur until the 1950's.[13, 20]

One of the most significant aspects of this recent development has been the active role of labor unions in fostering dental care plans. Until about 1950 unions did not play a particularly important part in the growth of prepayment dental plans, but after that time they shared sponsorship in more than half of the plans initiated.

Only about 259,000 persons, in 20 groups, were eligible for prepaid dental benefits through privately sponsored plans by the end of 1930.[14] These benefits were often minimal, and this listing includes any plan which offered clinical and radiographic examination and at least continuing emergency care. Ten years later the number of individuals included had increased to only some 317,000 persons. By mid-1963, however, the number of groups rose to 296 while the number of beneficiaries was boosted to 1,146,000. During the 33-year span, 1930 to 1963, the number of privately sponsored groups increased almost 14 times over, while the number of beneficiaries more than quadrupled. (In addition to those covered by privately sponsored prepaid dental care plans in 1963, an additional 340,000 persons were eligible for dental care financed by public welfare agencies and provided through dental service corporations in three states.)

Dental plans have expanded in coverage as well as numbers. In the early days of prepaid dentistry only about one third of the groups provided coverage for dependents as well as for members. In the late 1940's and through the 1950's, more and more groups were initiating dental plans which included dependents. As of 1960, well over half of the programs in operation included coverage for both members and dependents. By 1963, the ratio had gone up to nearly two thirds.

The scope of benefits provided in prepayment plans varies widely, but the trend is toward more comprehensive coverage. In order to identify these trends, the 1963 data on dental care plans were separated into three categories: (1) "Minimal" plans, which included diagnostic, surgical, and emergency care benefits but did not include restorations; (2) "Basic" plans, which offered more complete dental care including restorations but excluding dentures; and (3) "Comprehensive" plans, which offered benefits included in the first two categories, dentures, and, in many instances, other specialized services.[14] In 1930, 40 percent of the plans provided only minimal benefits, 20 percent included basic services, and only 40 percent had comprehensive benefits. By 1960, programs confined to minimal benefits had dropped to 11 percent of total plans; those in the basic category had dropped to 14 percent of the total; and programs offering more complete benefits, including restorations and dentures, had risen to 75 percent of the total. Apparently, no program started since 1960 has offered less than basic care as a benefit.

The trends identified in the 1963 survey have continued at an accelerated rate in the succeeding five-year period. The number of persons with some type of dental expense coverage rose from two to 5.2 million. The latter represented 2.6 percent of the population—a significant increase over the 1960 figure of 0.4 percent. All told, 933 plans (in 41 states, the District of Columbia, and Puerto Rico) were in operation at the beginning of 1969. Not surprisingly, the largest number of plans and enrollees were in the two most populous states. California's 249 plans covered nearly 1.9 million persons, while 1.16 million were covered by the 303 plans operating in New York in 1969. In general, the West had the largest number of persons covered and the South the least.[1a, 6a]

An even more marked expansion took place in the extent of

coverage. The inclusion of more benefits forced the Division of Dental Health to revise the categories of benefits for the Survey of Prepaid Dental Care Plans conducted in 1968.

This change means that plans currently listed as comprehensive are exactly that. The scope of services in the dental insurance policies studied in 1968 were:

SCOPE OF DENTAL SERVICES*	PLANS
Minimal benefits	18
Basic benefits	111
Intermediate benefits	521
Comprehensive benefits	274
Other (mixed services)	9

Although plans with large numbers of participants tend to dominate the scene statistically, one of the characteristics of current developments is the increasing diversity in both sizes and types of plans. The Dental Health Insurance Committee of the Florida Dental Society compiled a summarizing manual which identified more than 60 different types of dental care plans in operation. The plans varied widely in size, scope of services, and administration. One interesting finding was that there were as few as 35 adults and 125 dependents covered by a single nationwide plan administered by the California Dental Service (a dental service corporation).[26]

Many contend that private plans for the group purchase of dental care are entering their period of greatest growth. They anticipate that the number of plans will increase, that the number of beneficiaries will grow, and that more comprehensive services will be available. Such developments are consistent with the general trend toward budget payment for a wide variety of goods and services. Now that a majority of the population has some type of protection against the costs of hospitalization and medical care, it seems natural to expect a growing interest in methods of budgeting expenditures for dental care. Although the exact rate of growth may not be predictable, there seems no doubt that the development of dental prepayment plans will be one of the most significant influences on the future of the dental profession—but it may well be through the public rather than the private sector.

Organization of Dental Care Plans

There are many differences in organized plans for the provision of dental care. These variations relate to the method of providing

---

*Defined as follows: *Minimal benefits* = diagnostic services, radiographs, clinical examinations, and emergency Rx for relief of pain. *Basic benefits* = minimal benefits plus prophylaxis, topical fluoride applications, routine fillings, and simple extractions. *Intermediate benefits* = basic benefits plus inlays, crowns, oral surgery, partial and/or full dentures, and space maintainers. *Comprehensive benefits* = intermediate benefits plus periodontal treatment, fixed bridges, root canal therapy, and orthodontics.

or obtaining service, the source of funds, administration, and the method used to reimburse the professional personnel providing care.

Beneficiaries may receive care in the offices of private practitioners. Among plans using this method are programs for indigents sponsored by departments of health or welfare, the plans financed by the Department of Defense for servicemen's dependents, and plans administered by dental service corporations, Blue Cross, or insurance companies. (A dental service corporation, like an insurance company, is not a plan as such, but a legal mechanism used to administer a plan. See page 224.)

Service under a dental care plan may be provided either through "open" or "closed" panels. An open panel is characterized by three features: (1) any licensed dentist may elect to participate; (2) the beneficiary has his choice among all licensed dentists participating; and (3) dentists may accept or refuse any beneficiary.[10] In a closed panel, beneficiaries may go only to those dentists who have agreed to provide services under the prepayment plan. Dentists must accept any beneficiary as a patient. Group-practice clinics may participate in a plan as the exclusive provider of service (closed panel) or on an equal basis with other practitioners in the area (open panel).

The most striking departure from individual practice is the dental facility which utilizes the services of salaried dentists. A significant number of individuals receives service from salaried employees of the federal government. Others receive service from clinical facilities sponsored by industry, labor unions, consumer cooperatives, and health and welfare departments. These facilities are almost always "closed panels," since service is limited to a specified group of beneficiaries, and these individuals have a limited choice of dentists. In the next chapter it will be pointed out that a major federal agency appears to be promoting the establishment of closed-panel clinics to provide care for the disadvantaged.

Plans also differ in their sponsorship, both for the source of funds and the method of administering the plan. Funds for service must come either from the individual patient or from some outside party, although the distinction is not always clear. Payroll deductions to cover the premiums for group purchase are actually individual payments. Similarly, if the premiums are paid as a fringe benefit by a company in lieu of a wage increase, they may be said to represent a payment by an individual. The net effect of these two methods of payment, however, is the same as if an outside party assumed the cost of care, since they remove payment for dental service from the area of immediate personal choice. For convenience, these methods of payment may be considered third-party payments, along with provisions for care made by governmental agencies, philanthropic organizations, industry, or industrial or union welfare plans. The plans which relieve the patient of the necessity of paying for treatment out of his own budget have possibilities for increasing utilization.

The mechanics of collecting funds, contracting for service, and handling reimbursements may be administered by various kinds of agencies. The most significant developments in dental payment have occurred in those plans administered by closed-panel group practices, dental service corporations, commercial insurance companies, and independent private nonprofit insurance organizations.

Closed-Panel Group Practice. For want of a more precise designation, the first mechanism for the provision of care may be termed "closed-panel group practice." In the early 1960's the largest number of persons enrolled in private dental care plans received service from this source.[13] Since then the number of persons enrolled in plans of this type has remained about the same. However, because of the rapid growth of commercial insurance coverage and dental service corporation coverage during this period, the proportion of persons receiving care in closed-panel clinics in private dental care plans has dropped from 57 percent in 1962 to 11 percent in 1968.[6a, 13]

Closed-panel group practice includes two types of organizational structures which, although similar in many ways, differ in one important aspect—ownership and ultimate responsibility. Nondental organizations such as consumer cooperatives, industries, and labor unions own and operate dental clinics staffed by employed dentists. Closed-panel clinics of this type have existed for many years but only in recent years have they experienced significant expansion. The early clinics tended to be small, frequently were staffed only by part-time dentists paid on an hourly or daily rate (often at minimum levels), and generally offered a limited range of services. Today a significant number of beneficiaries receive comprehensive dental care from clinical facilities owned by nondental organizations. Although the ultimate responsibility rests with the owner group, the professional direction usually is delegated to a clinic director so that, in actual practice, the administrative pattern may be little different from the private group practice. Salaries may be adequate to attract dentists of high caliber and the operation of the facility planned to ensure the highest standards of dental care.

Group practice is nothing more than the conduct of a practice by two or more dentists who share business staffs, facilities, and services.[10] Commonly, the dentists consult with each other about patient care and often work together in treatment—particularly where some members of the group are specialists. Net income is divided equally or prorated according to patient load, years of service, and specialty status. There is no relation between group practice, per se, and the group purchase of care, prepayment, or closed-panel operation. Unlike most solo practitioners, however, a group practice of any size has resources and manpower which make it feasible to offer contracts to consumer groups, and a number have done so.

The dental profession has viewed the widespread growth of

closed-panel group practice as a threat to the private practice of dentistry.[6] Participation in such programs, however, is not considered a breach of professional ethics, and it has been recognized that this mechanism for providing care will continue to exist. Of particular concern has been the growth of facilities owned by consumer groups employing salaried dentists. The profession has urged that the growth of these facilities be discouraged by the development of more effective plans utilizing private practitioners through dental service corporations or insurance companies.

Dental Service Corporations. The dental profession has developed the dental service corporation in an attempt to adapt its

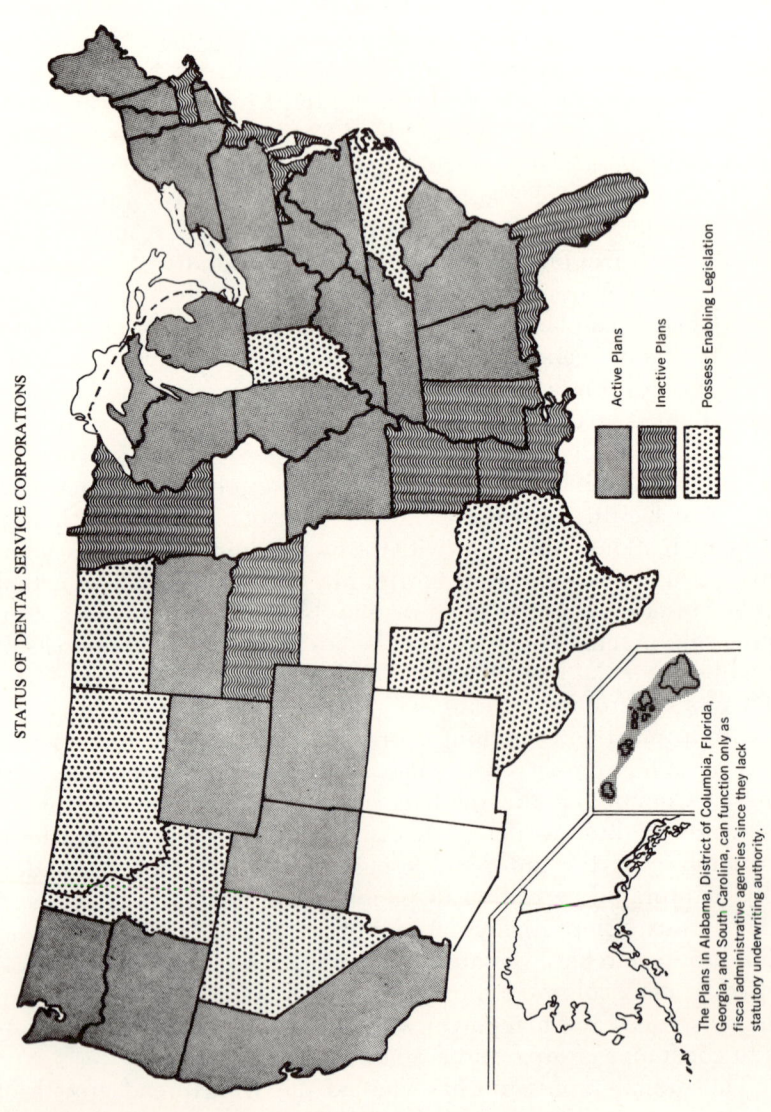

FIGURE 24a. The status of dental service corporations in the United States as of March 1969. (From Bonk[10]).

FIGURE 24b. The enrollment growth (people covered) of dental service corporations, 1960 to 1968. A comparison of Figure 24b with Figure 23 (page 212) shows the relatively small amount of people covered by dental service corporations. (From Bonk[1b]).

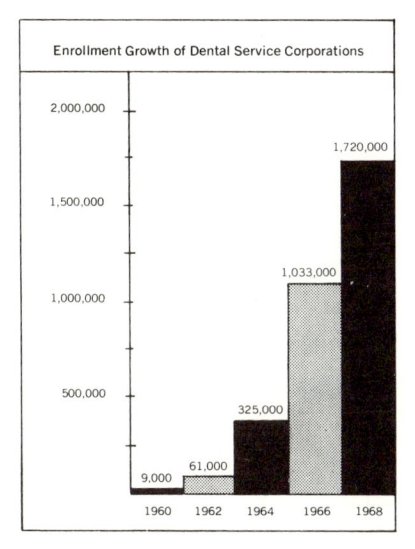

traditional patterns of practice to the demand for group purchase of dental care. Dental service corporations have followed the lead of the professionally sponsored community-wide "Blue Cross" and "Blue Shield" hospital and medical plans. Service corporations essentially are legal mechanisms through which participating dentists can contract to provide dental care to consumer groups. Ordinarily, the dental service agency is incorporated under the state laws governing either insurance companies or nonprofit corporations. Although technically independent of the dental society organization, the fact that the memberships of the corporation and the society are almost parallel ensures effective control by the profession. The corporation is, in effect, the business arm of the state dental society through which the society can assist in planning prepayment programs, administer the programs, and control the quality of care rendered. The flexibility of this mechanism permits the operation of almost any type of dental program (including closed-panel clinics if necessary); the provision of service in any locality where members of the dental society practice; and the coverage of any type of consumer group receiving benefits from labor unions, governmental agencies, industry, or institutions.

Dental service corporations represent an advanced development of the principle of meeting problems through collective effort. Negotiations take place between organization and organization, matching strength against strength, and holding the promise of equitable agreements to meet the needs of both the suppliers and the recipients of services. The individual dentist is not left to bargain alone with a powerful organization concerning his fees. The individual patient is not left to bargain alone in a field where he is incompetent to judge either the quality of the services rendered or the fair value of such services. The principles which the dental profession holds most basic, the free choice of dentist and the fee-for-service payment, can be kept intact.

Because of the obvious advantages that service corporations offer to the profession, they are developing rapidly. The first dental service corporation was organized in Washington in 1954. By mid-1963 there were seven in operation, and by 1969, there were 27 active service corporations providing coverage for about two million people.[1b, 24]

National Association of Dental Service Plans (Delta Dental Plans). A significant development in dental prepayment was the activation of the National Association of Dental Service Plans in June 1966. The organization was developed with the aid of staff from the American Dental Association (under the guidance of the House of Delegates), and its first efforts were financially underwritten by the Association, which still continues to provide substantial financial support in the form of loans and grants. Within a reasonable period of time, however, it became an autonomous agency supported and directed by the state dental service plans and dental societies who joined together to create the N.A.D.S.P.

During a period of rapid change, this national association has been able to exert the type of effective leadership that stimulated the development of effective local plans and helped to channel new group care programs through profession-sponsored agencies.

One of the major objectives that underlay the decision to establish the National Association of Dental Service Plans was to create a vehicle through which individual dental service corporations could participate in the underwriting of contracts covering beneficiaries in a number of different states.[17] A labor union or industry with workers in 10 or 15 states obviously would feel it necessary to provide reasonably comparable benefits in all geographic areas. However, a single service corporation is quite rigidly limited by statute to operate only within the political boundaries of the state in which it is chartered. This meant that state dental service plans were handicapped in competing in the "multistate market" where a substantial portion of current labor-management health care programs are developing. Through the national coordinating agency the state agencies can work together to tailor plans for this market.

The first such multistate plan was placed in effect on November 1, 1967, by the Northwest International Association of Machinists Benefit Trust to provide dental care coverage to 33,000 IAM mem-

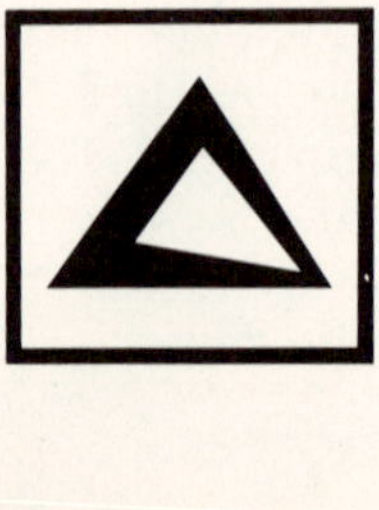

FIGURE 24c. The National Association of Dental Service Plans has developed this symbol for Delta Dental Plans, the new nationwide name for NADSP member groups.

bers and their dependents in an eight-state area. Since that time, other multistate plans have become effective.[1b, 18, 23]

Independent Nonprofit Insurance. In the 1950's, community-wide dental care prepayment plans were developed by nonprofit insurance corporations.[31] These organizations differ from closed-panel group practices and from dental service corporations because they are independent stock corporations unaffiliated with dental or consumer groups outside the field of health insurance. Unlike private commercial insurance companies they are nonprofit organizations. The successful independent dental insurance groups have resulted from the efforts of dentists and other community leaders to bring dental service within the reach of a larger number of individuals by making it a regularly budgetable expenditure. The initial development of independent dental insurance corporations was limited to the New York City area and, although individual enrollment was allowed, they provided primarily group coverage. The administrative structure and legal status of a nonprofit corporation provide perhaps even greater flexibility than the dental service corporation. Prepayment coverage has been offered on a service basis providing complete payment for dental care, on an indemnity basis with limits on the obligation of the plan, and in combination policies which give complete or partial coverage depending on the income of the family. An independent insurance company could also operate closed-panel clinics. Because the organizations of this type are not limited necessarily to the geographic area of a component or constituent dental society, they can sometimes offer coverage to a group of widely scattered beneficiaries more easily than a dental service corporation.

Commercial Insurance. Insurance companies have offered some degree of coverage for dental care as part of hospital and surgical policies. Quite commonly, benefits have been restricted to oral surgery procedures requiring hospital confinement. Not surprisingly, private companies approached the field of dental prepayment hesitantly because of the hazards of attempting to predict operating costs in an area where both actuarial and empirical experience has been limited. Nevertheless, some companies have initiated comprehensive group dental insurance plans.[1a] Several mechanisms for controlling the cost of care in these plans have been used. Often beneficiaries are required to meet all or part of the cost of initial care. Deductible provisions requiring the beneficiaries to pay a stated amount before being eligible for insurance payments and coinsurance features which limit the company's obligation to a certain percentage of the total cost are also used.

Since commercial insurance carriers expect to make a profit on their investment, the cost of providing coverage may be expected to be higher than for nonprofit agencies if both are equally efficient and attempt to provide equivalent benefits for the same group of beneficiaries. In health insurance fields, however, commercial carriers have been able to maintain a competitive position with professionally sponsored community-wide organizations by reducing selling and administrative costs through inclusion of health insurance in a comprehensive "package" plan, by aggressive promotion, and by covering only selected groups at premiums established on the basis of "experience rating" rather than "community-wide rating." Rates for insurance coverage are determined by past costs of providing service as related to such significant factors as age, sex, and socioeconomic status. If a private insurance company selects only groups with low needs for service and bases its rates on the experience of this group, it can offer lower premiums than a professionally sponsored plan which bases its rates on the experience of an entire community and feels morally obligated to offer coverage to high and low risk groups alike. Furthermore, if selected groups with a favorable experience are covered by the commercial group, the community-wide plans face the prospect of being forced to increase their rates and being priced out of the market. The dental service corporations, with the strong support of the dental profession, have demonstrated phenomenal growth in coverage in recent years. However, the number of persons receiving coverage for dental benefits under commercial insurance has increased more than twice as rapidly.[6a]

Commercial companies have no organizational tie with the dentists who provide service, and the profession has no voice in the determination of policy. Because of their independent status, the commercial companies usually provide coverage only on an indemnity basis. This means that the patient may go to any dentist and the practitioner is free to establish his own fees. It also means that the beneficiary cannot be certain that he is protected against the total cost of care. Furthermore, commercial coverage ordinarily does not encourage utilization of professional services.

Health Service Corporations. The health service corporations also have offered some dental coverage as part of hospital and medical policies—often limited primarily to services rendered in the hospital. A few Blue Shield organizations have started to offer prepaid dental care as an additional service to consumer groups, and the number may be expected to grow. The Blue Shield groups may be expected either to develop their own independent dental care plans or to contract with dental service corporations to provide dental service for customers of their medical plans.

Merits of Different Types of Plans

An important test of the value of a dental care plan is its ability to extend dental service of high quality to more people. Under some circumstances, particularly where groups of patients are concentrated in an area and loss of time from employment is of concern, a clinic installation may be more practical than a plan utilizing the offices of practitioners. This alternative is especially true of the military forces and in some industrial areas. Under many circumstances, however, a centralized clinic entails definite disadvantages because of the distances the patients have to travel for treatment.

An important element in public acceptability is whether the plan covers all costs of services or provides only set allowances — which may or may not meet the total charges. Under the latter plan the patient does not have complete protection and may not know until he arranges for the service how much balance he will have to pay. Moreover, it is an unhappy fact of life that, under such an indemnity arrangement, it is possible for a dentist, knowing the patient has insurance, to charge more than he otherwise would. For the profession the opposite feeling generally holds, since the indemnity type of insurance provides the least deviation from custom and requires no particular change in the financial structure of a practice.

An open-panel plan apparently is more satisfactory to those members of the public who have established a relation with a dentist in whom they have confidence and who, therefore, do not wish to change dentists in order to obtain service. Plans permitting free choice of dentists are also much more acceptable to the profession. Although some dentists may look askance at any form of closed-panel group practice, the major opposition has been to those in which dentists are employed on a salary and in which a clinic has been organized, equipped, and operated by a lay group, particularly a consumer or union group. It is feared that professional judgments may be overridden by economic or other considerations and that the dentists operating in these clinics will become mere technicians working on an "amalgam line." Although the acceptability of a plan to the profession is not the controlling factor, it may have an important bearing on the success and growth of dental plans.

It seems reasonable to believe that development of plans which make the purchase of dental care easier for the patient would lead more individuals to seek complete dental service. However, there is no evidence to date that easier methods of payment will, by themselves, bring about a large increase in the utilization of dental service unless the plan is of a type requiring no out-of-pocket expenditure by the patient. At present at least, the most important factor in increasing the amount of care will be the extent to which third-party funds — from government, industry, labor unions, and philanthropy — are available to purchase care for individuals.

Another important question in evaluating dental care plans is whether they are organized to provide an adequate range of services. A plan should offer complete services, with the possible exception of certain types of orthodontic care, and certainly cannot be considered adequate unless it includes provisions for preventive services such as topical applications of fluoride, prophylaxes, health education, and periodic recall. The professional aspects of the plan should be determined on the advice of representatives of the dental profession.

Mechanisms for "quality assurance" may violate the strong feeling of independence held by many dental practitioners. It seems apparent, however, that any conscientious administrator would feel compelled to insist that some method be utilized to ensure optimum standards of care to protect the consumers contracting for service. Utilized fairly and objectively, controls on quality can be of serious consequence only to the dentist whose incompetence makes questionable his right to practice regardless of the existence of dental care plans. One of the major attractions of dental service corporations to the profession is that, although they place some limitation on the relatively absolute freedom of dental practice, the profession itself, through its elected representatives, develops the mechanisms which will be of greatest mutual protection to dentists and consumer groups.

The most important factors in ensuring dental service of high quality are that a regular mechanism be established for the review of cases and that this review be conducted by dentists of established competence who are disinterested parties. Because of their close ties with the dental profession, service corporations are in an excellent position to operate a quality control program. A random sample of patients can be screened continuously throughout the year, and participating dentists who do not measure up to standard can be suspended. In this effort the corporation can have available the services of selected members of the profession in the entire area to serve as screening dentists and to serve on reviewing committees.

Quality control in a group practice may be enhanced by the pressures stemming from within the group to do as well as the best of its members. The integrity and standards of the most outstanding members often become the standard for the group. In addition, group practices may, and do, screen practitioners thoroughly before accepting them in the practice. The controls after acceptance, although they may be quite informal, consisting of "over the shoulder" surveillance and consultation, are real. Furthermore, there is no reason that formal review of selected cases cannot be conducted periodically by dentists from outside the group—as has been done.

In the indemnity plans usually offered by commercial insurance companies, there is no practical way to provide for a program of quality control since patients may go to any dentist they choose and the company merely indemnifies them for part of the cost of services.

The increasing concern for adequate control of the quality of care has been expressed by, among many others, the National Advisory Commission on Health Manpower. They strongly urged that the present system of granting lifetime licensure to practice be changed to one requiring periodic relicensure on the basis of evidence of continuing education. Those who did not choose to participate in acceptable educational programs would be required to submit to "challenge examinations."

Even more significant was the strong emphasis placed on stringent "peer review." The Commission recommended that:

> ... professional societies, health insurance organizations, and government should extend the development and effective use of a variety of peer review procedures in maintaining high quality health and medical care. These procedures should incorporate the following principles:
>
> Peer review should be performed at the local level with professional societies acting as sponsors and supervisors.
>
> Assurance must be provided that the evaluation groups perform their tasks in an impartial and effective manner.
>
> Emphasis should be placed on assuring high quality of performance and on discovering and preventing unsatisfactory performance.[22]

It has been pointed out that, all other factors being equal, the nonprofit organizations should be able to put a larger portion of the subscriber's premium into the purchase of care than can a commercial insurance company. In assessing cost, it is important to remember that an organized plan for the purchase of dental care does not necessarily reduce the cost of care. To whatever charges are currently being made for service must be added the cost of administration of a group plan. In fact, a successful group-purchase plan may increase the cost of dental care since a larger number of individuals will receive more comprehensive care. It is sometimes felt that costs can be controlled more closely in an agency-owned clinic. However, such installations require a considerable investment, which must be amortized. It has been demonstrated that costs can be predicted and controlled in programs utilizing dentists practicing in their own offices.

In the long run, dental service cannot be obtained on a "cut-rate" basis. If dentists in the community are utilized, resources adequate to remunerate them for their time are necessary or the more "successful" dentist will be unwilling to participate in the plan. If a clinic is utilized, salaries adequate to attract competent individuals must be paid to the dentists and their auxiliary personnel.

It is probably premature to attempt to define specifically the merits and shortcomings of the plans that have been proposed for the group purchase of dental care. Experience with dental payment plans has been limited, and many of them are still in the experimental stage. Even after a good many years of experience, it is evident that hospital and medical care plans are developing new approaches to the problems involved in the group purchase of care. Many problems remain to be solved, despite the wide experience that has been gained. There probably is no one approach that merits universal adoption. The value of a specific plan can be determined only by how well it meets the needs of the individuals or groups involved. Varying conditions in different localities will require different methods.

Utilization of Dental Care Plans

The cost of service, although an important deterrent to the utilization of professional treatment, is by no means the only factor. Educational attainment, levels of health knowledge, and cultural patterns are among the other influences which determine the extent to which individuals seek care. The group purchase of dental care will not ensure optimum utilization automatically, although it may be expected to increase the proportion who visit the dentist.

Studies of three dental care plans give an indication of the effect of third-party payment on the demand for care. The dental facility of the St. Louis Labor Health Institute, which offers routine dental care without charge to members of the Teamsters Union and their dependents, was utilized by 41 percent of the families and 27 percent of the eligible individuals during the study period.[8] An additional 15 percent of the individuals sought care from an outside dentist. Despite the elimination of financial impediments to complete dental care, less than half of this group visited a dentist even once during the year. The real significance of the Labor Health Institute data is not clear unless it is recognized that the beneficiaries had below average incomes and education. Only slightly more than one fourth of the membership had a high-school education, for example, in comparison with a national figure of more than 40 percent. The group contained a large number of older men and greater proportion of Negroes than the national average. This group, then, generally fell into the category of population usually considered relatively minimal users of regular dental care. Nevertheless, under a care plan which eliminated out-of-pocket costs for treatment, the utilization rates of this group were pulled up to approximate the national average. Furthermore, this level of effective demand was created without a strong program of dental health education and with but one clinical facility, and that was not conveniently located for all beneficiaries.

Another significant finding was that children were more likely to receive care than were their parents. Even in the families with the poorest education and the lowest income, half the children had seen a dentist during the study year and five out of six of these had received care at the Institute clinic. The study showed also that when one member of a family used the dental clinic the use of dental service by other members increased, so that the stimulating effect of dental prepayment appeared contagious.

Over 70 percent of the nearly 15,000 children eligible for dental care under the program of the welfare fund of the International Longshoremen's and Warehousemen's Union and Pacific Maritime Association visited a dentist each year during the first five years of operation.[21] Most of these children received complete dental care. Although utilization of dental services among this group of beneficiaries undoubtedly was increased merely by the availability of the dental care plan, administrators of the welfare fund have recognized that educational efforts are of vital importance if maximum benefits are to be realized from the program.

In fact, one of the significant strengths of prepayment plans is that they offer an excellent mechanism for effective programs of dental health education. Materials can be designed expressly to meet the particular requirements of particular groups. The use of appropriate educational methods may prove almost as important as lowering the cost barrier in persuading beneficiaries to seek the care they need. Since the entire group of eligibles is identifiable, effective use can be made of such materials as brochures and pamphlets, reminder slips inserted in pay envelopes, and a host of other possibilities exploited to influence eligibles to seek care. Workable systems of patient recall can be instituted with both sponsors and dentists taking part in order to attain the highest possible rate of utilization.

The highest utilization rate occurred in a prepayment plan covering persons who had enrolled voluntarily with the Naismith Dental Group.[29] In this plan, overall utilization was about 80 percent in each of three study years, a rate considerably above the national figures even for families with above-average income and educational attainment. More than 90 percent of the children five through 19 received service during the study period. Although it is apparent that use of services was higher in a plan in which enrollment was voluntary and continuing out-of-pocket expense for premiums was required, utilization still did not reach 100 percent.

Regardless of the variations in circumstances, it seems apparent that prepayment plans can result in substantial increases in demand for dental care despite their failure to achieve 100 percent utilization. It has been estimated that the number of individuals visiting a dentist annually will increase 20 percent with the institution of a prepaid dental care plan. Since the average amount of care received also will rise, the overall demand for service may be increased by as much as 100 percent.[12] The long-range impact of group-payment plans on utilization may be expected to be even greater. The increased number of children receiving routine care under the programs should raise the level of dental consciousness of the next generation of parents. Plans which include dental health educational efforts may be expected to bring about a marked change in attitudes toward dental care even among the adults of today. If the problem of payment has been eliminated, educational efforts to remove other blocks to seeking care should be much more effective.

BIBLIOGRAPHY

1a. Bock, W. B., and Sperberg, Mary J. Directory of prepaid dental care plans 1967. Washington, Government Printing Office, 1968. III + 309 p.
1b. Bonk, James. The dental service plan: an adventure in involvement. Am. Dent. A. J., 78:701-5, Apr. 1969.
1c. Bowles, G. E., chm. Report and recommendations of the Governor's Study Commission on Prepaid Hospital and Medical Care Plans. Lansing, Michigan Hospital Association, 1962. XXII + 72 p. (p. 1)

2. Council on Dental Care Programs, American Dental Association. Periodic fee surveys. Am. Dent. A. Reports of Officers and Councils, 109:10-1, 1968.
3. ———. Policies on dental prepayment. [Chicago], American Dental Association, 1968. 51 p. processed.
4. Council on Dental Health, American Dental Association. Budget payment plans for the individual purchase of dental care. I. Am. Dent. A. J., 55:446-51, Sept. 1957.
5. ———. Group dental health care programs. Chicago, American Dental Association, 1955. 97 p.
6. ———. Methods of payment for the group purchase of dental care; policies of the American Dental Association. Am. Dent. A. J., 60:485-91, Apr. 1960.
6a. Division of Dental Health, Public Health Service. Fact sheet; privately sponsored prepaid dental care plans. 1969. 1 p. mimeo.
7. Division of Dental Resources, Public Health Service. Budget payment plan of the Nevada State Dental Society. Washington, Government Printing Office, 1959. III + 18 p.
8. ———. Dental care in a group purchase plan; a survey of attitudes and utilization at the St. Louis Labor Health Institute. Washington, Government Printing Office, 1959. VI + 68 p.
9. ———. A dental society reports on budget payment. Washington, Government Printing Office, 1960. 28 p.
10. ———. Speaking of prepaid dental care; a glossary of terms. Washington, Government Printing Office, 1959. IV + 25 p.
11. Donabedian, Avedis, Axelrod, S. J., and Agard, Judith. Medical care chart book. 3rd ed. Ann Arbor, Bureau Public Health Economics, School Public Health, University Michigan, 1968. VIII + 240 p. (p. 217)
12. Evaluating Committee V. The impact of financing on demands for dental services. p. 175-84. (In Proceedings of the workshop on future requirements of dental manpower and the training and utilization of auxiliary personnel. Ann Arbor, University Michigan, 1962. 206 p.)
13. Health Programs Branch, Division of Dental Public Health and Resources, Public Health Service. Digest of prepaid dental care plans; 1963. Washington, Government Printing Office, 1964. III + 152 p.
14. ———. Unpublished data.
15. Hillenbrand, Harold. Detroit speech arouses wide-spread editorial comment. Am. Dent. A. Newsletter, 13:2, Dec. 15, 1960.
16. Kriesberg, Louis, and Treiman, Beatrice R. Public attitudes toward prepaid dental care plans: a summary. Chicago, University Chicago National Opinion Research Center, 1961. 19 p. mimeog.
17. Lassiter, H. C. Not-for-profit dental plans: NADSP concept. A paper presented before the 17th National Dental Health Conference, American Dental Association, Chicago, Apr. 22, 1966.
18. Machinists multistate program. Med. Care Rev., 25:112-3, Feb. 1968.
19. McBride, W. C. Contract dentistry. J. Dent. Child., 9:95-6, 3rd Quar. 1942.
20. Metropolitan Life Insurance Company. Industrial dental service. New York, Metropolitan Life Insurance Company, 1944.
21. Mitchell, G. E., and Ake, James. Five-year report on the dental program of the I.L.W.U.-P.M.A. Washington, Division Dental Health, Public Health Service. 20 p. + 13 tables. Unpublished.
22. National Advisory Commission on Health Manpower. Report of the National Advisory Commission on Health Manpower. Washington, Government Printing Office, 1967. 2 vols., vol. 1. VIII + 95 p.
23. National Association of Dental Service Plans. Multistate programs. Am. Dent. A. Reports of Officers and Councils, 109:173, 1968.
24. New California contract to provide coverage to 114,000. Dent. Health Highlights, 19:19-20, June 14, 1963.
25. New dental insurance plan offered, giving coverage to small employers. New York Times, p. 63, 68, Apr. 15, 1968.
26. Onychuk, N. G. Potential of dental prepayment. A paper presented before the 19th National Dental Health Conference, American Dental Association, Chicago, Apr. 8-10, 1968.

THE PURCHASE OF DENTAL CARE

27. Reed, L. S. Blue Cross and medical service plans. Washington, Government Printing Office, 1947. 323 p.
28. Smith, Q. M. Public attitudes toward prepaid dental care. Mich. S. Dent. A. J., 44:119-24, 128, Apr. 1962.
29. Smith, Q. M., Mitchell, G. E., and Lucas, Gertrude. An experiment in dental prepayment; the Naismith dental plan. Washington, Government Printing Office, 1963. IV + 31 p. (p. 3-4, 17-22)
30. Source book of health insurance data. New York, Health Insurance Institute, 1966. 88 p.
31. Washington Dental Service. The first national conference on administration of prepaid dental care programs. Seattle, Washington Dental Service, c1962. 153 p.

Additional Readings

A comprehensive report on the profession's prepayment system—Delta Dental Plans. Am. Dent. A. J., 78:700-19, Apr. 1969.
Avnet, Helen H., and Nikias, M. K. Insured dental care; a research project report. [New York], Group Health Dental Insurance, c1967. 371 p.
Denenberg, H. S. Prepayment dentistry and commercial insurance. Am. Dent. A. J., 67:830-42, Dec. 1963.
Division of Dental Resources, Public Health Service. The dental service corporation; a new approach to dental care. Washington, Government Printing Office, 1958. V + 70 p.
Dixon, F. G. Administration and management of a dental service corporation. Mich. S. Dent. A. J., 43:297-303,306, Nov. 1961.
Eilers, R. D. Actuarial services for a dental service corporation. Washington, Government Printing Office, 1967. V + 85 p.
―――. Problems confronting the organization and growth of a dental service association. Am. Dent. A. J., 67:842-54, Dec. 1963.
Follmann, J. F., Jr. Medical care and health insurance; a study in social progress. Homewood, Ill., Richard D. Irwin, 1963. XV + 503 p.
Gillespie, G. M. The role of the dental-service corporation in providing oral health for groups of consumers. J. Pub. Health Dent., 25:6-23, Jan. 1965.
Hoggard, F. M. The Michigan Dental Service Corporation; a review of objectives and operations to date. Mich. S. Dent. A. J., 44:42-9, 51, Feb. 1962.
Lambert, Camille, Jr., and Freeman, H. E. The clinic habit. New Haven, College and University Press, c1967. 191 p.
Melone, J. J. Prepaid dental care and employee benefits programs. Am. Dent. A. J., 67:855-61, Dec. 1963.
Mitchell, G. E., and Hoggard, F. M., Jr. The dental service corporation; organization and development. Washington, Government Printing Office, 1965. V + 64 p.
Mitchell, G. E., et al. Prepaid dental care ... a glossary. Washington, Government Printing Office, 1965. 28 p.
Pelton, W. J., and Rowan, J. C. Digest of prepaid dental care plans, 1960. Washington, Government Printing Office, 1960. VIII + 103 p.
Penchansky, Roy, and Safford, Beryl M. Prepayment for dental care: need and effect. Pub. Health Rep., 81:541-8, June 1966.

CHAPTER 12

PUBLIC DENTAL CARE PROGRAMS

Several million individuals are eligible to receive dental care from federal clinics and institutions. State and local welfare agencies, health departments, and philanthropic organizations provide care for additional millions. Public care programs for various segments of the population represent, therefore, a significant part of dental practice. Dental care is provided by public agencies to a variety of groups for a number of reasons. Knowledge of the characteristics of these public care programs can enable the profession to make good judgments about the appropriateness and quality of such programs. It may become increasingly important for the profession to be well informed on this subject, because public dental care programs are expanding. Some of these programs will complement private practice and strengthen present patterns of practice; others may seem to threaten the independence and security of the practitioner. Dentists and dental hygienists should be able to discern any functional differences among various care plans. Such discernment should help them to be objective in identifying those programs they wish to support and those that they consider not in the public interest and wish to oppose.

As professional people, dentists and dental hygienists cannot limit their efforts to opposing proposals as unsound. They have an obligation to identify areas of public responsibility that have been neglected and to recommend well-conceived programs to alleviate problems. The professional health worker has a vital stake in the problems of those individuals who, for a variety of reasons, are unable to obtain health care for themselves or their families. As a member of society, he shares the common concern of others for the general welfare of the population. As a member of a health profession, he possesses unique knowledge and skill which are needed to provide health care and to devise mechanisms to bring this care to greater numbers of people. And finally, since the dentist and dental hygienist earn their livelihood by providing professional services, they have an immediate personal interest in the mechanisms by which health care is provided and purchased.

Geiger has summarized succinctly the interrelation between the professional person and the society in which he lives.

> "The practice of medicine . . . is . . . a treaty with society." This is a fresh and startling phrase, and it cuts to the heart of the matter, for it asserts that medicine [dentistry] is, in its essence, a part of the one intricate social fabric that binds us all, personally as well as professionally. It is this fabric that unites us as men and dictates our responsibilities as human beings; and it is only within this social framework, similarly, that the physician [dentist] (or the scientist, or the teamster, or the teacher) can assess his role and define his particular responsibilities.[11]

DEVELOPMENT OF PUBLIC CARE PROGRAMS

An understanding of the factors which led to the development of public care programs provides an insight into the nature of the programs and clues about the direction that future development may take. Public medical care programs have developed as a response to specific problems, not because of an undifferentiated sympathy for the "unfortunate." Although some reformers may have been motivated by pure idealism in their efforts to focus attention on the unsatisfactory conditions that existed in their time, the public policy decisions that evolved from these efforts were influenced to a large measure by pragmatic considerations of public self-interest. Early efforts to care for the mentally ill, for example, apparently stemmed more from a desire to protect the community from the dangers of allowing the "demented" to roam at will than from concern for the welfare of those suffering mental illness. Similarly, early community efforts to provide care for acute illness attempted primarily to isolate the indigent sick and so protect the health of the more affluent members of society.

Although concepts of public responsibility for ensuring the security of individual citizens have undergone great changes, enlightened self-interest still plays an important role in determining the development of public care programs. More than a century after Dorothea Dix's crusade to humanize the treatment of the mentally ill, for example, the economic value to the community of providing prompt treatment has often appeared to be at least as large a factor in motivating the expansion of hospitals and community facilities as have purely "humanitarian" considerations.

In an attempt to identify the factors which were responsible for their initiation, Straus has analyzed the medical care programs operated by the federal government.[22] The conclusions drawn from this study also can be applied generally to the efforts of state and local governmental units.

In 1798 the United States Congress established the Marine Hospital Fund (forerunner of the Public Health Service) to provide medical care for merchant seamen. In so doing, the infant nation followed the precedent of other countries which, because of the need for a merchant fleet, provided medical service in order to maintain an adequate supply of efficient seamen. A number of other factors influenced the decision to establish this first organized medical care plan in the United States. Because of the nature of their employment, it was recognized that seamen were subject to special hazards to health and safety. These problems were compounded by the itinerant nature of their calling. At home on the high seas, few had an established residence on land. For this reason, they were denied access to the meager community resources that existed for the indigent sick. Rarely could they purchase services themselves, because they ordinarily did not accumulate any financial resources and few had family ties. Thus they were cut off from the sources of medical services usually available to others. In addition, the port cities viewed the seamen as a threat to the health of the entire community because of their potential for carrying communicable disease from one port to another and because of their inability to obtain medical care.

From this modest beginning, the medical care activities of the federal government have expanded steadily as additional groups of beneficiaries have been included. In the 1800's organized medical care programs were instituted for members of the armed forces, veterans, and American Indians. In the first four decades of this century the list of beneficiaries grew to include federal prisoners and persons suffering from leprosy and drug addiction. Since then others have been added. In analyzing the groups that have been eligible for federal health care programs, Straus has identified six conditions which influenced the decision to offer care:

 1. When federal public medical services are in the interest of national defense or economic production.
 2. When such services are required by dependents or "wards" who are the peculiar responsibility of the federal government.
 3. When the health of the nation appears endangered and public concern is aroused over the threat of disease.
 4. When it is expedient to provide medical care as a form of guaranteed security or reward for persons who are needed to perform dangerous or undesirable work in the interests of society.
 5. When working or living conditions of persons performing work in the interests of society involve extra health hazards or extra health problems.
 6. When persons are isolated (physically, socially, econom-

ically) from access to adequate private or local public medical services.[22]

Health care programs have increased both in the number of groups eligible for care and in the scope of services offered. The reasons for these increases are rooted in changes which have taken place during the growth and maturation of American society. Factors that are probably most important in determining the growth of the public health care plans have been changes in public attitudes and expectations, changes in the character of economic life and resulting modifications in the ability of individuals to meet their own needs, and changes in the nature of the health sciences.

A somewhat different analysis of historical trends would appear useful. This analysis will consider (1) the "Poor Law" era, when general health care services were at an absolute minimum and dental care was practically nonexistent, (2) the development of an organized public medical and dental service on a somewhat systematic basis from 1935 to 1965, and (3) the recently enacted legislation that has brought about major changes in an established pattern.

HEALTH (AND DENTAL CARE) PROGRAMS IN THE "POOR LAW" ERA: 1700-1935

The early development of public care programs in the United States quite naturally reflected the experience in England, and to a certain extent this influence lingers in some public attitudes. The earliest structured form of social services in Britain was conducted by the monastic orders during the eleventh to fifteenth centuries. These orders maintained a vast system of social relief, conducting hospitals for the sick and mentally ill and giving the poor money for food. In 1536 and 1539 Henry VIII dissolved these monasteries by two acts of Parliament. The result was to create widespread destitution. In an attempt to deal with this problem, the "Poor Laws" were established in 1601 by Queen Elizabeth. These laws made it the duty of the local community, for its own area, to set to work the able-bodied who lacked the means to maintain themselves, to apprentice destitute children to various craftsmen, and to provide for the poor, the lame, and the blind whose families were unable to support them.

The problems of the impoverished and the problem of dealing with them were both heightened at this time by the first effects of the industrial revolution, which was to transform an agricultural society into an industrial one. This change meant that a society in which there were closely knit, self-contained families in isolated local communities who held themselves responsible for the care of their own poor and unfortunate became a highly industrialized urban society, with the problems of mass unemployment, starvation, and poor living and working conditions beyond the ability of any small group to handle. The voluntary migration to the cities encouraged overcrowding, disease, and epidemics. Women and children suffered severe hardships in the mines and factories.

The "Poor Laws" were an attempt by Parliament to deal with problems of social deprivation. At the start of the industrial revolution in 1760, however, these laws dealt only with the relief of destitution, which was as far as the state went in its feeling of responsibility for the personal well-being of its citizens. At this time the economic doctrine of laissez-faire was widely accepted, and this, combined with the Malthusian theories of population growth, allowed the governing classes to rationalize away any need to interfere to improve the lot of the poor.[9]

Malthus, in 1830, wrote that the growth of the population would exceed the expansion of the food supply. The growth of the population needed to be checked either by moral restraint or by the inroads of starvation, disease, war, or other disaster, all of which he grouped under the heading of "misery and vice." He advocated delayed marriage and continence as the preventive measures necessary but held that only the threat of misery would stimulate the masses to exercise this restraint. The source of terrible living conditions was not the result of unjust socioeconomic conditions, but of the natural laws of a "benevolent Creator, which, while they furnish the difficulties and temptations which form the essence of such a stage [of worldly probation], are of such a nature as to reward those who overcome them, with happiness in this life as well as in the next."[17]

Given this view, public welfare programs that were as degrading as possible and that maintained recipients at the level of misery were sanctioned by considerations of both public policy and the Almighty. Often-expressed criticisms about public welfare today (for example, that it encourages laziness or illegitimacy) would seem, in part, to reflect lingering traces of the writings of Malthus as well as the "Puritan ethic."

The earliest welfare efforts of colonial times quite naturally paralleled those of England and Europe in the 1700's. But again, changes in society in the United States—as in the rest of the world—brought about the gradual development of a variety of institutions to aid the needy. It is hardly necessary to review the evolutionary transitions that took place as America grew from a primarily agricultural economy clustered along the Atlantic seaboard to a nation of 50 states, wealthy beyond previous dreams, highly industrialized, and with the majority of the population living in urban centers.* The gradual

---

*An excellent review of the factors which have influenced the development of public welfare services has been given by Wilensky and Lebeaux and by Wickenden and Bell. Also suggested as recommended readings (at the end of this chapter) is a sampling of articles and reports which should form a part of the background information of any well-informed health practitioner. *The Report of The National Advisory Commission on Civil Disorders* in particular is recommended.

disappearance of the frontier territory signaled also the gradual disappearance of the frontier philosophy that every man could be sufficient to meet his own needs. Through the years there has been an increasing public concern for security against the unpredictable hazards of life and a greater recognition of an obligation to other members of society. There has also been a development of more economic equality and the growth of a large "middle class." In this context, government at all levels has played an increasing role in regulating what appeared to be excesses in private competition, in ensuring certain minimum standards of protection for all, and in providing a channel through which individual charity and concern could be institutionalized and made more effective and efficient.

The changes in the economic and social structure also modified the ability with which some segments of the population could cope with the problems of everyday living. As social organization became more complex, however, families and individuals became less self-sufficient. Increasing industrialization, in itself, has made the life of some individuals more difficult. For example, many adults of limited intelligence who could find employment as day laborers in the rural economy of a century ago could find no place in today's complex industrial society. Currently, dislocations created by the automation of industry illustrate how individuals who are willing and able to work may become unemployable because the skills they possess are no longer needed. As the standard of living of the population rises, the general concept of the requirements essential for life naturally rises also. As such societies evolve and advance, private and religious charities may no longer be adequate to handle the needs of all those who fall below the accepted idea of the minimum requirements. In this case, societies may develop new methods of ensuring that the basic needs of all their members are met. Eventually a social philosophy may be adopted which calls for the establishment of a minimum floor of economic security for all individuals, and agencies (such as voluntary health and welfare organizations and official departments of welfare) develop in an attempt to ensure that no group falls below this level.

The area of health services is one that has experienced great changes in public expectation. Even the very wealthy received but minimal medical care in colonial days. Through the 1800's there was little scientific knowledge about disease, and the standards of medical practice were low. Lawrence Henderson, the distinguished medical authority, noted that "it was about the year 1910 or 1912 when it became possible to say of the United States that a random patient with a random disease consulting a doctor chosen at random stood better than a fifty-fifty chance of benefiting from the encounter."[13] When effective health care was generally unavailable, the provision of medical care for the disadvantaged did not become a significant public issue.

To a large degree, the advances in scientific medicine have themselves created problems involved in providing health services for those segments of society unable to purchase them. The development of new knowledge and medical skill has created a new level of minimum needs and has presented society with new problems in meeting these needs. Furthermore, these advances in health care have occurred at a time when public concepts of the minimum level of need have risen rapidly. Medical care is considered by many to be the right of every individual, not the privilege of the wealthy.

Dentistry did not play a significant part in the early development of public medical care programs. Although a few public clinics were established on a voluntary basis by dentists as early as the 1850's, public dental care facilities remained almost nonexistent for many years. The Public Health Service, for example, did not employ dentists on a regular basis until 1919.[21] Until relatively recent times, the major health problem was to reduce death from infectious diseases. Oral health was of relatively little concern in the period when the population was decimated periodically by typhoid fever, diphtheria, cholera, and smallpox.

In recent years, with the major killers of the past under control, the health professions and the public have been able to devote their efforts to the control of chronic diseases, the rehabilitation of the handicapped, and the attainment of the maximum potential for productive living for every individual. As the nature of health problems changed, complete oral health care—in contrast to mere relief of pain and infection—has, in the minds of many, evolved from a luxury to a basic component of complete health service. As a result, there has been increasing public interest in obtaining more comprehensive service for themselves and in providing at least minimum dental service to the indigent.

PUBLIC WELFARE, MEDICAL AND DENTAL CARE PROGRAMS: 1935-1965

The year 1935 was a landmark in the history of governmental health programs, for it marked the passage of the original Social Security Act by the Roosevelt-dominated Congress. In the first place, the Act created a compulsory system based on employee-employer contributions to provide income maintenance for the elderly—a plan called social insurance by some and a payroll tax by others. The program was administered at the federal level and because of the use of separate payroll deductions did not compete for funding with other programs operating from general tax revenue. A subsequent section will discuss how this program was changed, 30 years later, to include the financing of physician and hospital services.

By the same act, a new mechanism was developed to support welfare and public health services. For the first time these areas of concern were assumed as a national responsibility. However, unlike the Social Security system, the administration of the new health and welfare programs remained at the state and local levels through a system of grants-in-aid. (A grant-in-aid is an appropriation of monies by the Congress to be used in a cooperative effort with the states for a particular purpose.) Both health and welfare programs were on a categorical basis. In this system Congress made funds available for certain *kinds* of health problems and certain *kinds* of people needing income support. The patterns of providing health and welfare services are changing now with great rapidity. To understand the significance of some of these changes, it is necessary to understand the established pattern of some 30 years' duration that is in the process of rapid evolution.

PUBLIC DENTAL CARE PROGRAMS

Federal Programs

Agencies of the federal government have participated in public dental care programs both by providing care directly and by providing financial assistance and consultation to the states and local communities.[27] The largest single group of individuals who have been eligible for dental care directly from the federal government are the military personnel (and, in limited instances, their dependents), who receive care from installations under the Department of Defense. The second largest direct care program has been operated by the Public Health Service to provide service for merchant seamen, members of the Coast Guard, American Indians and Alaskan natives, inmates of federal penitentiaries, and others. Immediately after the Second World War, the Veterans Administration had an extensive public dental care program, providing service to veterans both through government clinics and by purchasing care from private practitioners. The regulations governing eligibility were quite broad at first but were later tightened to include eligibility only for "service-connected" dental disabilities. With the passage of time, the dental program dwindled. Most of the service now provided by this agency is offered to inpatients in veterans' hospitals.

The American system of constitutional government is based partly on maintaining a balance between the power and responsibilities of the federal government and the governments of the states. In attempting to maintain this balance of power, the United States Congress frequently has been faced with an uncomfortable dilemma. Problems have arisen which — although they involved areas of responsibility that seemed traditionally to rest with the states—clearly appeared to be national in scope and to be of such major extent that they could not be handled by units of state government alone. Several decades ago, this dilemma was met partially by the development of a mechanism for the use of earmarked "grants-in-aid."

Monies were allocated among the states according to a specified formula. In order to receive these grants, the states had to expend their own funds for the same objectives as those supported by the grant-in-aid—often in the ratio of one dollar from state or local services to two dollars from federal sources.[12] In addition, a state had to comply with a few general regulations designed to ensure that the money was expended for the purpose for which it was appropriated, that proper accounting methods were maintained, and that personnel were employed on the basis of merit, not political affiliation.

It has been claimed by some that the grant-in-aid mechanism was an important factor in strengthening the effectiveness of state and local governmental operations. Still others have asserted that it has permitted an attack on problems of national scope without violating the sovereignty of the states. Grants were allocated on the basis of a formula which took into account the relative wealth of the state and its special problems, as well as the population. Grant-in-aid funds were awarded to the states, not to local communities. Depending upon the philosophy of government within the boundaries of each state, the funds could be used primarily to provide service directly from the state level or they could be distributed for use in supporting services administered at the local level.

Four constituent agencies of the Department of Health, Education, and Welfare have administered federal grants-in-aid which have been used to support public dental care programs.[8] The Public Health Service and the Children's Bureau both have made grants to states to support health department services which may or may not (depending on local custom and practice) have included the operation of public dental care programs. The Social Security Administration has supported state and local welfare agencies which underwrite health services to recipients of public welfare. The Office of Vocational Rehabilitation has supported programs for the rehabilitation of the handicapped—programs which often include the provision of dental care when it is important to the rehabilitation of an individual.

STATE AND LOCAL PROGRAMS

Administration of Dental Care Programs. Because the autonomous authority of state government largely has been preserved, the administration of public dental care efforts has differed widely from one area to another. Institutions (such as prisons or hospitals for the mentally ill), which usually represent a significant segment of public care activities in the state, may be autonomous or may be assigned to a department of health or welfare, a department of corrections, or a department of institutions. All states have vocational rehabilitation and crippled children's service agencies, but, again, they may exist as autonomous units or be assigned to some other agency in state government. Administrative responsibility for special segments of the population, such as residents of institutions or children with specific handicaps, is not too difficult to determine. The major confusion about the administrative responsibility for public dental care is in the area of providing services for the indigent — primarily in differentiating the responsibilities of departments of public welfare from those of departments of public health.

Part of the misunderstanding arose because the public and the health professions did not recognize differences in the purported basic objectives of public health agencies and public welfare agencies, and perhaps because they did not, the distinction became more and more blurred both in practice and in administrative organization as more and more states merged their departments of health and welfare. If these distinctions are not recognized, the health department may be viewed as an agency primarily concerned with the provision of care for certain segments of the population — particularly the indigent. The dental profession's view of the different objectives of the two types of public agencies was summarized in a statement adopted by the House of Delegates of the American Dental Association:

> Public welfare services are distinguished from public health services in that:
> a. public welfare services are primarily concerned with meeting emergencies created by the lack of funds to provide essential living requirements.
> b. public health services are directed toward attempts to help people help themselves and are concerned with the promotion of optimum health and the prevention of disease among all segments of the population.[6]

This differentiation is clear in principle but considerably less so in practice, since the participation of health departments in care programs has varied widely from one jurisdiction to another.* Some dental public health programs have provided no care; some have provided care to indigent children only; yet others have spent almost their entire budgets on treatment for the indigent or disadvantaged. These diverse patterns have been influenced by tradition in the

---

*The problem is further compounded by the distribution of the health needs. Modern public health programs seek to promote optimum health for the entire population. Yet those who find it most difficult to obtain health care (such as the indigent) are often those whose needs for care are the greatest. Thus an agency which strives to maintain a balanced program emphasis is confronted by the paradox pointed to by Anatole France: "The law, in its majestic equality, forbids all men to sleep under bridges, to beg in the streets, and to steal bread — the rich as well as the poor."[10]

ABBREVIATIONS:

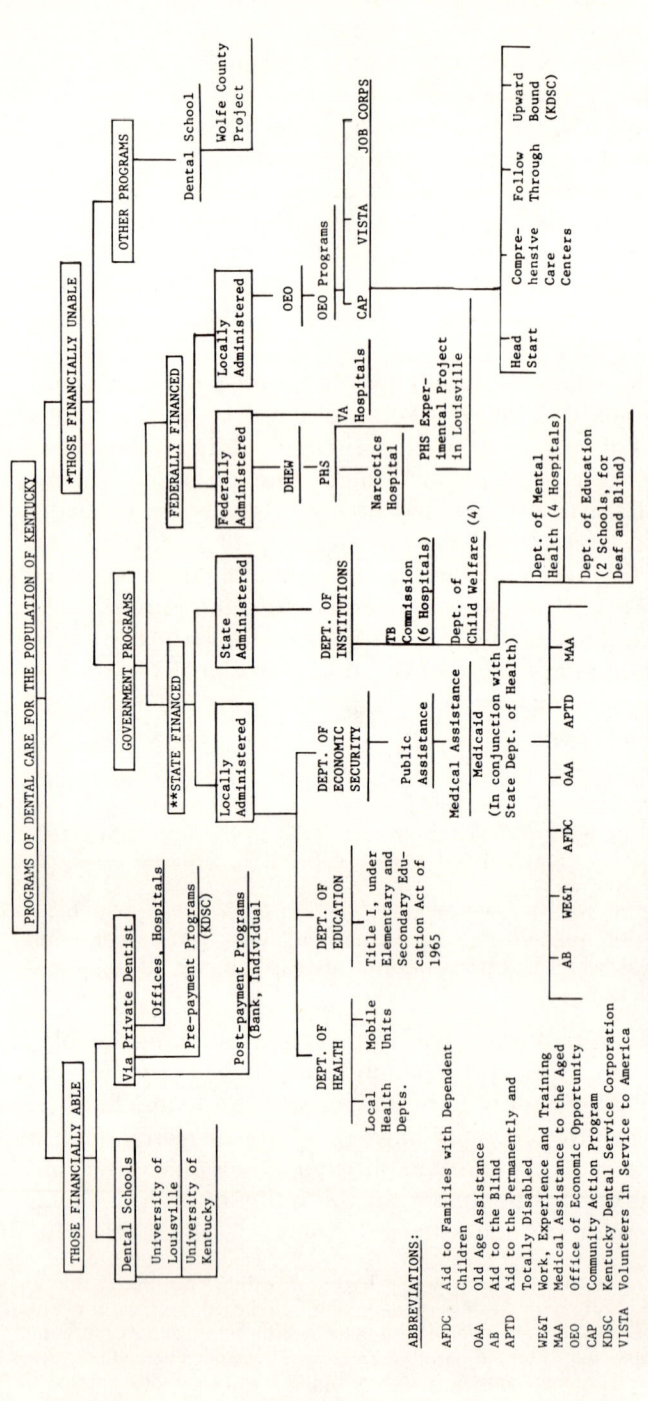

AFDC Aid to Families with Dependent Children
OAA   Old Age Assistance
AB   Aid to the Blind
APTD Aid to the Permanently and Totally Disabled
WE&T Work, Experience and Training
MAA   Medical Assistance to the Aged
OEO   Office of Economic Opportunity
CAP   Community Action Program
KDSC Kentucky Dental Service Corporation
VISTA Volunteers in Service to America

*Because of the scope of some of these programs, some people who are financially able may also be included.
**It should be remembered that almost all state funds originally come from the Federal Government, but in these programs the state serves as the middleman for funds.

FIGURE 25. One of the major characteristics of public dental care programs is their diversity. This chart indicates the variety of organized dental care efforts in one state in 1968. (Rodriquez, Mario, Chinea, Jose, and Kaplis, Norma. A survey of some dental care programs in the state of Kentucky: the extent to which care under these programs is available to indigent Kentucky children. [In Young, W. O., Fishman, S. R., and Shannon, Jean, eds. 1967-68 community dentistry fellowship program: summary and students' reports. Lexington, University Kentucky College Dentistry, 1968.])

jurisdiction concerned, by the particular needs of the area, and by the attitude of the dental profession. The variation in programs also has reflected philosophical differences among public health workers concerning the proper role of the health department in the provision of medical or dental care.

The establishment of a public care program traditionally has involved two basic decisions on public policy which have been determined by the legislative or executive authority in the particular jurisdiction. The first has related to the establishment of a care program—and its financing—for a specific segment of the population. The second basic decision has been to determine what agency of the local, state, or federal government would be assigned the responsibility of administering the program. In many jurisdictions, this administrative decision has been that medical and dental care programs might be more effectively administered by a health agency than by a welfare agency. In these cases, however, the care program was only one segment of a total program directed toward improving the health of the entire public.

The basic role of health departments in the provision of care has been summarized by the American Public Health Association: ". . . public health departments have an obligation and an unusual opportunity in the field of medical [dental] care. This is especially true in the prevention of disease and disability. Whether or not the public health agency participates in or actually administers medical care services, it should exert leadership in setting standards, in promoting quality and efficient use of resources through health education, demonstration and research."[24]

Eligible Groups and Scope of Services. The basic policies* of the American Dental Association on public and private responsibility for financing dental care are: (1) "Dental care should be available to all regardless of income or geographic location as rapidly as resources will permit. Private and community programs should provide

---

*The policies of the American Dental Association reflect the conviction that oral health services are important to the health and well-being of all individuals. These policies (whether concerned with dental care, education of the public, prevention of disease, support of research, or the government of the profession) follow the "principle of subsidiarity." Commenting on the application of this principle, Hillenbrand has said:

"This principle holds that the responsibility for the development and conduct of any program should rest with the smallest unit which has the capacity, and is willing, to carry out the obligation. . . . The principle of subsidiarity further holds that responsibility should not pass from the lower to the higher levels except for the strongest of reasons.

"This principle should not be construed, however, to place responsibility on the higher orders only in the most unusual circumstances. There are many programs which, by their very nature, require the energy and resources of a group rather than of an individual. Examples that come readily to mind are fire protection, police protection and the safeguarding of water and food supplies. In these areas, the individual and the family have placed their responsibilities in the hands of a community so as to insure a more effective service. . . . All of this philosophizing is by way of trying to identify the real responsibilities of the dentist, the component society and, in sequence, the constituent and national societies."[16]

for priority treatment, prevention and control of dental disease in children, and for the elimination of pain and infection in adults."[6] And (2) "... dental health should be the concern, first, of the individual, then the family, the community, the state and the nation in that order."[16]

INDIGENTS. Although it has been accepted widely, in theory at least, that society has a responsibility to provide dental care for the needy, the amount of dental care available to indigent families and those with marginal incomes varies considerably and is often nonexistent. Because of a lack of public programs adequate to meet the need, a significant part of the population has received no more than relief of pain and emergency extractions and can expect an early loss of teeth. Many individuals probably could not obtain even this minimum level of service.

An important factor was that grants-in-aid have been available to support assistance programs only for specific categories of needy individuals. By 1950 these categories included the blind, dependent children, the permanently and totally disabled, and the aged.[2] Those who did not qualify for aid under one of these four categories—even though they might be equally needy—were included in a catch-all program known as "general assistance," financed entirely by state and local funds. Health services could be, and often were, included in the assistance provided for those who could qualify for aid under these programs. In practice, however, many communities found the need for public welfare services so great, and their financial resources so limited, that only minimal amounts of basic medical service could be offered. Furthermore, those with marginal incomes—the "medically indigent," with incomes large enough to exclude them from public assistance but too small to meet the costs of medical care—could receive little help.

HANDICAPPED CHILDREN. In every community there are children who have unique dental problems resulting from or complicated by intellectual, physical, or emotional handicaps. The dental problems of handicapped children are unique for two reasons. The very nature of the handicap often makes it difficult to perform dental procedures. For this reason, the dentist providing service frequently must have skills and knowledge not usually taught in dental school, and there must be available special facilities, such as hospital and outpatient clinics, where premedication and general anesthesia can be used when indicated. In many areas neither the dentists with special training nor the special facilities for treatment are yet available. These dental problems are further complicated by the fact that the financial resources of the family frequently have been drained by the necessity of meeting a variety of special costs, such as for rehabilitative services, braces and appliances, extra assistance in the home, and special education and training. Even families with moderate incomes find it impossible to purchase all the services they need, and dental care is frequently one of the rehabilitative services which is ignored.

Children with oral clefts present some of the greatest needs for dental rehabilitation. The complete or partial failure of the segments of the lip and the roof of the mouth to unite creates a grotesque facial deformity and destroys the partition between the oral and nasal cavities. Unless therapy is successful, these individuals go through life with deformed noses, tightly scarred lips, mutilated palates, incoherent speech, and lack of a functioning dentition. Successful therapy requires the solution of a series of complicated clinical problems by a coordinated effort on the part of many specialists. Dentists play a key role in the team approach to therapy in guiding the development of the dental arches and facial pattern during growth, in constructing speech appliances which compensate mechanically for tissue deficiencies, and in maintaining the strategic natural teeth which are vital to rehabilitation therapy, proper appearance, and speech.

The cost of such extensive rehabilitation service is beyond the reach of all but a few families. As a result, most children with clefts have received care through state programs which provide services to crippled children or through private philanthropic organizations. In addition to financial assistance to meet the cost of rehabilitation services, effective team operation requires an organizational structure that can be provided best by a health department, medical school, teaching hospital, or rehabilitation center.

All state crippled children's service programs have provided services for children with oral clefts. (These programs have been administered by independent state agencies, by state departments of welfare, health, or education, or by universities and have been financed cooperatively by state funds and grants-in-aid from the U.S. Children's Bureau.) Furthermore, a number of rehabilitation centers offer this service either through contract with the official rehabilitation agency in the state or on a private basis. In addition to comprehensive rehabilitation services, routine dental care has been provided at no cost for children in most of these programs when their families were unable to bear the cost. The preservation of the natural teeth is of such vital importance to successful orthodontic treatment, surgery, and speech therapy, for example, that any rehabilitative program for these children should include routine dental care. A 1964 survey indicated that at least 41 states offered dental care as part of their rehabilitative services.[28]

Deformities of occlusion not associated with oral clefts can be considered a handicapping or "crippling" condition. Crippled children's service programs have been hesitant to provide treatment for malocclusion because of the shortage of orthodontists and the costliness of the service. The financing of public orthodontic treatment programs is complicated by the fact that some deviation from "normal" occlusion occurs frequently and there is no precise method of differentiating a malocclusion of minor significance from a severe dentofacial deformity. Despite these problems, the number of states including "disorders of occlusion, eruption, and tooth development" in their definition of crippling conditions eligible for care rose from only nine in 1950 to 26 in 1960, and the number of children receiving treatment through crippled children's service programs increased from 746 to 3,156.[20] In addition, some children have received treatment through dental divisions of state health departments, particularly in New York, which pioneered in the development of public orthodontic programs.[4]

Public orthodontic care programs limit service to severe problems found in children whose families cannot finance private care. The definition of what constitutes a "severe" deformity usually is developed in conjuction with an advisory committee of orthodontists, since these definitions must be broad and somewhat subjective. A consultant orthodontist or an advisory committee usually is utilized to review the children referred for treatment and to make the final decision as to eligibility.

Many mentally retarded children require special management technics in the dental office or in the hospital if restorative dental care is to be accomplished.[1] In the past, many retarded children were institutionalized at an early age, but today increasing numbers live at home during the formative years. The growing number of mentally retarded individuals in the community is due to a number of factors, including: (1) a longer life expectancy because of the availability of antibiotics and modern medical care; (2) the realization that many children have a better opportunity to develop what inherent potential they have if they can remain in the security of their own homes; and (3) the fact that the increasing numbers of mentally retarded individuals have overwhelmed the capacity of institutions for custodial care.

Cerebral-palsied children (including those who may show evidence of some retardation) have a variety of problems that complicate treatment.[1] The major difficulty stems from the frequency with which these children suffer extraneous dyskinetic movements of portions of or the entire body, making it difficult to perform mouth hygiene procedures and requiring special methods of stabilization to provide effective dental treatment. The difficulties in rendering service to the paraplegic or the quadriplegic are obvious. Other handicapped children who present special management problems are those suffering from muscular dystrophy or emotional disturbances.

In contrast to the relatively extensive provisions made to care for the dental needs of children with oral clefts, the oral health status of other handicapped children generally has been neglected. Until rather recently, community resources to assist in the provision of dental service for these individuals were quite rare. However, the dental problems of handicapped children have received increasing attention. A number of state dental divisions and crippled children's service programs have provided dental care as part of other rehabilitative services offered to children with specific handicaps. Throughout the United States, dental schools, teaching hospitals, rehabilitative centers, and outpatient clinics have established facilities to provide the special services necessary. Voluntary agencies, including the Society for Crippled Children and Adults (Easter Seal), the United Cerebral Palsy Association, and the National Association for the Mentally Retarded, have taken an active interest in the development of more adequate facilities and have established special clinics in a number of communities.

CHRONICALLY ILL ADULTS. The problems of providing dental care to chronically ill adults and to the aged are quite similar to those which complicate the treatment of handicapped children. Because of age, long neglect, or the debility caused by illness, the oral health status of these individuals frequently is poor. The treatment needed to restore the mouth to normal is often not obtained because of the lack of special facilities to provide treatment and because the illness and disability have exhausted the financial resources of the individual and his family. In a large measure, the current practice of dentistry is based on the premises that patients are ambulatory and can come to the dental office, that they are in fair physical condition, and that they have finances adequate to pay for care. Those potential patients who do not meet these criteria often find it difficult, if not impossible, to obtain dental treatment. The number of chronically ill and aged in the population of any community may be expected to increase, and the problem of providing dental care for the homebound and residents of nursing homes can be expected to be of increasing significance to the public and to the dental profession.

A Public Health Service demonstration project has pointed the way toward the development of effective community programs to meet the dental needs of the aged and the chronically ill.[7] Prevalence studies of more than 3,300 chronically ill patients in Kansas City indicated that almost eight out of 10 needed treatment. Of these, more than half were mentally and physically able to receive treatment if proper facilities were available. Dental services were provided either by transporting patients to a central clinic or by taking the dentist to the home, where specially designed portable equipment made it possible to perform routine restorative dental treatment.

The lessons learned in this project have not, to date, been applied widely throughout the United States. Because of the size of the problem and the necessity for organized effort to meet the need on a community basis, dental care for the majority of the chronically ill and the aged probably will not be a reality until official health and welfare agencies assume the responsibility of organizing and financing such programs.

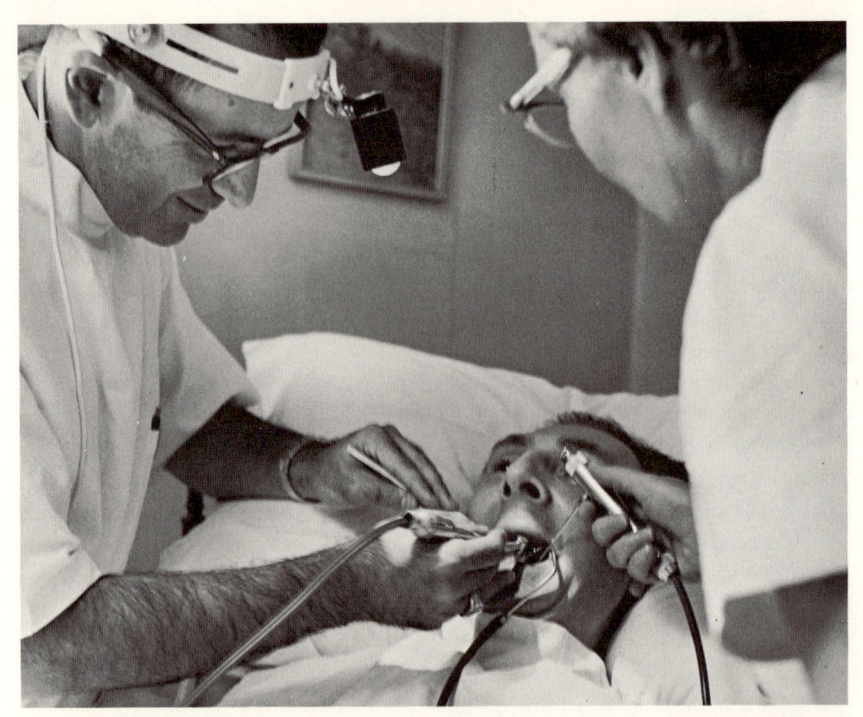

FIGURE 26. Dental treatment being provided for a homebound patient in the Kansas City project. (Courtesy Division of Dental Health, Public Health Service.)

THE INSTITUTIONALIZED. State and local agencies have assumed direct responsibility for a large number of individuals who are institutionalized in hospitals, prisons, and institutions for the care of the mentally retarded. It is estimated that more than one million persons are confined to these types of institutions—a patient load exceeding the population of each of 14 states.[26]

When an individual enters a state institution for the treatment of mental illness or tuberculosis, it would seem that the state should assume the responsibility for providing complete health care. Similarly, when an individual is imprisoned, the state should assume the responsibility for providing the minimum necessities for normal living, including medical care. If dental care is an essential health service, not an elective luxury, an institutional program cannot be considered adequate unless provisions have been made to provide dental service of high quality for the residents. A lack of proper dental services would seem to violate the moral obligation assumed by the state when a person is institutionalized.

Unfortunately, dental services in the institutions of a number of states are minimal—frequently limited to emergency care. The Council on Dental Health of the American Dental Association has urged all state dental societies to survey institutional dental services and to work to improve their caliber. The Association has recommended that responsibility for the dental care in all institutions in a a state be centralized in a single agency under professional dental supervision.[5]

The dentist in practice should be willing to assume professional responsibility for the oral health of the handicapped, the chronically ill, and the aged. In some instances, at least, dentists are hesitant to care for children with oral clefts because of the unusual technical problems sometimes encountered and for cerebral-palsied children because of difficulties in management. Similarly, patients with tuberculosis or mental illness may sometimes find it difficult to find a dentist willing to provide care, even when their physicians have indicated that treatment is safe for both the dentist and the patient. Even the aged may not always be welcomed in some dental offices, because they require extra care in management and because they often need additional time and attention from the dentist to alleviate their fears and anxieties. As a member of a healing profession, the dentist would seem to have at least two obligations. First, he should use his knowledge and skill to restore oral health and function to all those who seek his services — particularly those who are handicapped or ill. Many of these individuals, however, are not now able to seek his services. Therefore, the dentist's second obligation would appear to be to work with other dentists and the public to mobilize community resources for the provision of assistance to those who cannot help themselves.

WELFARE, MEDICAL AND DENTAL PUBLIC CARE PROGRAMS: 1965-

The 89th Congress (1965-1966) enacted more legislation with implications for the field of health than all 88 previous congresses. A wide variety of actions were taken affecting and effecting many agencies and programs. At the time this chapter is being written it is difficult to predict the exact size and shape of the changes taking place.

Some of the programs described earlier will not be modified greatly in the coming decade, particularly services for federal beneficiaries, handicapped children, and the institutionalized. The major impact of the new legislation will affect the Social Security system, recipients of public welfare, the organization of departments of health, and the funding of local health programs.

Social Security System. The best known health measure to be enacted in 1965 was the Medicare amendment (Title 18) to the basic Social Security legislation, which created a compulsory basic "insurance" plan for the aged, for hospital and related care, and a voluntary plan for physicians' services and other medical and health services. The most fundamental characteristics of the hospital plan are that participation is compulsory, benefits are by entitlement, not by need, and it is financed by its own payroll deduction.

For the first time in this country, a significant segment of the population is covered by a compulsory program that pays for the cost of health care regardless of economic need. The janitor and the company president are entitled to the same benefits if they are over 65. Since the cost of the program does not compete for regular tax dollars at either the state or federal level, it appears that it would be relatively easy for the number of beneficiaries and the scope of services to be increased. For example, the Secretary of Health, Education, and Welfare can ask that health services under Social Security be extended to cover all handicapped individuals at the same time that other federal agencies are engaged in a hectic effort to cut billions of dollars from ongoing programs to help reconcile a limited tax increase against the cost of an overseas war.

Public Welfare

For many years public welfare payments were made directly to recipients only. The size of the monthly check was determined by a formula which attempted to determine "minimum costs" for living, including housing, clothing, food, and—presumably—medical care. The total dollar amounts were ordinarily so low that most individuals could have afforded only limited emergency care. Furthermore, the choice was left to the recipient about whether to buy health care or some other item that he judged to be a "necessity."

A significant breakthrough in meeting health needs came with the passage of the so-called Kerr-Mills bill, which was an attempt (supported by both the American Dental Association and the American Medical Association) to meet the health care needs of the indigent aged. Although its sponsors had high hopes for its effectiveness in meeting the needs of this segment of the population, performance was disappointing: relatively few states elected to participate, and even those that did offered a fairly restricted range of services. (The passage of the bill actually preceded the 1965 date, but its major influence came later.) However, the Kerr-Mills plan introduced to the public welfare system the use of "vendor payments"; that is, payments directly to those who provided service.[18] This procedure removed payment of health care from the area of elective choice by the recipient. The plan also served as the predecessor to the major changes brought about in the 1965 amendments to those sections of the Social Security Act relating to public welfare programs —Title 19, a new program commonly referred to as Medicaid.

The controversy over Medicare (Title 18) tended initially to obscure the significance of its companion legislation. Whereas Medicare (Title 18) specifically excludes dental care except under rare circumstances, Title 19 is of much more immediate relevance to the dental profession because it promises to bring about major increases in dental care services financed from public funds. The Title 19 amendment was designed to implement the provision of comprehensive health care (including dental care) on a gradual basis over a 15- to 20-year period. The states were allowed some latitude in deciding the pace with which they would move into the health care field. However, the Congress made the eventual implementation almost mandatory by ruling that federal matching funds (grants-in-aid) would be cut off unless states met certain deadlines.[23]

In general, the pattern has been to offer minimum basic health services to those in the categories eligible for cash payments—the blind, dependent children, the permanently and totally disabled, and the aged. Customarily the scope of services to be offered is next broadened. Finally, services are provided for the "medically indigent": those who have an income sufficient to disqualify them from receiving cash payments. States had the right to implement all or part of the program immediately after passage of the law and a number did so. In order to continue receiving the federal grants which pay for the major share of the entire public welfare program, the states must have implemented at least part of the program by 1970. By July 1, 1975, all states must provide comprehensive health care for all indigent and medically indigent persons.

It is possible that the Congress may relax the timetable for the implementation of the entire program of health services if the states find it difficult to assume their share of the cost, as has been so in several instances. Nevertheless—give or take a few years—it seems clear that the health professions are faced with the task of providing comprehensive care to a large segment of the population that has until now received only minimal emergency service.

DEPARTMENTS OF HEALTH

Current programs of state and local health departments have been greatly influenced by the availability of grants-in-aid appropriated by the Congress to attack special health problems. Under this system generous appropriations might be available for heart disease control, for example, but little for improving the sanitation standards of restaurants. In many areas program priorities were also strongly influenced by the views of the health practitioners in the area. This influence was often exerted directly through membership on the board of health that established policy directly. In other areas this influence was exerted less directly through pressures on or persuasion of the physicians, dentists, or nurses working for the department.

It is to be expected that this pattern will be changed considerably by the impact of the "Comprehensive Health Planning and Public Health Service Amendments of 1966" (P.L. 89-749). Instead of grants-in-aid earmarked for specific programs, the states will now receive one lump sum, "block grants," to assist them in providing "comprehensive public health services." In order to establish priorities at the state level, separate grants are made to establish and support state planning councils, and in some instances, local or area councils. The councils are to be composed of representatives of state health agencies, nongovernmental organizations and groups concerned with health, and consumers of health services. The *consumers* of health services must constitute a *majority* of the council.

During the coming decade, the health professionals will increasingly find that the final decisions about establishing and maintaining health programs will not be theirs, but will rest in the hands of knowledgeable laymen. If the recommendations made by physicians and dentists are reasonable and clearly in the public interest, they will probably be accepted. If these recommendations are shortsighted and self-serving, they will probably be rejected.

Local Health Program Funding

The state health department (and in large cities, the local health department) traditionally has been the unit for the planning and implementation of dental health programs. In some areas, local school boards have also used tax revenue to provide both educational and corrective dental services. In either instance a tradition has been established and the dental profession usually has known who was providing services and the character of these services.

Such is no longer true, and the profession frequently finds it difficult to know what kind of public programs are being planned, or even who is planning such efforts. There are now a variety of funding mechanisms that may be made available directly from the federal government to local agencies, often to nonhealth-oriented organizations. Several types of grants designed to strengthen elementary and secondary school programs may include dental care at the option of local officials. Similarly, the local programs funded by the Office of Economic Opportunity usually include the provision of dental treatment in one way or another. Often grant applications are prepared by local people and funded by Washington agencies without prior consultation with the dental profession. In the future, members of the profession will need to become much more knowledgeable about the activities of local agencies if they expect to be in a position to offer timely and appropriate consultation.

Neighborhood Health Centers

One of the developments most disturbing to organized dentistry has been the establishment of Neighborhood Health Centers by the Office of Economic Opportunity. These centers are designed to offer a full range of comprehensive health services to the residents of the poverty area in which they are located. The residents of the area are involved in planning for the center's operation. The centers are staffed by salaried physicians, nurses, social workers, dentists, and a variety of aides and auxiliaries.

The development of this concept has apparently committed the O.E.O. to the provision of care for a large number of people in what are essentially "closed-panel" clinics staffed by salaried personnel. The officials contended that private practice cannot adapt to meet the health needs of the poor, who have special problems of ignorance, lack of transportation, and suspicion of existing agencies.

It is also contended that the Neighborhood Health Center concept results in more efficiency, better control of quality, less expense, and a less fragmented type of service, brought to the consumer near his home and under one roof. Better continuity and comprehensiveness of services are also claimed. Furthermore, the planners point out that private health practitioners are rarely located in the ghettoes of the inner city where the disadvantaged are.

Spokesmen for organized dentistry have pointed out:

> O.E.O. betrays an excessive reliance on public sector technics in health care delivery in an apparent belief that the private practice system is too inflexible, or private practitioners too unwilling, to make a genuine contribution to this endeavor. In the short run, this reliance has already led O.E.O. into championing a technic that, whatever its value in some circumstances, may well be questionable as a permanent or total solution to the given problems.
>
> It is neither equitable nor sensible to discount in advance, without offering it a full opportunity to participate, the private practice system that encompasses most of the nation's health service potential.[3]

Other spokesmen for organized dentistry have claimed that there is no proof that the Neighborhood Health Center is less expensive or more efficient. They contend further that if the disadvantaged are to be brought into the "mainstream" of American life it will not be through public clinics with the old stereotype of long waits on hard benches and impersonal treatment, but through the traditional medium of private practice, where the bulk of dental care is now rendered. They also question shifting the short supply of dental personnel from their already established practices to public clinics.

There are obviously merits and demerits to both systems. Already some 40 to 50 Neighborhood Health Centers have been established in major cities. Whether they will continue, be modified, or be abandoned, and to what degree dentistry will be involved, are

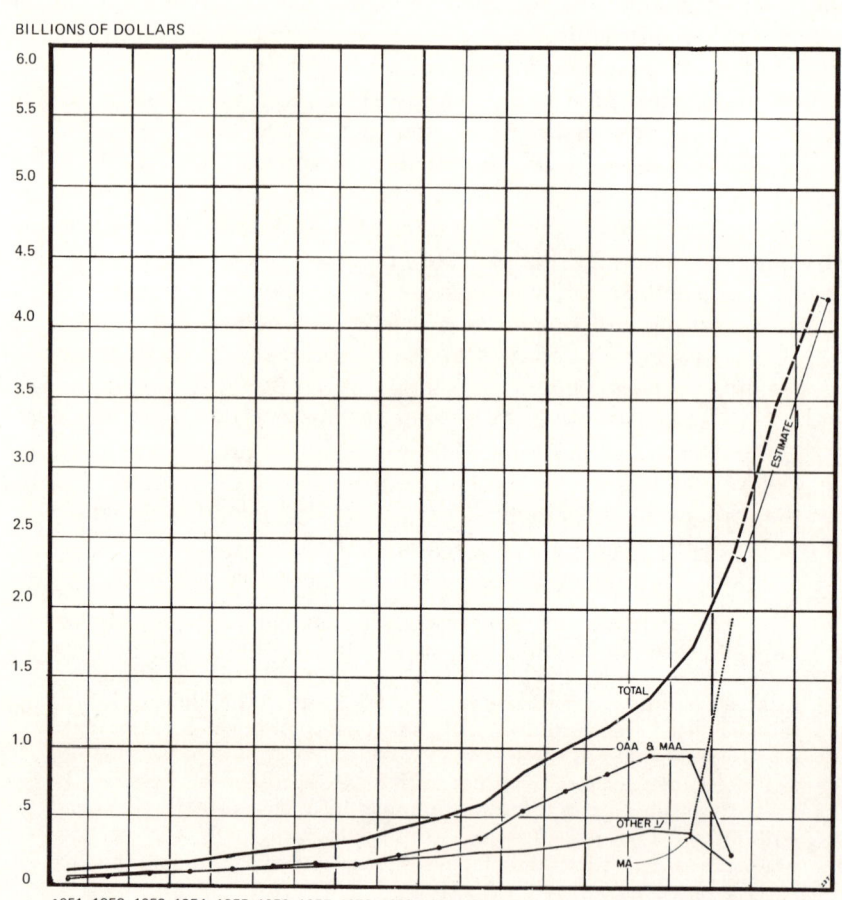

FIGURE 27. The growth of federally assisted payments to the providers of health services. [Abbreviations refer to: Aid to the Blind; Aid to the Partially and Totally Disabled; Aid to Families with Dependent Children; General Assistance; Old Age Assistance; Medical Assistance to the Aged; and Medical Assistance.] This chart dramatically demonstrates both the rapid growth of public care programs and the shift from the categorical aid programs to the broad coverage under Title 19. (Source: Department of Health, Education, and Welfare, Budget Justification FY 1969)

[1] AB, APTD, AFDC, and GA.

difficult to predict. Probably the Centers will be continued in some modified form and in combination with some form of the private practice of dentistry as it is now known, possibly with some government-assisted system of prepaid financing. In any event, it is wise for the dental health practitioner to remember that for each one of him there are 2,000 members of the public. Therefore, he must be both responsive and responsible in his dealings with the public of his community.

FUTURE DEVELOPMENT OF PUBLIC DENTAL CARE PLANS

One of the consistent trends in the development of modern societies has been an increasing governmental concern for the lives of its citizens. Participation by governmental agencies in health affairs has expanded rapidly, particularly since the First World War. There are good reasons to believe that governmental activity in health affairs may continue to increase, possibly at an accelerated rate.

As the caliber of available medical services has improved, medical and hospital costs have been pushed higher and higher. Advances in technology, the development of new and expensive drugs, the need to utilize a wide range of specialists' services—in fact, virtually all the developments which have contributed to improved care—have meant more expensive care and, consequently, greater urgency in finding ways to finance it. Increased medical knowledge and skill have helped to create a sharp rise in the need and demand for health care. The increase in longevity has resulted in a larger number of older people in the population and an increase in morbidity and disability— especially mental illness and various types of chronic disorders—the areas in which medical science is still least effective. As a result, improved levels of health have intensified the problem of payment for medical service. Furthermore, as previously stated, public attitudes toward health care have undergone revolutionary changes and many now apparently view medical care as a civic right, not as a private luxury. All of these factors have contributed to the public interest in the organization of health services and to the resulting political pressures. Although dental care is not as immediate an issue as hospitalization and physicians' services, any pattern established in medicine may be expected to influence dentistry.

Increasing governmental participation in health affairs, particularly the growth of care programs, has been viewed with concern by many members of the health professions. Many dentists have feared that public care programs for various segments of the population might expand gradually until they include all citizens. If so, the United States would join the large group of nations that provide tax-supported health services under a nationwide health system. Reports from other countries have convinced many members of the dental profession in the United States that such plans apparently are detrimental both to the public and to the profession, that they may become exorbitantly expensive, and that the control and regimentation which may be imposed on the profession encourage mediocrity.*

Whether or not a form of state medicine eventually may be adopted in this country may depend to some degree on the actions of the health professions, but the final decision will be made by the public. Eventually those arrangements that are seen by the public as necessary to secure services deemed sufficiently valuable will probably be adopted. A Secretary of the Canadian Dental Association, reflecting experience in a nation where the dental profession is facing threatening political pressures, has pointed out:

> ... a crisis in health services has been building up on a worldwide basis, particularly during the last two decades, and the climax has been reached in every developed country save two or three. If action from outside the profession is to be avoided it will be necessary for constructive efforts to be made within the profession. In the light of experience elsewhere, acceleration of all activities in solving existing problems is essential. In doing so the interests of both those who receive the services and those who provide the services must be understood and protected. The great difference between now and a few years ago is that decisions related to the methodology of health services have become two-party agreements whereas formerly, alteration was determined by the profession alone.[15]

It does appear that the health professions will not prevent the development of state medicine in this country merely by expressing opposition to any change in the status quo. The best opportunity may lie in the development of plans to meet the health needs of the public

---

*The dental profession has opposed compulsory health insurance vigorously and usually with clarity and precision. The same clarity of thinking frequently has been lacking in much public debate over the proper role of government in health affairs. Although the term "socialized medicine" may originally have been valuable in defining certain aspects of public life, it has been so widely misused that it may contribute to misunderstanding rather than clarification. Many dentists and physicians seem to use the term "socialized medicine" to define any type of activity with which they are not in agreement.

Probably few practitioners are opposed to all "socialized medicine." Socialized medicine is defined as: "Administration by an organized group, a state, or a nation of medical and hospital services to suit the needs of all members of a class or all members of the population by means of funds derived from assessments, philanthropy, taxation, or other sources."[14] Compulsory health insurance, included in this definition, is opposed by most dentists. Other forms of "socialized medicine," such as the care provided by the good ship *Hope* or the health care provided soldiers in Vietnam, would appear so clearly desirable as to be noncontroversial.

The type of governmental intervention most feared by the dental profession apparently is *state medicine,* defined as: "Administration and control by the national government of medical and hospital services provided to the whole population and paid for out of funds raised by taxation."[14] Dentists who are opposed to *state medicine* might well say so and leave the use of fuzzy terms such as "socialized medicine" to those who are ignorant of their meanings.

through a variety of mechanisms that preserve the greatest degree of independence for the profession. In some cases it may be desirable to lend active support to governmental efforts to meet health needs that cannot otherwise be attacked effectively. Obvious examples of these types of efforts are the provision of dental care for the indigent, the support of dental research, and the strengthening of public health programs of prevention and health education. In addition to supporting positive programs in these areas, the American Dental Association has urged its membership to support voluntary programs to meet the dental health needs of certain segments of the population through cooperative mechanisms, such as dental service corporations.

The challenge to the dental profession was summarized by Patton in 1961 while he was president of the American Dental Association: "The greatest danger . . . is not the invasion of health fields by the government, but, rather the loss of leadership by the health professions. We have the heavy responsibility to demonstrate the faults of certain proposals or plans, to suggest alternatives that will better meet the needs of the public interest. . . . The profession must be both watchful and constructive."[19]

ADA DENTAL HEALTH PROGRAM FOR CHILDREN

The American Dental Association did move to provide the type of leadership called for by Dr. Patton. The House of Delegates at the 107th Annual Session of the Association adopted a proposal for a "Dental Health Program for Children." The objective of this program was stated as follows:

OBJECTIVE: The objective of the American Dental Association Dental Health Program for Children should be to make the benefits of an organized program of dental health education, preventive dentistry and dental care available to all children, particularly the needy and underprivileged.

This objective should be attained by the application of the following principles:

1. All dental services should be provided which are necessary to prevent disease and to restore and maintain oral health.

2. Guidance and consultation at local, state and national levels should be made available by the profession, through dental associations, in the planning, operation and evaluation of the program.

3. There should be full cooperation in planning, operating and financing the program between private and public agencies at local, state and national levels.

4. The scope of the local program should be determined at the community level and should be based on the general standards which have been established through the state and national programs.

5. The use of all preventive measures should be en-

couraged and an incentive program for the intensive promotion of the fluoridation of public water supplies should be established.

6. Increased support should be provided for research in all procedures and programs for improving the dental health of children.

7. All preschool and school children, through the age of 18 years, should be included in the program and existing resources should be made available on a priority basis to the younger age group.

8. The initial program in each community should be expanded on a planned and systematic basis to include additional age groups of the school population as rapidly as experience and resources permit.

9. The dental health education components of all local, state and national programs should be expanded.

10. Every individual should be encouraged to develop increasing responsibility for his own dental health and parents should be motivated to full responsibility for the dental health of their children.

11. The services of private practitioners and of all existing resources and facilities should be utilized fully in the operation of the program.

12. The right of freedom of choice by both the patient and the practitioner should be preserved.

13. The highest quality of dental services should be available to all.

14. The opportunities for the basic and continued education of dentists and dental auxiliaries should be expanded as needed in order to insure an adequate supply of qualified personnel for the program.

15. The use of the voluntary prepayment and postpayment programs for the purchase of dental care for children should be expanded.

16. Priority consideration should be given to reimbursement for professional services on the "usual and customary fee" basis.

17. Fiscal responsibility for the dental care of nonindigent children and families must continue to lie with the individual, the family and private and voluntary agencies.

18. The terms indigent and dental indigent, for the purpose of this program, should be defined by appropriate state agencies in accordance with existing state laws and regulations in full consultation with representatives of the dental profession.[25]

It was recommended that the program be initiated with a series of pilot or exploratory programs to provide the experience necessary to predict the cost and to develop appropriate administrative mechanisms. It was suggested, therefore, that project grants be made available by the federal government to start such experimental efforts. Essentially the plan would call for the establishment of comprehensive prepayment insurance for all children in the community. Initially only selected groups would be offered coverage, but as the backlog of treatment needs was reduced and manpower shortages eased, additional groups of children would be added. The cost of the prepayment premiums for indigent children would be met by public funds made available on a matching basis between the federal and the state agencies. It was hoped that the wide variety of different agencies at the federal level that provide some type of dental benefit could pool their efforts into a single source of funds for the national plan. Parents who were not indigent would be allowed and encouraged to purchase dental care for their children on a prepaid basis also. Hopefully, all members of selected groups of children would have complete protection against the cost of routine dental care.

It is difficult to predict the extent to which this ambitious proposal may be accepted by the administration and the Congress. The initial course has been a cautious one involving a proposal for a minimum of funding for experimental programs. It is not clear whether or not the principles of giving priority to children, on an incremental basis—both of which are in conflict with the current legislation setting up Title 19—will be incorporated into law. Finally, the various federal agencies that include dental care among their programs will probably be reluctant to surrender their existing programs in order to put together the united effort called for by the American Dental Association.

A proposal for a national dental health plan for children would develop a long-range comprehensive partnership between the profession and the federal government. In making the proposal, the Association has moved into the potentially hazardous frontiers of pioneering new relations between the health professions and government. Experience in the United States has indicated that such partnerships can be satisfactory and fruitful. The partnership between the academic community and the National Institutes of Health is an indication of the strength that comes from a properly developed relation. Similarly, the space program is a remarkable tribute to the effectiveness of the partnership between government appropriations and administration and the free enterprise initiative and drive of the American business community. Other attempts at forming such a partnership have been less successful—sometimes for both sides.

Some hold that the American Dental Association has courageously taken a gamble with the future of the profession. The Association has recognized that the interaction between the profession of dentistry and government can only become more and more involved with the passage of time. It has learned the lessons obvious in the observation of changing currents in politics and the social scene. It has wisely determined that the greatest chance to develop a partnership that would be mutually beneficial to the profession and the public would be to take the initiative in beginning the dialogue and cooperative effort, rather than to wait until it was overtaken by the developments of time. Now, only time itself can reveal whether this course of action was appropriate.

BIBLIOGRAPHY

1. Album, M. M., ed. Proceedings of the workshop on dentistry for the handicapped. Philadelphia, (University Pennsylvania), 1958. 121 p.
1a. Advisory Committee on Intergovernmental Relations. A Commission report;

intergovernmental problems in Medicaid. Washington, Government Printing Office, 1968. XIV+ 122 p. (p. 20).
2. Bierman, Pearl. Dental health care in public assistance programs. Am. Dent. A. J., 54:189-94, Feb. 1957.
3. Bishop, E. M., and Christensen, H. M. Dentists and the war on poverty: a discussion on Neighborhood Health Centers. Am. Dent. A. J., 75:45-54, July 1967.
4. Bushel, Arthur, and Ast, D. B. Rehabilitation programs for the dentally physically handicapped child. Am. J. Pub. Health, 43:1156-61, Sept. 1953.
5. Council on Dental Health, American Dental Association. Dental care programs in state institutions. Am. Dent. A. Tr., 99:100-1, 1958.
6. ———. Official policies of the American Dental Association on dental health programs. Chicago, American Dental Association, c1957. 77 p. (p. 7, 8, 49)
7. Division of Dental Public Health and Resources, Public Health Service. Dental care for the chronically ill and aged; a community experiment. Washington, Government Printing Office, 1961. VI+ 54 p.
8. Easlick, K. A., ed. The administration of local dental programs. Ann Arbor, Continued Education Service, School Public Health, University Michigan, c1963. VIII + 278 p. (p. 16-23)
9. Eastep, P. B. Development of dental care programs for the children of Great Britain and the United States. Lexington, University Kentucky, College Dentistry, 1968. VIII + 139 p. Typed thesis.
10. France, Anatole. In Crainquebille (Cited in Seldes, George, comp. The great quotations. New York, Caeser-Stuart: Lyle Stuart, c1960. XI + 892 p.) (p. 254)
11. Geiger, H. J. Social responsibility of the physician. Scient. Mo., 85:89-94, Aug. 1957.
12. Gerrie, N. F. Grants-in-aid in federal-state dental public health program relationships. Am. Dent. A. J., 54:182-8, Feb. 1957.
13. Gregg, Alan. Challenges to contemporary medicine. New York, Columbia University Press, 1956. 120 p. (p. 13)
14. Gove, P. B., ed. Webster's third new international dictionary of the English language, unabridged. Springfield, Mass., Merriam, c1961. 56a + 2662 p. (p. 2162, 2229)
15. Gullett, D. W. The meaning of the present. Am. Col. Dent. J., 27:213-21, Dec. 1960.
16. Hillenbrand, Harold. The 1960 workshop on prepaid dental care; part II. Mich. S. Dent. A. J., 42:366-72, Oct. 1960.
17. Malthus, Thomas. A summary view of the principle of population. p. 13-59. (In Three essays on population [a Mentor Book]. New York, New American Library World Literature, 1960. X + 144 p.)
18. Mitchell, G. E. Patterns and prospects in public assistance dental care. Am. Dent. A. J., 68:76-82, Jan. 1964.
19. Patton, C. H. Report of president. Am. Dent. A. Tr., 102:9-16, 1961.
20. Saffian, Sadie. Program trends in crippling conditions, 1950-1960. Washington, Government Printing Office, 1962. 40 p.
21. Schmekebier, L. F. The Public Health Service. Baltimore, Johns Hopkins, 1923. 298 p. (p. 66-7)
22. Straus, Robert. Medical care for seamen; the origin of public medical service in the United States. New Haven, Yale, 1950. XVI + 165 p.
23. Summaries of recent legislation affecting dentistry. Bethesda, U.S. Department Health, Education, Welfare, Public Health Service, Division Dental Health, 1968. n.p.
24. Technical Development Board, American Public Health Association. Public health role in medical care. Am. J. Pub. Health, 50:569-70, Apr. 1960.
25. The American Dental Association Dental Health Program for Children. Chicago, American Dental Association, n.d. 30 p.
26. U.S. Bureau of the Census. Statistical abstract of the United States, 1967. 88th ed. Washington, Government Printing Office, 1967. XII + 1050 p. (p. 79, 164)
27. Young, W. O. Dental health. p. 5-94. (In Hollinshead, B. S., dir. The survey of dentistry; the final report. Washington, American Council Education, c1961. XXXIV + 603 p.)
28. Young, W. O., and Mink, J. R. Dental care for the handicapped child. Rehabilitation Lit., 26:98-103, Apr. 1965.

Additional Readings

A nation within a nation. Time, 91:24-32, May 17, 1968.
Bergner, Lawrence, and Yerby, A. S. Low income and barriers to use of health services. New Eng. J. Med., 278:541-6, Mar. 7, 1968.
Drew, Elizabeth B. Going hungry in America; government's failure. Atlantic, 222:53-61, Dec. 1968.
_____. Reports; Washington. Atlantic, 223:4-14, Jan. 1969.
Division of Dental Resources, Public Health Service. The dental service corporation in a public assistance program; a report from Washington State. Washington, Government Printing Office, 1959. VI + 50 p.
Hawkinshire, F. B. W. Thoughts and feelings about poverty; a brief summary of two workshops on understanding the underprivileged child. Chicago, American Dental Association, (1969). 82 p. + appendices.
Herzog, Elizabeth. About the poor; some facts and some fictions. Washington, Government Printing Office, 1967. 85 p.
Irelan, Lola M., ed. Low-income life styles. Washington, Government Printing Office, 1966. VIII + 86 p.
Kerner, Otto, chm. Report of the National Advisory Commission on Civil Disorders. New York, Bantam, 1968. XXV + 609 p. + charts. (paperback)
Ralston, R. M., ed. Sources; a Blue Cross report on the health problems of the poor. Chicago, Blue Cross Association, c1968. 64 p.
Schorr, Lisbeth B., and English, J. T. Background, context and significant issues in Neighborhood Health Center programs. Milbank Mem. Fund Quar., 46:289-96, July 1968 (Part 1).
Somers, H. M., and Somers, Ann R. Doctors, patients, and health insurance. Washington, Brookings Institution, c1961. XIX + 576 p.
Time essay; Welfare and illfare: the alternatives to poverty. Time, 92:25-6, Dec. 13, 1968.
Wickenden, Elizabeth, and Bell, W. Public welfare; time for a change. New York, Office University Publications Columbia University Press, c1961. IX + 124 p.
Wilensky, H. L., and Lebeaux, C. N. Industrial society and social welfare. New York, Russell Sage, 1958. 401 p.

CHAPTER 13

DENTAL MANPOWER RESOURCES

Today, the ability of the profession to discharge its responsibilities is threatened by a potential, if not real, shortage of personnel as well as by maldistribution. Unless dentistry can cope with increasing demands for service, pressure groups may be expected to urge the use of less trained personnel in ways which may not seem appropriate to the dental profession. The graduating dentist has a particular interest in the study of dental manpower resources, since he must choose a location to establish practice. The relative supply of dentists varies widely from state to state and from city to city. As a result, some areas consistently suffer a lack of dentists; others may have more dentists available than are needed to satisfy public demand regardless of regional or national shortages. The selection of a location to establish practice should be guided partly by a knowledge of the relation between the demand for service and the supply of professional personnel.

SUPPLY OF DENTISTS

TRENDS IN RELATIVE SUPPLY[*]

The census of 1850, the first in which dentists were enumerated separately, listed 2,900 dentists serving a population of 23

---

[*]The relation between the number of dentists and the population to be served may be calculated on the basis of the number of *active* dentists, the number of *practicing* dentists (excluding those active dentists engaged full time in teaching, research, or government service), or *all* dentists. Ratios based on the number of active dentists are comparable with data from the U. S. Census. Historical trends can be expressed

million—one dentist for every 8,000 persons.[24] During the last half of the nineteenth century the profession expanded rapidly, its membership swelled by those trained as apprentices or in the growing number of dental schools. By 1900 the number of dentists had more than tripled and the count of persons per dentist had dropped to about 2,550.

For the next three decades the profession continued to grow more rapidly than the population, and by 1930 the country had the most favorable ratio of persons per dentist ever attained: one dentist to 1,728 persons. The year 1930 marked a sharp turning point, and from that year to date the relative supply of dentists has declined.

The reversal of the trends in dentist supply was caused initially by changes in dental education. Soon after the first dental school was established in 1840, the recognition that a school was a potential source of profit spurred a rapid increase in educational facilities. Perhaps as many as 150 dental schools, both good and bad, were established from 1850 to 1920.[24, 33] Many operated only for short periods of time, but some, particularly those affiliated with universities, have remained in operation to this day. The period of rapid growth came to an end as the profession moved to improve the quality of dental education and eliminate substandard programs. The efforts of the Dental Education Council (formed in 1909 and the predecessor of the Council on Dental Education) culminated in 1926 when a minimum of one year of college was required prior to entrance into a four-year professional curriculum. The publication of a four-year study of dental education by William Gies in the same year hastened the demise of the proprietary school—the last such institution became a public trust in 1929.[33]

Strengthening the dental curriculum reduced the number of graduates, both by eliminating substandard schools and by lowering the number of potential students who could meet the entrance requirements and the demands of the course of study. Shortly thereafter, the impact of the depression cut still further into dental school enrollments. During the 1930's, not enough dentists were graduated to replace those lost by death or retirement but, because of the decelerated birthrates during this period, the number of persons per dentist rose only to 1,870 by 1940.

The diminishing supply of dentists became particularly apparent when large numbers of practitioners were withdrawn from the

---

most easily by counts of active dentists (excluding those in the federal service, since they do not serve the civilian population) taken from census enumerations and estimates of the Division of Dental Health of the U. S. Public Health Service.[22, 23, 38–44] Counts of all dentists, although showing a slightly unrealistically larger supply, reflect essentially the same relation between the supply of dentists and the population. Data based on the total numbers of dentists, developed by the Bureau of Economic Research and Statistics of the American Dental Association from listings in the *American Dental Directory*, are of particular value because they provide more detailed current information on such factors as distribution by counties and number of specialists.

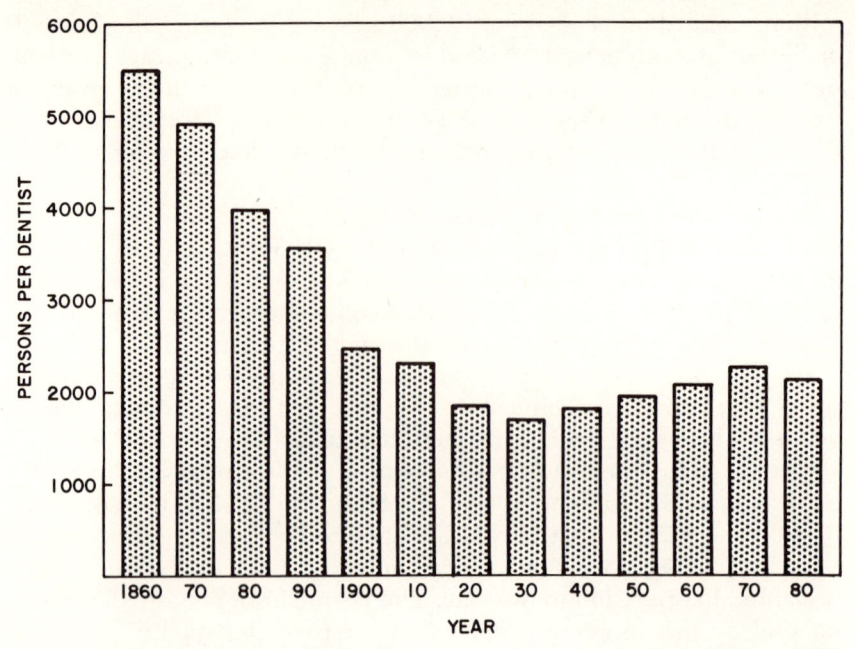

FIGURE 28. Number of persons per active dentist in the United States, 1860-1980. (Division of Dental Public Health and Resources, Public Health Service;[23] Division of Dental Health, Public Health Service;[22] Morrey, L. W. Dental personnel. Am. Dent. A. J., 32:131-44, Feb. 1, 1945; U.S. Bureau of the Census.[38-44])

civilian population to meet the military requirements of World War II. The extreme shortages that resulted were alleviated only partially by the return to peacetime conditions, first because a new prosperity had increased demand for care and then because of the population growth resulting from the wartime rise in birthrates.

A major effort has been made since the war to expand educational facilities to match population growth and increasing per capita demand. During the two decades between 1945 and 1965, for example, the total dental school undergraduate enrollment almost doubled, going from 7,300 to more than 14,000. Although these efforts were sufficient to maintain a reasonable balance between supply and demand, the relative supply of dentists has continued to decline. It is estimated that by 1970 the number of persons per active dentist will climb to 2,219, a sharp contrast to the 1930 figure of 1,729.[22]

DISTRIBUTION

The relative supply of dentists varies widely, ranging in 1960 from 1,151 persons per active dentist in the District of Columbia to 5,512 in South Carolina.[23] Eighteen states had a smaller count of persons per dentist than the 1960 average for the continental United States of 2,177, while 32 had a larger number. In general, the north-

DENTAL MANPOWER RESOURCES 269

PERSONS PER DENTIST - 1970

SOUTH CAROLINA	
ALASKA	
MISSISSIPPI	
GEORGIA	
NORTH CAROLINA	
NEW MEXICO	
ALABAMA	
ARKANSAS	
LOUISIANA	
TEXAS	
WEST VIRGINIA	
KENTUCKY	
VIRGINIA	
NEVADA	
OKLAHOMA	
ARIZONA	
TENNESSEE	
NORTH DAKOTA	
MARYLAND	
DELAWARE	
NEW HAMPSHIRE	
MAINE	
SOUTH DAKOTA	
INDIANA	
KANSAS	
WYOMING	
FLORIDA	
VERMONT	
OHIO	
IDAHO	
MISSOURI	
RHODE ISLAND	
MICHIGAN	
MONTANA	
IOWA	
ILLINOIS	
PENNSYLVANIA	
CALIFORNIA	
WISCONSIN	
COLORADO	
NEW JERSEY	
NEBRASKA	
UTAH	
CONNECTICUT	
HAWAII	
MINNESOTA	
MASSACHUSETTS	
WASHINGTON	
NEW YORK	
OREGON	
DISTRICT OF COLUMBIA	

UNITED STATES 2,219

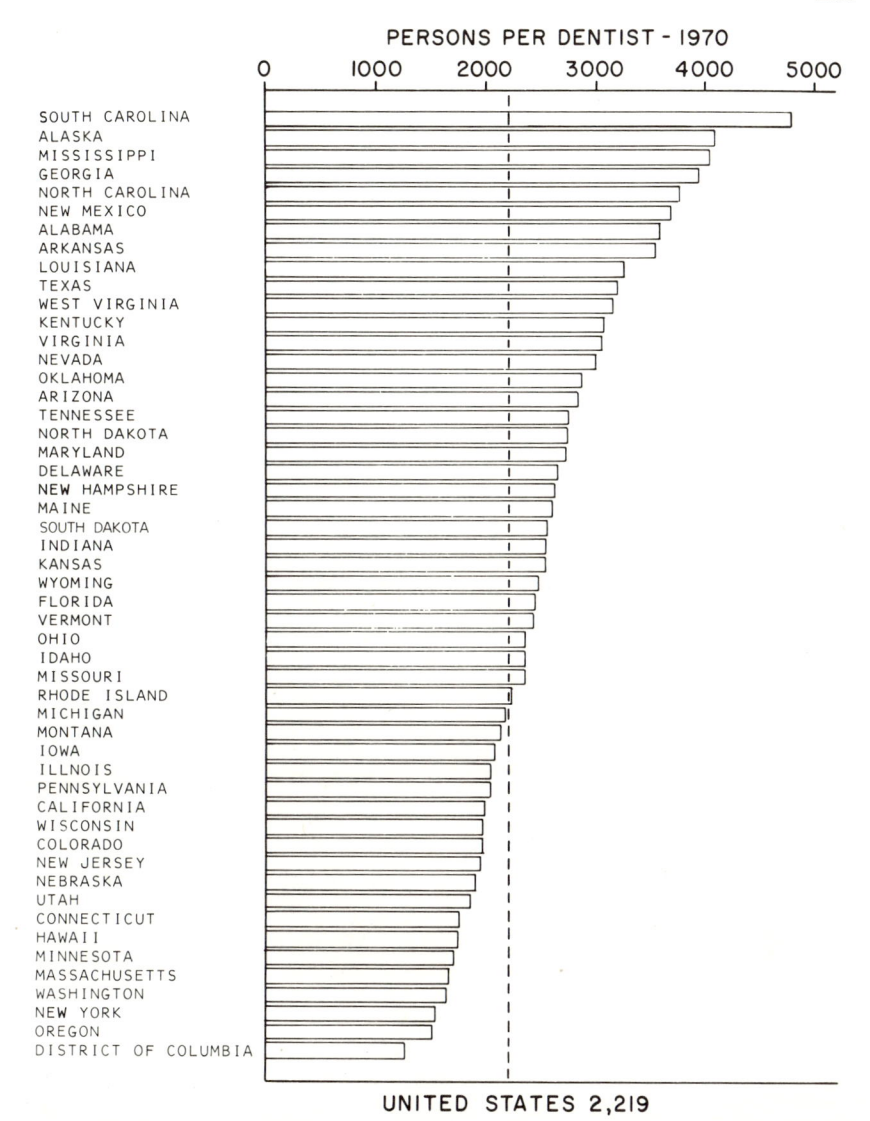

FIGURE 29. Estimated persons per active dentist by state, 1970. (Division of Dental Health, Public Health Service.[22])

eastern and far western states had the most adequate supply, while the southern states had the least satisfactory. In fact, all but two of the 15 states having more than 3,000 persons per dentist were located in the upper and lower South and the Southwest.

Fortunately, there is evidence of modest improvement in the *distribution* of dentists. From 1950 to 1960 the number of persons to be served by each active nonfederal dentist in the United States increased by eight percent, from 2,016 to 2,178. During this decade, however, the relative standing of the regions with the least adequate supply (upper and lower South) improved, and the number of persons

TABLE 30. NUMBER OF PERSONS PER DENTIST BY REGION, 1950-1970[*]

	1950	1960	PERCENT CHANGE 1950-60	1970	PERCENT CHANGE 1960-70
United States	2,016	2,178	8.0	2,219	1.9
Great Lakes	1,812	2,103	14.2	2,148	2.1
Midwest	1,912	2,190	14.5	2,276	3.9
Mid-Atlantic	1,539	1,687	9.6	1,816	7.6
New England	1,694	1,849	9.1	1,837	−0.6
Lower South	3,919	3,610	−7.9	3,297	−8.7
Upper South	3,702	3,132	−15.4	3,143	0.4
Far West	1,692	1,833	8.3	1,918	4.6
Rocky Mountain	2,120	2,147	1.3	2,043	−4.8
Southwest	3,258	3,294	1.1	3,097	−6.0

[*]Division of Dental Public Health and Resources, Public Health Service;[23] Divsion of Dental Health, Public Health Service.[22]

per dentist dropped by 15.4 and 7.9 percent. In the Southwest, the region with the second highest count of persons per dentist, the 1950 ratio of population to dentist of one to 3,258 remained stable, increasing by only 36. The regions which lost the most ground were the Great Lakes and Midwest. Although the count of persons per dentist rose by 14 percent during the decade in these states, the relative supply of dentists remained higher than the national average.

This trend has continued in the 1960's. It is estimated that from 1960 to 1970 the average number of persons to be served by each dentist will increase by about two percent. The regions where a substantial improvement in the relative supply of dentists is predicted are those that had high counts of persons per dentist in 1950 and 1960 (lower South, Southwest, and Rocky Mountain). In contrast, the region where the relative supply is expected to decline most sharply is the region that had the lowest number of persons per dentist in both 1950 and 1960 (Mid-Atlantic).[22]

Variations in the relative supply of dentists occur at all levels, local, state, and regional. The distribution of dentists, particularly in states and regions, is probably influenced by the availability of educational facilities, since dentists tend to locate within the area in which they received their training.[35] (The nation's 55 dental schools are located in only 32 states, the District of Columbia, and Puerto Rico.[12]) The supply of dentists also reflects, in part, variations in demand for service. Thus, areas with low educational levels and below average per capita income tend to have a smaller relative supply of dentists. Rural areas tend to be less adequately served than urban areas because of at least three factors. First, counts of the population living in areas classified as rural include many who reside in or near metropolitan areas and have ready access to professional services. Second, the demand for care is often lower in rural areas. Finally, dentists and

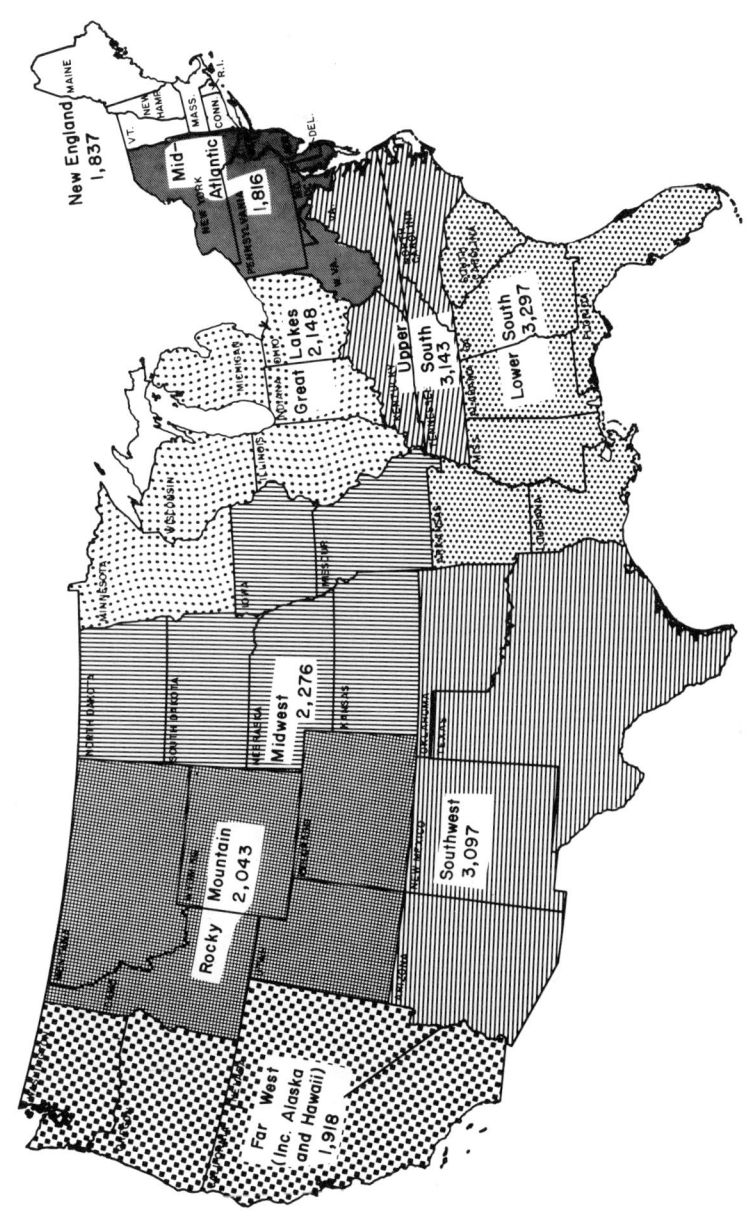

FIGURE 30. Estimated persons per active dentist by region, 1970. (Division of Dental Health, Public Health Service.[22])

their wives are understandably attracted by the cultural and social advantages of larger cities and are thus less likely to locate in rural areas.

Dental Specialists

The early development of dental specialists was quite informal. Some dentists took graduate training, or a residency, before limiting their practices. Others undertook a formal "preceptorship" by working in the office of a qualified specialist and under his direction. Still others merely developed additional skills through practice, short continuing education courses, and study of the literature. When one of these individuals was confident of his own skill (and his ability to secure referrals from other practitioners), he would announce to his former patients and colleagues in the profession that he was limiting his practice to a certain area of dentistry. Varying patterns developed as each specialty developed and matured relatively independently. Examining boards to certify specialty competence came into being, as well as specialty societies (such as the American Academy of Pedodontics and the American Association of Orthodontics) that maintained educational and experiential qualifications for membership. In addition, 10 states established specialty licensure following examination by the state board of dental examiners.

During the early 1960's, the American Dental Association attempted to develop an overall pattern which would be both logical and equitable. Technical control of specialty designation was achieved in two ways. First, the Judicial Council (with the approval of the House of Delegates) ruled that one could not announce that his practice was limited to a special area of practice unless he met the educational requirements set by the Council on Dental Education (and the House). In 1961, the House of Delegates established that the basic preparation for all specialties would require a minimum of two years of academic studies leading either to a certificate or a degree.[17] During a transitional period, four different methods of qualification for the right to announce limitation of practice were recognized: (1) certification as a diplomate of one of the eight American boards authorized by the Association; (2) possession of a specialty license from one of the 10 state boards that examine in the specialty fields; (3) completion of two years of advanced academic studies in an approved program; and (4) exclusive limitation and ethical announcement of such limitation prior to 1965.[18] In all cases the individual must limit his practice exclusively to the specialty. Today criteria for those entering a specialty is full-time limitation in addition to either the completion of two years of advanced study or specialty licensure by a state board.

Examining boards have been established (under guidelines set by the Council on Dental Education) in each of the eight areas of specialty practice recognized by the profession: dental public health, endodontics, oral pathology, oral surgery, orthodontics, pedodontics, periodontology, and prosthetics. Certification as a diplomate by one of the American boards is not a prerequisite for limitation of practice. The purpose of a board is to provide leadership in the elevation of standards for the practice of the specialty and, through examination and certification, to recognize those individuals who have demonstrated unusual competence.

More than 9,000 recognized specialists are expected by 1970.[22] The actual number of dentists in limited practice is higher than available data indicate. A special 1965 study, for example, showed that there were about 4,000 dentists who had "informally limited" their practices, in addition to the some 6,700 meeting the established criteria for listing in A. D. A. publications.[37] These individuals are those who limited their practices prior to 1965 without seeking other types of recognition. Presumably the number of "informally limited" dentists will dwindle with time as their ranks are thinned by death and retirement.

The number of additional specialists being added by graduate schools and residencies will result in marked increases in the numbers of recognized specialists. The projected 1970 figure of 9,600 is in marked contrast to the 2,808 identified in 1955, just 15 years previously.[4] The number of specialists will continue to rise at a faster rate than the general dentist population. About seven percent of all active dentists were identified as specialists in 1965. It is predicted that the percentage of specialists in the profession will double (to 14.4 percent) by 1975 and increase threefold (to 22 percent) by 1985.[37]

Trends in the population growth and the pattern of dental health care suggest that even these increases may be insufficient to provide adequate specialist services. Although there is probably a much greater "need" than "demand" for orthodontic care, that demand is increasing at a steady rate. The development of new dental care plans with emphasis on the young intensifies the need for greater numbers of pedodontists. The character of pedodontic practice will change with more widespread fluoridation, but any decrease in dental treatment needs will be balanced by increases in the number of individuals under 18 as well as by rising per capita utilization. The retention of teeth due to fluoridation, as well as the increase in the number of elderly persons, should have an impact on oral pathology, oral surgery, periodontics, endodontics, and prosthetics — an impact which would seem to ensure increased demands for service. The need for public health dentists already exceeds the supply, and the development of new governmental programs will result in even more critical shortages of individuals with a background in administrative dentistry.

The need for specialists may become particularly apparent as dentists in general practice feel the pressure resulting from increases in demand. Experience suggests that dentists who have time available often perform some services done by specialists, such as treating children or doing minor oral surgery. When these dentists become busy, they prefer to send more of their "problem patients" and patients with special problems to the specialists. It is quite possible, however, that the dentist in general practice in the 1970's may find it difficult to obtain assistance for any except the most difficult problems. The possibility of this occurrence would suggest the need for greater emphasis (both in dental school and in continuing education) on the treatment of periodontal diseases, management of minor deviations from normal occlusion, performance of uncomplicated surgical procedures, and handling of children who present management problems. The bulk of oral health care has been the responsibility of the general practitioner and it appears that it will remain so.

FUTURE NEEDS

To Meet Population Growth

One of the significant characteristics of American history has been the steady growth of the population. Population growth, an important influence on the development of the nation in the past, is a major factor influencing the future course of industry, government, and the professions.

Population change is the result of interaction among births, deaths, and net migration. The census of 1790 enumerated 3.9 million persons living in the 17 states along the Atlantic coast.[47] Since that time the population has increased steadily, passing 200 million persons for the first time in this decade.[46] Immigration, a significant factor in population change in the early history of the country, now plays a minor role, but births have consistently exceeded deaths by a wide margin and life expectancy has risen steadily.

The population increases of past decades provide a basis for future expectations. The Bureau of the Census has issued four projections of population growth through 1980, based on various assumptions regarding the future birthrate.[45] The estimate most commonly accepted (Series I-B) indicates that between 1965 and 1975 the population will grow from 196 million to 223 million—an increase of 27 million persons. By 1985, an additional 40.8 million persons will have been added to the population to be served by the dental profession, for a total of more than 260 million.

Because the dangers of future manpower shortages have been recognized, federal funds have been made available to assist in the construction of new dental and dental hygiene schools, to renovate existing ones, and to support expanded faculty and student enrollment. There is a lag of at least a decade, however, between the authorization of a new school and the graduation of a significant

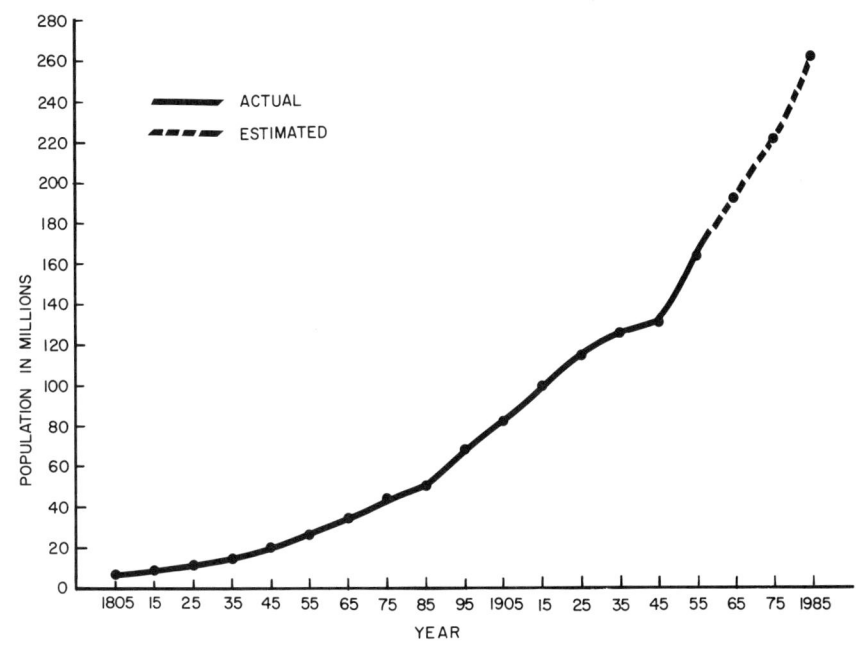

FIGURE 31. Population of the United States 1805-1955, and estimated population (Series I-B) to 1985 (U.S. Bureau of the Census.[45-47])

number of students. Even with existing schools, shortages of both funds and qualified faculty, as well as delays in construction, limit the speed with which larger enrollments can be accepted. The continued high level of population growth will mean that the increased number of graduating dentists may be able to accomplish only a stabilization of the relative supply of dentists. It is estimated that the 1980 count of persons per dentist will drop only to 2,090.[22]

To Meet Increased Demand

Overwhelming as the demand for dental care just to match population growth may be, there is evidence that this problem will be compounded by a rising per capita demand for care per se. Chapter 10 pointed out that the percentage of the population visiting the dentist annually, as well as the yearly expenditures for dental care per person, has risen steadily during the past three decades. The increasing educational and income levels of the population—two factors closely associated with demand for service—indicate that these trends will continue, probably at an accelerated pace.

In addition to the rising demand resulting from these clearly predictable changes in the characteristics of the population—the "automatic market"—other changes in the pattern of demand may be anticipated from the growth of governmental and other types of dental payment programs. Chapters 11 and 12 summarized the factors which point toward the rapid expansion of third-party payment plans which, by removing the barrier of immediate patient payment, may bring about increases in the utilization of dental services.

Fortunately for the dental profession, changes in dental demand in recent years have come about slowly as the result of factors that have a long-range impact. Changes in the attitude of individuals toward the value of oral health, for example, do not occur overnight, but move in a moderate and steady progression. The profession has been able to increase productivity and adapt to past rises in service demands. It must be recognized, however, that these factors which increase demand have a pyramiding effect and that the maximum impact has not been realized fully. Furthermore, the minor increases in demand that have resulted from experimental payment programs have had as yet little effect on overall utilization rates. The combination of factors creating greater total demands for care may be expected to "snowball" in the coming decades. All available evidence suggests that the number of dentists anticipated in the future may not be able to increase productivity (under present patterns) sufficiently to meet the demand for care.

MEETING THE DEMAND FOR CARE

Reducing Dental Needs

There are a number of procedures available for the partial prevention of dental disease. The reduction of dietary sugars, topical application of fluoride, the addition of fluorides to the diet of children by prescription of tablets or concentrated solutions, and the use of a fluoride dentifrice, for example, have been demonstrated to reduce the occurrence of oral disorders. Although these methods of prevention have proved to be effective for those conscientious individuals who utilize them systematically, they have never been adopted by a large enough proportion of the population to bring about measurable reductions in the overall occurrence of dental disease.[25, 27, 31] The only preventive procedure that has demonstrated the ability to reduce dental diseases significantly in large population groups is fluoridation of community water supplies.

Despite its proven effectiveness, fluoridation probably will not make a major impact on dental needs — partly because of widespread failure to utilize the procedure. Previous chapters have pointed out the difficulty in gaining public acceptance of fluoridation. Even if universally adopted, the procedure cannot be expected to make a major impact on dental manpower requirements.

Although the role of water fluoridation in reducing the attack of dental caries has been clearly determined, the extent to which lifetime treatment needs are reduced is debatable. With advancing age, dental caries accounts for a smaller share of the total dental needs than does periodontal disease. One of the major benefits of a reduced caries attack is the longer retention of the teeth. This very benefit actually may increase rather than reduce the lifetime treatment needs by necessitating the provision of time-consuming services such as crowns, bridges, and partial dentures, rather than full dentures. Furthermore, the need for routine prophylaxes and diagnostic services, as well as for treatment of periodontal disease, can be expected to continue in a group having a low caries rate long after edentulousness has overtaken those with a high rate of caries attack. Although water fluoridation may reduce the treatment needs of a child population, it is doubtful that this may be expected for the total population.

Increasing the Supply of Dentists

The major task, if a manpower shortage is to be avoided, would seem to be to create additional facilities for the education of dentists. The problem can be stated simply but not solved readily. The capacity of dental schools now expected to be in operation in 1970 will, at most, merely approximately maintain current ratios of supply.[22] An even greater expansion would be necessary to allow for increased per capita demand. Meeting these goals would require a level of financial support for dental education far greater than has ever existed to date for the construction of new schools and the expansion of existing ones. New sources of funds for dental education (and for other health sciences) may ease the financial plight of educational institutions. It is doubtful, however, that educational facilities can be expanded rapidly enough to compensate for both population growth and increased demand. Furthermore, even if sufficient numbers of new schools could be constructed, there is no assurance that competent faculties could be obtained to staff the institutions. In addition, the mounting costs of dental education and competition from other, perhaps more glamorous, occupations make it increasingly difficult to recruit sufficient numbers of qualified students. The goal of educating a sufficient number of dentists to match population growth (making no allowance for increased demands) is probably the highest that can be anticipated reasonably. Even this goal will not be achieved unless members of the dental profession recognize its importance and support efforts to increase training facilities, provide adequate financing for dental education, recruit and educate dental teachers, recruit dental students, and obtain scholarships and loans to help meet the cost of dental education.

Increasing Productivity

It is evident that the efficiency and productivity of the average dental practice have been increasing, since rises in the per capita use of dental services have occurred at a time when the amount of dentist-time available per person has declined. As a result, the profession has not fallen behind in its ability to meet the demand for dental care to date. During the past 30 years the volume of services provided by the average dentist has more than doubled, and in recent decades it has increased at the rate of three to four percent each year.[34]

It is doubtful that dentists can accelerate the pace of productivity increases, or even maintain past rates of growth. In fact, the profession is probably reaching a peak of average efficiency. The initial surge of productivity which occurred during the early 1940's probably reflected the fact that dentists who previously had free time became busier. In relatively few sections of the country can this type of increase be expected again. Another important factor, starting even in this period, was the rapid growth in the use of commercial dental laboratories, which assumed greater responsibility for the mechanical aspects of prosthetic service. Again, it is doubtful that any sizeable additional increases in productivity will result from more widespread use of laboratory technicians.

Great changes in dental practice have occurred in the past decade including improved efficiency of office design, the use of high-velocity vacuum for the evacuation of oral fluids, and the development of high-speed cutting instruments. These changes, particularly high-speed equipment, have resulted in increased productivity. At present there is no indication that further major increases in productivity may be anticipated from the use of improved dental equipment. By 1958 almost 60 percent of all practicing dentists already were utilizing high-speed or superspeed equipment, a figure that must have risen to nearly 100 percent currently. There is no certainty of the development of other types of equipment that will promote productivity to a degree comparable to high-speed handpieces.[10]

A considerable part of the increased productivity noted during the past 30 years has been due to the greater use of auxiliary personnel. The percentage of dentists employing at least one auxiliary person rose from 65.6 in 1950, to 82.6 in 1962, and to 89.9 in 1964. During this period the percentage of offices employing more than one auxiliary also increased.[5,6,9]

The increasing use of auxiliary personnel appears to hold the greatest promise for future increases in productivity of the average dentist. Although the trend toward the utilization of greater numbers of auxiliaries will probably continue and result in further increases in productivity, it may be expected that a saturation point eventually will be reached. Some dentists do not have the education or the temperament to utilize additional personnel. There will always be concentrations of dentists in certain desirable places, and many dentists will not be busy enough to utilize additional aides. It should be noted, however, that the saturation point in increasing productivity through the utilization of auxiliaries might be postponed indefinitely if present patterns of utilization change, and if there is a shift in the philosophy of dental practice.

UTILIZATION OF ANCILLARY AND AUXILIARY PERSONNEL

Dental Hygienists

Although the profession of dental hygiene is relatively young — in fact, it was the year 1914 that saw the establishment of the first training course — it has gained wide acceptance as an integral part of dentistry. The role of the hygienist assumes growing importance as dentistry becomes increasingly oriented toward preventive services, particularly those directed toward diseases of the gingiva and supporting tissues in the mouth. The hygienist also extends the services of the dentist to more patients by relieving him of those professional duties for which she has been trained and licensed, and allowing him to devote all his time to those services which only he is trained to do. It has been estimated that the amount of dental care could be increased by 25 percent if dental hygienists were utilized to the maximum extent.[36]

Educational facilities for dental hygienists have grown rapidly, particularly during the past quarter century. In 1946 the 17 schools then in operation graduated 403 hygienists. Ten years later the number of schools had grown to 35 and the graduating class had more than doubled.[36] The 61 schools in operation in 1968 graduated more than 1,700 dental hygienists.[19] The number of schools is expected to rise to 90 by 1970. Total enrollment will nearly double during the five years from 1965 to 1970, going from 3,800 to 6,300.[15]

One of the significant recent trends in hygiene education has been a shift in the type of sponsoring educational agency. Most of the early dental hygiene schools were opened in conjunction with institutions that trained dentists at the undergraduate or graduate level. Even as late as 1950, such schools were the sponsors of 19 of the 26 dental hygiene programs.[14] By 1967, however, only about half (30) of the hygiene programs were associated with dental institutions. Of the 57 listed in that year, 14 were in junior or community colleges, 10 in four-year colleges, and three in vocational or technical schools.[15]

Despite the somewhat limited professional life of women, the number of active hygienists has risen relatively rapidly. During the 1950's the number almost doubled, going from 6,500 to 11,400. The supply of hygienists rose to 16,000 in 1966, and it has been estimated that as many as 42,000 may be employed by 1975.[11]

Although the profession is growing in size, dental hygienists serve only a fraction of dental practices. In 1964, for example, only 19 percent of practicing dentists utilized a hygienist either full- or part-time, and only 11 percent employed one full-time.[5] There is no arbitrary rule of thumb that can be used to measure the total number of active dental hygienists who could be used effectively. A reasonable goal would be for all areas of the United States to match the supply of hygienists now available in the most adequately supplied region. To do so would require an expansion of educational facilities far beyond anything thought of today.[49]

The dental hygienists who are practicing are distributed very unevenly. The erratic distribution reflects the great regional variations in the rate of development of the profession. These differences are illustrated most dramatically by the fact that more than 35 years elapsed between the establishment of the first one-year hygiene school and the time when all states legally recognized the profession. As late as 1955, two thirds of all dental hygienists ever graduated were trained in the Northeast region—the area where the profession originated and where the first schools were established.[36]

Because hygienists do not engage in solo practice, it is primarily the dentists' recognition of their value, not the public demand for care, that determines the growth and development of the profession. In areas where dental hygiene started early, it has had time to develop maturity and strength, but in other areas the profession is almost in its infancy. As a consequence, there has existed an unusual relation between the supply of hygienists and the demand for their services by the dental profession. In states with a relatively large number of dental hygienists the demand exceeds the supply, whereas in other areas a very few hygienists seem to satisfy the demand evidenced by the dentists. The latter situation reflects the fact that dentists have not had the opportunity to employ hygienists and are therefore not accustomed to using their services.

Over and above the concern of expanding productivity to meet demands for service, the dental practitioner has a personal stake in the utilization of hygienists and in the development of additional schools to ensure an adequate supply. A dental hygienist increases the net income of a practice both by the services she renders directly to patients and by freeing the dentist from time-consuming and relatively unremunerative tasks so that he is free to concentrate on the more demanding types of service that command higher fees. Patient education, coupled with an effective recall system, builds a dental practice, increases the proportion of patients who will accept complete restorative service, and contributes to the dentist's professional satisfaction.

Dental Assistants

The more than 84,000 dental assistants working in the United States are important factors in the provision of dental care.[5] Their precise role in dental practice, however, is not easy to describe. Unlike dental hygiene, a profession with definite educational requirements and legal responsibilities, dental assisting is a vocation that is difficult to define. The first dental assistants, employed in the late 1800's, were trained on the job by their dentist-employers and their duties were confined to receiving patients, performing "housekeeping" chores, and handling clerical and bookkeeping procedures. Today many dental assistants follow the pattern of their predecessors of a century ago. Only a small minority of assistants have received any type of formal training. Although no comprehensive studies of the functions of active dental assistants are available, it is accepted generally that many function only in the limited role of receptionist, clerk, and "housekeeper."

On the other hand, the use of well-trained assistants to perform a wide variety of functions is increasing rapidly. The most important addition to her duties is that of assisting at the chair where she serves virtually as a second pair of hands for the dentist. She (or a second assistant) aids the dentist in the securing of radiographs (in some

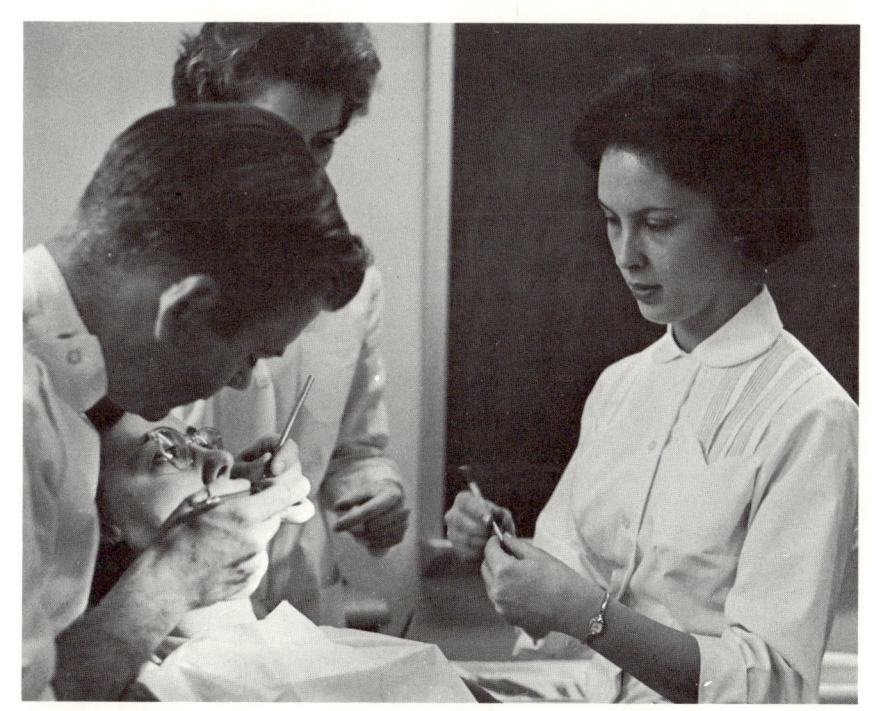

Figure 32. The use of "chair-side" and "roving" dental assistants. (Courtesy Division of Dental Health, Public Health Service.)

cases exposing the film herself under the dentist's supervision), develops, mounts, and labels the film. The assumption of additional responsibilities, again under the dentist's direction, for making appointments, handling financial arrangements, and ordering supplies are important functions of the effective assistant. In recognition of the variety of skills demanded of a dental assistant, formal training programs have been organized, minimum standards of preparation have been adopted, and a program of certification has developed as a joint effort of the American Dental Assistants' Association and the American Dental Association.[21]

To function effectively a dental assistant should be trained adequately—if possible, in an accredited program; if not, by correspondence or after-hour instruction while employed. She should be paid adequately for the important duties she is expected to perform. In most practices these duties should be shared by more than one person to permit chairside assisting without interruption.

Unfortunately, many dentists do not utilize assistants effectively. Almost one fourth of the dentists employed no assistants in 1961. More than half utilized only one assistant or only part-time assistants. Less than 10 percent utilized two or more assistants or receptionists.[9] Furthermore, the salaries paid are not high, averaging only $50.00 to $79.00 a week. Only one out of 10 reported an income of over $80.00 per week in a 1960 survey conducted by the Survey of Dentistry.[32] It should be noted that these figures are based largely on responses from members of the A.D.A.A.—a group likely to represent the most stable and best remunerated segment of the field.

Yet the evidence is clear that the employment of assistants is associated with both the productivity and the income of a dental practice. The 1962 Survey of Dental Practice reported that dentists with two full-time employees saw a quarter more patients in a year than did those with one.[8] Dentists with two chairs and two assistants reported a net income about 60 percent higher than those with only one chair and one assistant.[7]

Dental Laboratory Technicians

The services of dental technicians are utilized by nine out of 10 dentists in the United States.[9] The relation between a conscientious dentist and technician is a productive one in which the dentist utilizes his skills for diagnosis, treatment planning, design, and prescription of an appliance, while the technician performs the mechanical tasks necessary to fabricate the appliance. Through constant repetition the technician develops great accuracy and speed in technical procedures and relieves the dentist of time-consuming functions. The majority of dentists are conscientious in utilization of laboratory technicians, and most technicians follow ethical procedures and carry out the directions they have received from dentists. Unfortunately a minority of dentists and technicians have created problems by failure to observe ethical standards. In these cases dentists have abdicated their responsibility to make an accurate diagnosis, to design and prescribe the indicated appliances, and to ensure that the appliances are satisfactory. On the other hand, technicians, overconfident because of their skill in mechanical procedures, have attempted to deal directly with the public and offer a service for which they are not qualified by training or experience.

Every practitioner has an ethical and moral responsibility to fulfill his proper function of making an accurate diagnosis and giving specific detailed instructions in writing for the laboratory procedures to be carried out by the dental technician. By so doing, the productive relation between dentistry and the dental laboratory craft will be preserved, the productivity of dental practice will be maintained, and the public will receive truly professional prosthetic service.

Future Role of Auxiliaries

Although the utilization of auxiliary personnel has expanded greatly in the past half century, there has been no appreciable break with the tradition which, with the exception of the very limited responsibilities assigned to the hygienist, permits only the dentist to perform clinical services for a patient. Maximum increases in productivity from the use of auxiliary personnel may be anticipated only if the profession studies ways in which additional technical procedures can be delegated to lesser trained personnel. The gradual acceptance of the hygienist to perform oral prophylaxes and the use of dental assistants to expose and develop x-rays indicate that such delegation can take place without diluting the quality of dental care. That the delegation of even these relatively minor segments of practice has been done reluctantly is indicated by the fact that as late as 1968 dental hygienists in 27 states were still legally prohibited from going beneath the margin of the gums when doing a prophylaxis.[13]

Dentists have been much more hesitant to delegate responsibility for patient care than have been their colleagues in medicine. A nurse, for example, routinely gives injections of biologicals and medications in the physician's office, but in the dental office the only dental personnel permitted to use the hypodermic syringe is the dentist himself. Modern hospital and medical care would be virtually impossible if physicians had been as hesitant to delegate selected types of patient care as are dentists.

A consideration of the delegation of clinical duties to personnel who have not had education comparable to a dentist has aroused controversy within the profession. Dentists in the United States view with grave misgivings the "dental nurse scheme" that has existed in

New Zealand for many years and is now being adopted in several other countries. The New Zealand "dental nurses" are not, in fact, dental auxiliaries. They are actually limited practitioners who provide for children a restricted range of dental procedures with minimal, or token, supervision from fully trained dentists.[48] Understandably, most dentists in the United States question the underlying assumption that less knowledge and skill are required to care for the developing dentition of a child than the care of an adult. Similarly, the activities of dental technicians who attempt to deal directly with the public, the so-called "denturists" or "bootleg laboratories," have created a feeling of apprehension on the part of the dental profession.

Consideration can be given to expanded clinical duties of auxiliary personnel without becoming involved in the development of inadequately trained individuals dealing directly with patients. Just because the nurse is permitted to remove sutures, give injections of biologicals, and administer immunizations does not mean that she attempts to set up an independent practice and offer her services to the public without supervision from a physician-employer. Similarly, the fact that the dental hygienist is permitted by law to perform oral prophylaxes and apply fluorides topically has not meant that members of this profession have attempted to provide services for the public without the supervision of a dentist.

The role of dental auxiliaries in dental practice is undergoing a thoughtful reappraisal. The House of Delegates of the American Dental Association has urged dental schools and the federal services to conduct experiments to determine the proper functions of dental hygienists and of dental assistants.[30] Several significant studies have been developed in response.

Experimental Studies. In 1963, the Royal Canadian Dental Corps reported a pilot study on the utilization of auxiliary personnel with advanced training which established a precedent for studies in the United States.[3] The study was to determine whether "clinical technicians" or "dental therapists" (somewhat equivalent to dental hygienists) could undertake additional responsibilities and be employed effectively under conditions existing in the average clinic of the Corps.

The plan went through three phases. The baseline identified productivity under the normal staffing ratio of one dental officer and one assistant. During the next phase a second operating room and an additional assistant were added, resulting in a 37.4 percent increase in productivity. When a "therapist" with advanced training shared the clinical duties, productivity was 99.1 percent higher than for the two-man team and 61.7 percent higher than when two assistants were used conventionally in two operatories.

The "clinical technicians" or "dental therapists" chosen had previously had 34 weeks of formal training and three and a half years of experience. During an additional 16 weeks of training they were taught application of the rubber dam; placing and removing of matrix bands; packing, carving, and finishing amalgam restorations; and placing and finishing cements. Experience with the "clinical technician" functioning at this level was satisfactory, and their use was recommended throughout the Corps.

The United States Navy reported a similar study in 1964, using experienced corpsmen with additional clinical and practical training of seven weeks' duration.[16] The control team consisted of a dental officer and two technicians who operated at one chair using conventional procedures. One experimental team consisted of a dental officer and three technicians who operated at two chairs, with the technician inserting the restorative material in teeth prepared by the dental officer. The second experimental team consisted of four technicians and a dental officer utilizing three chairs, with the technicians performing the same functions. During the 12-week investigation the productivity of the two experimental teams was increased proportionately with the additional technician. The quality of the restorations was judged by independent examiners (from both dental practice and dental schools) to be at least equal to, and perhaps better than, the quality now produced in the average civilian dental office in the United States.

The Division of Indian Health of the Public Health Service conducted a limited study using dental assistants to perform similar expanded clinical functions.[1] Relatively little increase in productivity was noted, primarily because of limited training and clinical facilities that were inadequate to utilize the services of a dentist and two auxiliaries when all were attempting to provide clinical services. The primary focus of the study, however, was to evaluate the quality of restorations placed after preparation of the tooth by the dentist. Independent evaluations by two dentists not connected with the Division showed that the restorations placed by the dentists were rated "unsatisfactory" approximately as often as those placed by the dental assistant. This finding is not particularly surprising, since the dentists had been responsible for training their assistants in the expanded functions and had also checked finished restorations before dismissing a patient.

One of the most comprehensive studies has been conducted at the University of Alabama, using carefully selected female high school graduates who received clinical and didactic instruction for a 24-month period.[29] After this training they were allowed to take impressions for study casts; place and remove rubber dams; place and remove temporary restorations; place and carve amalgam, silicate, and acrylic restorations in previously prepared teeth; and apply final finish to and polish these restorations. They are referred to as "dental therapists."

The control group for the evaluation of the quality of service was a group of advanced dental students working in a special "dental assistants utilization" clinic. Careful precautions were taken so that the dentists who evaluated the finished restorations (outstanding private practitioners not connected with the dental school) could not know whether patients had been treated by an advanced dental student or a dental assistant. Similarly, the instructional staff did not know the findings of the evaluation until the major share of the data had been collected.

The dentists who were asked to evaluate the quality of the restorations placed by the dental auxiliaries followed detailed written criteria. For the various aspects evaluated, the proportions of the clinical procedures judged excellent were consistently greater for the specially trained auxiliaries than for the dental students — differences that were usually statistically significant. The proportions of unacceptable procedures were small and sometimes favored the dental student and sometimes the auxiliary, most often the auxiliary.

Similar experimental programs have been done in a variety of other settings. The Public Health Service is carrying out a major study of expanded duties of auxiliaries in a special Development Center in Louisville. At the University of Minnesota an experimental program to train a special auxiliary for use in pedodontic practice has been established.[20] The same institution has initiated a one-year training program "to determine the tasks that are presently performed by a fully trained orthodontist that can be delegated to a lesser trained technician." The training includes record preparation, appliance construction, appliance maintenance, patient education, and laboratory procedures.[19] The Division of Indian Health is planning additional studies, as are a number of dental schools.

The experience to date has consistently shown that auxiliaries who are properly trained and supervised can perform a variety of clinical functions efficiently and well. These findings parallel experience in at least two other countries. The New Zealand dental nurse, providing routine care for children after two years of training, has generally been accepted as providing restorations of good quality. (The criticism of the program has related to other factors, such as administrative patterns, the lack of adequate training for diagnosis and treatment planning, and the failure to correct this deficiency by direct supervision from a dentist.) In 1957 the General Dental Council of England approved an experimental program of two years to train the so-called "New Cross Auxiliary" (named after the hospital where the training program was located).[28] They were to provide routine restorative and preventive dentistry for children but *only* working in school clinics and under the *immediate* supervision of a fully trained dentist. Evaluated carefully after six years, the experiment was judged a success and the use of this type of auxiliary made a permanent part of the school dental service.

Projecting the Future

It is difficult to predict the exact role that dental auxiliaries will play in the practice of the future. It does seem reasonable to expect that students who use this edition of the text will be graduated and licensed to practice under laws that are more permissive than any that have been in existence since dentistry won, in the mid-1800's, the right to have practice regulated. Only broad trends can be considered here. For information about current developments in auxiliary utilization the student is referred to the *Journal of the American Dental Association.*

The mechanism that will be used to bring about more liberal usage seems clearly to lie in changing the nature of the laws that regulate the practice of dentistry and the role of state licensing boards. Most laws have been negative in their approach. After defining who may practice dentistry or dental hygiene, they ordinarily have proceeded to give lengthy, detailed lists of clinical services that can be performed only by a dentist. The acts have most frequently defined limited approved functions permissible by the dental hygienist under the direction of a dentist with the specific provision that she may do no procedures that are not mentioned in the law.

In 1968, Conway pointed out that the law in 27 states did not allow the hygienist to "clean" other than the clinical crown, while 23 states permitted her to operate below the crown but only to remove deposits from directly beneath the free margin of the gingiva.[13] So restrictive have been the laws that few state boards of dental examiners have even had the right to modify current practices by issuing rules or regulations.

The 1967 House of Delegates of the American Dental Association asked state dental societies and state boards of dental examiners to revise their practice acts to eliminate serial listings of permissible duties and to give the examining boards authority to issue rules or regulations defining appropriate responsibilities of the dentist and his auxiliary.[2] Once the general pattern of rigidly restrictive legislation has been eliminated, the dental profession will need to be prepared for an orderly, systematic shift in the pattern of auxiliary utilization. This shift will be guided by an increasing emphasis on the responsibility of the dentist for dental patient care and a reduction in legal restraints on the ways in which he can organize his practice to provide this care. It will be necessary for dental schools to prepare their students for this increased responsibility of supervision so that the most efficient and safe utilization will be made of the expanded roles and functions of auxiliaries. Dental hygiene and dental assisting schools will need to reorganize their curriculums in order to prepare their students for the new roles. Dentists, dental hygienists, and dental assistants already in practice will need postgraduate courses in this regard, also.

No clear pattern is emerging in regard to the expanded role of dental hygienists vis-à-vis dental assistants. Some contend that hygienists should expand their roles in the direction of patient education, preventive procedures, and periodontal therapy, while assistants turn in the direction of restorative procedures. Others indicate that a third type of auxiliary—not definitely named as yet, but "dental therapist" has been suggested—will emerge. Still others maintain that the extension of duties should go first to the dental hygienist because of her relatively extensive preparation and because she is already licensed to provide intraoral services. Some thoughtful observers of the New Zealand dental nurse, the New Cross auxiliary, and of the current American auxiliaries contend that none of these patterns can be imposed upon or maintained in—as the case may be—the United States. Rather, they suggest that a new pattern of auxiliary utilization will have to be developed through evolutionary procedures—a pattern specific to the United States and its culture and needs.

There are rather clear indications of the nature of the clinical responsibilities that will eventually be delegated. In the planning of the Alabama study, reviewed earlier, tasks to be delegated "were selected because they were reparable and could be corrected or redone without excessive harm to the patient's oral health."[29] An editorial in the same issue of the *Journal of the American Dental Association* endorsed the concept of limiting delegated functions to those of a "reversible nature."[26] Following this line, discussion of auxiliary utilization among informed dentists has increasingly centered on three types of procedures that could *not* be delegated to trained auxiliaries: (1) diagnosis and planning of treatment, (2) the cutting or severing of soft or hard tissues, and (3) prescription of drugs or appliances.

Conway recently presented a suggested model for a dental law which combines increased permissiveness in usage of personnel and control of professional conduct by regulation rather than by serial lists of forbidden actions:

> Licensed dentists may assign to their employed dental hygienists or assistants intraoral tasks that do not require the professional competence or skill of the employer-dentist, subject to the following conditions:
> 1. The performance of intraoral tasks by dental hygienists or assistants shall be under the direct supervision of the employer-dentist.
> 2. None of the following procedures may be assigned to a dental hygienist or assistant or to any other person not licensed to practice dentistry.
>   A. Diagnosis, treatment planning and prescription (including prescriptions for drugs and medicaments or authorizations for restorative, prosthodontic or orthodontic appliances).
>   B. Surgical procedures on hard and soft tissues within the oral cavity or any other intraoral procedure that

contributes to or results in an irremediable alteration of the oral anatomy.

The board of dental examiners shall issue rules or regulations specifying the tasks that licensed dentists may, under the authority of this act, assign to (1) dental hygienists and (2) dental assistants.

The practice of dental hygiene shall consist of those prophylactic, preventive and other procedures that licensed dentists are authorized by this act and dental examining board rules or regulations to assign only to their employed licensed dental hygienists. The dental examining board shall issue rules or regulations defining the procedures that may be performed by licensed dental hygienists engaged in school health activities or employed by public agencies.[13]

The public has granted to the dental profession the sole right to provide oral health care. This right carries with it the serious responsibility to be prepared to provide this care when it is sought. As a growing population seeks an increasing per capita level of dental service, the profession faces one of the most serious challenges in its history. Fortunately, most leaders of dentistry are beginning to demonstrate once again that the profession has the courage and imagination to meet the new challenges of a changing society.

Bibliography

1. Abramowitz, Joseph. Expanded functions for dental assistants: a preliminary study. Am. Dent. A. J., 72:386-91, Feb. 1966.
2. American Dental Association policy on expanding dental auxiliary functions. Am. Dent. A. J., 76:1052, May 1968.
3. Baird, K. M., Purdy, E. C., and Protheroe, D. H. Pilot study on advanced training and employment of auxiliary dental personnel in the Royal Canadian Dental Corps: final report. Canad. Dent. A. J., 29:778-87, Dec. 1963.
4. Bureau of Economic Research and Statistics, American Dental Association. Facts about states for the dentist seeking a location; 1956. Chicago, American Dental Association, c1956. 34 p. (p. 7)
5. _____. 1965 survey of dental practice; IV. Professional expenses, auxiliary personnel. Am. Dent. A. J., 72:1181-6, May 1966.
6. _____. Survey of the dental profession; 1950. II. The dentist and certain aspects of his training and practice. Am. Dent. A. J., 41:376-82, Sept. 1950.
7. _____. The 1962 survey of dental practice. X. Summary. Am. Dent. A. J., 68:133-5, Jan. 1964.
8. _____. The 1962 survey of dental practice. VII. Number of patients and patient visits. Am. Dent. A. J., 67:533-8, Oct. 1963.
9. _____. The 1962 survey of dental practice. IV. Professional expenses; auxiliary personnel. Am. Dent. A. J., 66:868-76, June 1963.
10. _____. The 1959 survey of dental practice. VI. Use of high speed equipment; prescriptions written. Am. Dent. A. J., 61:520-3, Oct. 1960.
11. Bureau of Health Manpower, Public Health Service. Health manpower perspective: 1967. Washington, Government Printing Office, 1967. IX + 81 p. (p. 7, 13)
12. Bureau of Membership Records, American Dental Association. 1968 American dental directory. Chicago, American Dental Association, c1968. R154 + 939 p. (p. R7-R13)
13. Conway, B. J. Modifications of dental practice acts which will legalize expansion of auxiliary duties. Am. Dent. A. J., 76:1050-2, May 1968.
14. Council on Dental Education, American Dental Association. Dental students' register, 1950-51. Chicago, American Dental Association, n.d. n.p. (Table 10)
15. _____. Development of the profession's capacity for the training of dental auxiliary personnel. Am. Dent. A. J., 75:941-7, Oct. 1967.

16. Council on Dental Education, American Dental Association. Appendix I, Greater utilization of dental technicians. II. Report of clinical tests. Am. Dent. A. Tr., 106:45-54, 1965.
17. ———. Specialists and specialties. Am. Dent. A. Tr., 102:219, 1961.
18. ———. Qualifications for examination by specialty boards. Am. Dent. A. Tr., 106:390-3, 1965.
19. ———. Dental auxiliaries. Am. Dent. A. Reports of Officers and Councils, 109:30-6, 1968.
20. ———. Utilization and training of dental hygienists and dental assistants. Am. Dent. A. Tr., 108:43-4, 1967.
21. ———. [Report.] Am. Dent. A. Tr., 101:21-49, 1960.
22. Division of Dental Health, Public Health Service. Unpublished data.
23. Division of Dental Public Health and Resources, Public Health Service. [Background information.] p. 115-33. (In Proceedings of the workshop on the future requirements of dental manpower and the training and utilization of auxiliary personnel. Ann Arbor, University Michigan, 1962. 206 p.)
24. Division of Dental Resources, Public Health Service. A study of dental manpower requirements in the West. Boulder, Colorado, Western Interstate Commission Higher Education, (1956). IX + 247 p. (p. 19-23)
25. Dollar, M. L. Estimate of the effects of fluoridation, improved equipment, and additional auxiliary personnel on dental manpower requirements. p. 475-82. (In Hollinshead, B. S., dir. The survey of dentistry; the final report. Washington, American Council Education, c1961. XXXIV + 603 p.)
26. Expanded functions for dental auxiliaries. Edit. Am. Dent. A. J., 75:563, Sept. 1967.
27. Galagan, D. J. A public health dentist looks at topical fluorides today. J. Dent. Child., 26:164-72, 3rd Quar. 1959.
28. General Dental Council. Final report on the experimental scheme for the training and employment of dental auxiliaries. London, Spottiswoode, Bulbantyne, 1966. 100 p.
29. Hammons, P. E., and Jamison, H. C. Expanded functions for dental auxiliaries. Am. Dent. A. J., 75:658-72, Sept. 1967.
30. House of Delegates, American Dental Association. [Resolution 10-1960-11.] Am. Dent. A. Tr., 101:208, 1960.
31. Jordan, W. A., et al. The Askov dental demonstration; a ten-year study of a community dental health program, 1948-1958; final report. North-West Dent., 38:444-65, Nov. 1959.
32. Kesel, R. G. Dental practice. p. 95-238. (In Hollinshead, B. S., dir. The survey of dentistry; the final report. Washington, American Council Education, c1961. XXXIV + 603 p.)
33. Mann, W. R. Dental education. p. 239-422. (In Hollinshead, B. S., dir. The survey of dentistry; the final report. Washington, American Council Education, c1961. XXXIV + 603 p.)
34. [Moen, B. D.] Population per dentist, 1960 to 1980. Am. Dent. A. J., 64:700-6, May 1962.
35. Pelton, W. J., Pennell, E. H., and Pennell, Maryland Y. Location of dentists in relation to dental school attended. Pub. Health Rep., 70:1237-41, Dec. 1955.
36. Pelton, W. J., Pennell, E. H., and Vavra, Helen. Health manpower source book. 8. Dental hygienists. Washington, Government Printing Office, 1957. V + 87 p. (p. 1-7)
37. The need, demand, and availability of dental health services; report of study group I. Am. Col. Dent. J., 35:188-202, Apr. 1968.
38. U.S. Bureau of the Census. U.S. census of population, 1960, Volume 1, Chapter C. General social and economic characteristics. Washington, Government Printing Office, 1962. XLVII + 147 p.
39. ———. U.S. census of population, 1950. Volume II. Characteristics of the population. Washington, Government Printing Office, 1953. XI + 486 p.
40. ———. U.S. census of population, 1940. Volume II. Characteristics of the population. Washington, Government Printing Office, 1943. XIII + 977 p.
41. ———. U.S. census of population, 1930. Volume V. General report on occupations. Washington, Government Printing Office, 1933. IV + 591 p.
42. ———. U.S. census of population, 1920. Volume IV. Occupations. Washington, Government Printing Office, 1923. 1309 p.

43. U.S. Bureau of the Census. U.S. census of population, 1910. Volume IV. Occupation statistics. Washington, Government Printing Office, 1914. 615 p.
44. _____. U.S. census of population, 1900. Volume II. Population. Washington, Government Printing Office, 1902. CCXXIII + 754 p.
45. _____. Current population reports; series P-25, no. 375; revised projections of the population of states, 1970 to 1985. Washington, Government Printing Office, 1967. 110 p. (p. 18)
46. _____. Statistical abstract of the United States, 1967. 88th ed. Washington, Government Printing Office, 1967. XII + 1050 p. (p. 5)
47. _____. Historical statistics of the United States, colonial times to 1957. Washington, Government Printing Office, 1960. XII + 789 p. (p. 7)
48. Walsh, J. P. The dental nurse. Am. Col. Dent. J., 32:62-9, Apr. 1965.
49. Young, W. O., and Stearns, Patricia. Current challenges to the philosophy and objectives of dental hygiene education. J. Dent. Educ., 26:222-7, Sept. 1962.

Additional Readings

Public Health Service. Third National Conference on Public Health Training; August 16-18, 1967; Report to the Surgeon General. Washington, Government Printing Office, 1967. V + 112 p.

Public Health Service, National Center for Health Statistics. Health manpower; United States—1965-1967. Washington, Government Printing Office, 1968. IV + 56 p. (p. 26-32)

_____. State licensing of health occupations. Washington, Government Printing Office, 1968. VI + 171 p.

_____. Health resources statistics; health manpower and health facilities, 1968. Washington, Government Printing Office, 1968. VII + 260 p. (p. 59-70)

Report of the National Advisory Commission on Health Manpower. vol. I. Washington, Government Printing Office, 1967. VIII + 95 p.

Simmons, J. H. Summary of the Workshop on Dental Manpower, "Meeting the dental needs in the 1970's." Am. Col. Dent. J., 36:28-33, Jan. 1969.

Section Five

DENTAL HEALTH EDUCATION

CHAPTER 14
Dental Health Education

"Mrs. Kirkpatrick, I want you to do a good job of keeping it clean around that bridge. Be particularly careful around the pontic. We want that tissue tone maintained, and we don't want any recurrent caries around the three quarter on that abutment on the second bicuspid, do we?" asked Dr. Graham, as he was washing his hands following the cementing of a fixed bridge for Mrs. Kirkpatrick. He failed to see Mrs. Kirkpatrick's expressive shrug of the shoulders and interpreted her muffled grunt as acknowledgment that she had understood him. He then moved on to the next operatory and Mrs. Kirkpatrick attempted to puzzle out what he had meant while at the same time biting down hard on multiple cotton rolls as the cement set.

Dr. Graham believes that he has a responsibility to educate his patients about dental health and is confident that he fulfills this function adequately. Since she has only a vague idea of the meaning of words such as "pontic," "tissue tone," and "three quarter," Mrs. Kirkpatrick probably does not feel that she received a clear explanation—to say nothing of being educated or motivated to practice good oral hygiene.

CHAPTER 14

DENTAL HEALTH EDUCATION

There is ample evidence of the need for more effective dental health educational efforts. In a nationwide survey, for example, 60 percent of the respondents felt that ". . . some people are just born with good teeth and others are not—and there is not much anyone can do about it."[17] One fourth of the respondents in another survey were of the opinion that " . . . a toothache does not necessarily require the attention of a dentist since it will often disappear by itself."[1] The actions of patients soon make it clear to most dental and dental hygiene students that the public is not well informed about dental health. Ignorance about dental health and firmly held misconceptions about dentistry will characterize many of the patients that the practitioner will serve after graduation.

Members of the dental profession have unique opportunities for dental health education available to them both in the private office and in the community setting. (The community setting encompasses not just the schools, but also the entire realm of professional groups, official and voluntary agencies, service groups, hospitals, industries, and special community groups such as the chronically ill and aged.) The thesis that the profession does not make full use of its opportunities is supported by a study of the characteristics of dental practices.[18] Less than 60 percent of the dentists interviewed even claimed that education of patients was a routine measure in their offices. Yet other studies indicate that 85 to 95 percent of all dentists surveyed were of the opinion that dentists themselves had the prime responsibility to educate the public in matters of dental health.[1, 18] Nor are dental hygienists apparently doing the job of health education that they could. A survey of practicing dental hygienists showed that almost two thirds stated that they devoted less than 30 percent of their time to instructing patients in correct diet and oral hygiene habits; over one quarter spent only 10 to 19 percent of their time in this activity.[13]

Furthermore, the study of dentists' attitudes indicated that only one quarter of the dentists surveyed took part in school health programs. Of the dentists reporting, 37 percent stated that they had promoted or are promoting projects of fluoridation; but when questioned further, only two percent claimed to have participated in the organization of the fluoridation movement in their communities.

Perhaps others should share the responsibility, too. Most health departments, both state and local, do not have the staff and resources to conduct comprehensive educational efforts, or even to offer assistance to all the other agencies that should be participating. The school provides an excellent setting to teach children about oral health, yet few systems have a formal health educational curriculum which includes suggested teaching approaches and outlines specifically for dental health education. The opportunity for further development of health educational programs in the schools is shown by the fact that more than half of the school principals responding to a questionnaire indicated that they would like help in improving their dental health educational programs.[31]

DENTAL HEALTH EDUCATION DEFINED

What is dental health education? Does it mean an intensive publicity campaign during National Children's Dental Health Week? Or is it an occasional lecture to a high school assembly or the showing of dental health films in the schools?

There are many academic definitions of health education, but perhaps it might be defined simply as *the provision of health information to people in such a way that they apply it in everyday living.* The information can be provided either to the individual on a one-to-one basis or to groups of people in the community setting. Dental health education is only one facet of the total educational stimuli that are constantly being presented to the individual or the community. The important word in this definition is "apply." The measure of effective health education is in the application, the translation of knowledge into action. For instance, 90 percent of a representative sample of the population indicated that a person should go to the dentist regularly.[6] Perhaps many of them would say, at least twice a year. It is known, however, that only about 40 percent of the people get into the dental office in any one year. Certainly members of the dental profession may be expected to recognize the value of regular dental care, but not all dentists seek care routinely. Knowledge is not enough; knowledge must be translated into desirable practices.

The same is true about the dentist's knowledge of health educational practices and methods. Knowing that he should educate his patients does not mean that he does so. Knowing what he wants his patients to understand does not mean that he knows how, when, or where he should provide the information to them. Therefore, it would seem that the primary objective of any dental health educational program is to stimulate and motivate practicing dentists and dental hygienists (and dental assistants) to provide information about dental health to their patients and the community in such a way that it will be translated into desirable patterns of action. Furthermore, the action recommended should be reasonable.

SOME BASIC PRINCIPLES OF HEALTH EDUCATION: CONTRIBUTIONS OF THE SOCIAL SCIENCES*

In order to provide health information in a way that will motivate individuals to apply it in everyday living, it is necessary to understand something about the factors which influence human behavior. What a person will learn and the actions that he will take toward the maintenance of health or the treatment of disease are determined by his attitudes and his motivation. It should be noted that just as a teacher cannot make the student learn, members of the dental health team cannot directly motivate the patient or the community. Motivation, like learning, is a process which involves multiple complex factors. As one social psychologist has pointed out:

> ... we do not and cannot motivate people. No hope, procedure, training program, gimmick or sermon can motivate a human being. Human behavior springs from the energy created by the individual's organism. Our job is to provide or to create an environment that will release this energy.[3]

In order to learn about how the environment that will stimulate individual or group motivation might be created, recent studies by social scientists, which may have provided some insight about the determinants of human behavior, should be examined.

Conditions Leading to Action

There are certain conditions under which individuals may take actions to regain or preserve their health. In the first place, people

---

*Much of the material on the contributions of social science to insights into human health behavior is based on conversations with and the writings of I. M. Rosenstock, Ph.D., Professor of Public Health Administration; D. P. Haefner, Ph.D., and S. S. Kegeles, Ph.D., both Associate Professors of Public Health Administration; and C. A. Metzner, Ph.D., Professor of Medical Care Organization; all of the School of Public Health, The University of Michigan. A selected group of their pertinent publications is included in the references at the end of this chapter.

with obvious symptoms of disease ordinarily will act to regain their health, if, as will be noted later, they feel there is an action that they can take which will be effective. This type of action may be considered to result from high motivation, and little persuasion or education from the outside may be necessary.

More sophisticated knowledge about health and considerable persuasion are required if action is to be taken under the second condition—that apparently well (asymptomatic) people will act to prevent illness. The contrast between these two levels of effort is illustrated by those patients who will seek service from a dentist only when they have a toothache and those who are willing to return regularly for periodic examinations and treatment.

People also may take a health-related action for a nonhealth reason. Some of the most powerful motives for following proper health practices are not related to health at all. Studies on social pressures indicate that groups exert powerful influences on their members to conform to group standards.[5, 15] Koos, for example, found that some mothers sought the services of a pediatrician not because they were convinced that their children needed routine medical supervision but because they wished to conform to the accepted standards of their social group.[14] Probably the initial motivation for learning to brush the teeth, or even to visit the dentist periodically, is not primarily a direct concern about dental health but rather a desire to conform to standards set by the family and friends.

If dentists and dental health educators can find more than one reason for their patients to carry out a certain health action, the chances obviously are increased that the patients will do it. Dentists and dental health educators who merely appeal to the health motive are failing to tap the richness and variety of human motivation and longing. Dental health practices will be taught more effectively if they are related to a variety of factors and not just "health." More effective learning takes place in learning one's culture through the process of socialization. The child who takes a step closer to "civilization," for example, by brushing his teeth regularly, is rewarded with love and affection not only by his parents but also by the members of his family, other adults, playmates, and the school system. Pressures to conform stem from all these sources.

Crucial Factors

In order to take a voluntary preventive health action, the individual or the group must have a readiness and willingness to act. Readiness should imply the physical, social, and emotional capability to act. Factors such as fatigue, for example, may influence or be a barrier to readiness.

In addition to the capability to act, the concepts of reinforcement and continuity are crucial. In the educational process, whether in the private office or in the community, these concepts simply mean that the dental health educator needs to understand what the patient already knows and build from there; and as the dental health educator builds, he or she reinforces—that is, repeats—the communication stimulus in different ways at different times. The educational factors of readiness, continuity, and reinforcement are all interrelated.

Whether or not an individual will act to preserve his health also depends on his judgment of its value in contrast to other things that he wishes to do. Hochbaum has noted, "Health motives present only a very small aspect of the vast and complex motives of man. . . . As often as not, health motives are the weaker ones among such competing motives. . . ."[11] Where there is a conflict of interests, for example, the person must decide that seeking dental care to preserve his teeth is more important to him than purchasing shoes for the children, buying a new TV set, or spending his free time bowling or playing golf. This decision will be conditioned by an assessment of the relative importance of the barriers to seeking care, such as cost, fear, past unpleasant dental experiences, or the difficulty in getting an appointment.

Among the other important factors that help determine an individual's action about health are three crucial—and highly subjective—beliefs: (1) that one is susceptible to a particular disease; (2) that the disease would be severe if it should occur; and (3) that there is an action which can be taken that would be effective in reducing one's susceptibility to the disease or the severity of the disease should it occur.[10, 16, 20, 22]

Because dental caries starts early in life and affects the majority of the population, most individuals probably recognize their susceptibility to this disease. Because of the widespread ignorance about periodontal diseases, however, many individuals may not recognize their susceptibility to the attack of these conditions. Mere recognition that the disease could occur, however, is not likely to motivate action unless the individual feels that such an occurrence would have serious consequences for him. There is some evidence, however, that people without symptoms are more likely to make a voluntary prophylactic visit to the dentist than they are to obtain tests for tuberculosis or cancer on a purely voluntary basis in the absence of symptoms.[9]

The assessment of the seriousness of a disease is related to two factors—the clinical severity of the disease and the possible interference with the things a person wants to do. Most people probably do not view dental diseases as being clinically severe.* Still, they may appear serious to the individual because he dreads expense and feels

---

*Robbins found that 11 percent of the respondents in a survey considered dental diseases "very serious" as compared with 30 percent for tuberculosis; 39 percent, polio; 41 percent, mental illness; 50 percent, heart disease; and 83 percent, cancer.[19]

that regular care will reduce the cost, he might suffer social disapproval from bad breath or unsightly teeth, his income might suffer from unsightly anterior teeth, he fears the loss of part of his body, or he dreads the inconvenience of dentures.

Even if an individual believes that he is susceptible to the disease, and feels that it would have serious consequences for him, he may still neglect to do anything about it. The third crucial belief that determines whether an individual will seek treatment is that he must feel there are actions which can be taken to prevent or alleviate the condition. Of course, the action or cure must not be seen as worse than the disease. If a person believes that dental diseases may be prevented, that the dentist has the skill to control the diseases that do occur, and that it is possible to maintain the natural dentition, he may seek regular preventive care. On the other hand, if the loss of teeth is thought to be inevitable, the person sees no point in seeking other than emergency treatment for the relief of pain and infection. It has been pointed out that more than half of the individuals questioned by the National Opinion Research Center agreed with the statement, "Some people are just born with good teeth and others are not—there is not much anyone can do about it." It is apparent that this failure to recognize the effectiveness of dental services in controlling dental disease is an important deterrent to seeking dental care.

The Role of Mass Media

Dentists sometimes urge their dental society or the American Dental Association to purchase television time "to get dental health education across to the public." The social sciences can answer some of the questions about the strengths and weaknesses of the media of mass communication (such as radio, television, and newpapers) in contrast with personal, face-to-face efforts. Rosenstock has summarized these findings in the form of principles:[21]

> 1. Mass communication methods are more effective in providing information and a favorable background climate than in stimulating behavior. Personal solicitation is a more effective method of obtaining a specific response.[4]
> 2. Groups of differing educational and social status show different patterns of use of the mass media. Even when exposed to the same medium, individuals with different educational backgrounds differ in how much and what kind of material they learn. For example, in a review of studies on response to polio vaccination campaigns, it has been shown that upper educational groups rely on certain mass media to a greater extent than groups of lower education. Moreover, even within the same medium the two groups listen to and learn different things. Groups of high social and educational status tend to obtain more of their health and science information from impersonal communication media, while those of lower social and educational status tend to obtain more of their health information from personal, face-to-face contacts.[23]

3. Communications often flow through a two-phase process. Occasionally communications intended for a target audience do not reach them directly. Rather, the information is received by a middle man who may be called an "influential person" or an "opinion leader" who in turn transmits selected aspects of the message to the ultimate audience. Thus, while health information transferred through the mass media may not reach the target group for whom it is intended, it may reach a group of opinion leaders to whom the target group looks for advice. However, the opinion leader transmits only what he wishes to transmit.[12]

4. A corollary to these points is that *individuals and groups differ in their acceptance of and reliance on various communications* and the degree of acceptance may vary from situation to situation. In studies of the 1957 influenza epidemic, it became clear that the general public relied on newspapers and radio for information about the ... epidemic but they relied on their physicians for *personal* information on the threat to themselves and their families.[24]

5. *The power of mass communication to influence behavior is limited.* ... One would hardly expect unmotivated people to perceive, let alone be influenced by, outside communications, or strongly motivated people to be moved by information that conflicts with their beliefs. ... .[7]

In addition, it should be pointed out that the dental patient is also limited by his ability to read, to hear, and to understand the vocabulary of the dental communication.

Advertising vs. Health Education. Not surprisingly, many dental and dental hygiene students are impressed by the success of advertising in accomplishing its aims through the use of mass communications media. Actually, advertising is not as successful in creating changes in behavior as it may appear. To measure the success of advertising, one must consider the goals of commercial enterprise. Even the largest corporation rarely needs to capture more than five percent of its potential market to show huge profits; often one percent will do. Dentists and dental health educators on the other hand are after an almost impossible goal. They want 100 percent of the people to enjoy the benefits of fluoridation, to visit the dentist regularly, and to achieve optimum dental health. Thus, in dental health, goals are necessarily set much higher than in commercial enterprise.

It is also important to recognize that advertisers frequently deal with motives which people already have — such as the desire for food or pleasure. In this situation, the main requirement for selling is for the advertiser to provide some incentive or appeal for acquiring *his* product rather than his competitor's. Frequently used incentives include free samples, colorful packaging, contests, and other such devices. Dentists and dental health educators, on the other hand, are more frequently dealing with patients or potential patients who may not be motivated, especially if they are not currently suffering from, or are not aware that they have, some dental illness. The problem here is to teach new motives, a task which is more difficult than that of selecting an appropriate incentive or appeal.

Consider the kinds of action consumers are urged to take in commercial advertising in contrast with dental health education. The advertiser normally has it within his power to make the act of purchasing a product simple, convenient, and pleasurable. He may even offer prizes or free samples. The dentist or the dental health educator is faced with a more difficult task of asking people to submit to procedures which are often inconvenient, uncomfortable (if not painful), expensive, and time consuming.

The advertisers' target groups also should be considered. Advertisers can use media which will reach the groups most likely to purchase their product. Ordinarily, a highly advertised product is addressed to a particular audience, frequently, the economically advantaged family, the very group which *does* rely on mass media for its information. Unlike dental health education, advertising rarely directs its campaigns to the total public. Reaching a large heterogeneous group is necessarily more difficult than reaching a small homogeneous group.

In short, one must conclude that advertising has a far more reachable goal than does dental health education—in advertising, even modest success can make fortunes.

To summarize, mass communication methods may be useful in setting a favorable climate for a recommended dental health action. But where a specific dental health *action* is desired, personal, face-to-face communication, even solicitation, is recommended, since it has been found to be effective in stimulating the desired behavior.

The implications for dental health education should be obvious. Each dentist, dental hygienist, and dental assistant should utilize every opportunity in his day-to-day, face-to-face, personal contacts with the public, his friends, and his patients to stimulate interest in dental health and to improve public knowledge.

DENTAL HEALTH EDUCATION IN THE DENTAL OFFICE

Dentists have unique opportunities for dental health education. Most educators and communicators have concluded that education and communication are best conducted on a one-to-one basis at a time when something that is real and has meaning is happening to the person who is being educated. Sandell has stated flatly, "The most effective dental health education can be accomplished in the dental office by dental personnel . . . the dentist in his office has the finest educational opportunity available, if he will but use it."[25] The most powerful, most effective method of influencing people is through face-to-face communication, which may be defined simply as "to talk with someone and to get him to talk back with you." It has been hypothesized that a "Madison Avenue advertising man would forego his luncheon martinis for the chance to 'push a dental product' through the medium of the face-to-face contact which 90,000 dentists have with at least 72,000,000 patients annually. Organized dentistry has something that Madison Avenue cannot buy for any price."[27]

Sandell also has pointed out that the dentist has the knowledge necessary to advise the patient concerning dental health and that he has the skills required to provide the treatment that is needed.[26] But if the patient is reluctant to accept the advice and treatment, there is little that the dentist can do. The dentist's knowledge and his ability to provide dental care of high quality far exceed the public's willingness to accept such treatment.

Interpersonal Relations

The most important factor in determining the effectiveness of patient education is the personality and attitude of the dentist, the dental hygienist, and the dental assistant. Traeger's admonition to physicians is relevant to the dental profession:

> A basic change in the doctor's attitude is necessary.... The doctor must recognize that he lives in a changing world; one in which people don't want to be condescended to; people just don't want to have their disease cured—they want a permanent relationship with their physicians [dentists]; they don't want a "general practitioner"— they want a "personal physician [dentist]."
>
> A doctor must discover a new kind of dignity—not based on pretense. He must cease to be a "medicine man." The patient wants to be allowed to participate.... He doesn't want to be treated as a medical [dental] illiterate. The patient is going to other sources for information only because he is not getting it from doctors. Medical [dental] people ... should disseminate knowledge themselves rather than have others do it.[28]

There are several personal qualities which, if not essential, are at least important to the conduct of patient education. First, the dentist and dental hygienist must have an honest and sincere interest in and concern for the health of their patients. Second, they must understand people and know something about human behavior. Third, if practitioners want to understand other people, they must first understand themselves. A dentist who understands, recognizes, and accepts his own weaknesses, his unfulfilled objectives, his threatened prestige, his hurt pride, his fears of the unknown, and his accumulated tensions is more likely to treat his patients with sympathy, dignity, and respect. For him, patient education should be easy.

Educational efforts involve a two-way relation between the practitioner and his patient and are a part of every dental experience. The educational aspects of treatment procedures can be good or bad, depending on the effect on the patient. In the process of the examination of a new patient, the doctor recommends a prophylaxis and complete radiographic examination. If the patient responds negatively (saying that his last dentist didn't clean his teeth or take x-rays and he thinks it isn't necessary now), the doctor's integrity has been challenged, and he may feel the urge to dismiss the patient. To do so, of course, would not help the situation — or the patient. The preferable course is to explain to the patient, in a friendly manner, the importance of these two procedures and perhaps, if necessary, give him time to think it over. It is well to remember that a patient's understanding of, and his attitude toward, dental health and dental treatment depend largely on his past experience, home environment, education, and sense of values.

In planning treatment, the dentist must be prepared to offer services which, at first glance, may seem to be less than ideal. Ethically and morally, the dentist is obligated to make every effort to relieve pain and infection. If the patient refuses further care, the dentist should attempt to persuade him to seek optimum oral health, but not unreasonably. The patient's goal of personal oral health may be considerably less than the ideal, and the dentist may have to be content at this time to take but one small step toward his own ideal goal. At a later appointment perhaps he can initiate the next step. The dentist's ideal may never be achieved, but if a realistic goal can be attained for that patient, a valuable service will have been rendered.

Changing an individual's attitude toward dentists, dental health, or dental care is not a simple, fast procedure, since these attitudes are a result of many previous associations and experiences. The patient who questions the dentist's advice is not necessarily being difficult or obstinate. Unreasonable as they may appear, his actions probably are based on what he feels is sound judgment; changing them will not occur easily or automatically.

Educational Opportunities

It should be recognized that patient education begins with a person's first contact with the dental office — usually with the receptionist or the dental assistant who answers the telephone. If the assistant answers the phone with a warm, vibrant, pleasant voice (the one the telephone companies call "the voice with a smile"), a favorable climate is achieved at the beginning. If the patient has a question or two over the phone about his dental condition (which probably prompted the call in the first place), the manner and the competence with which the dental assistant answers the questions are important factors. Therefore, the dentist has an obligation to see that his assistant has at least a basic knowledge about dentistry and oral health practices. If it is a question that she cannot answer, she should be willing to obtain the answer from the dentist and call the patient back.

The next contact of the patient with the dental office is usually in the reception room. The timeworn jokes about the ancient, dog-eared copies of the *National Geographic* in dentists' reception rooms unfortunately reflect a condition that still exists. The reception area in the dental office should have attractive, informative, dental health educational materials conveniently displayed. They should be up-to-date, cover a broad range of dental subjects of pertinence to the potential patient, and be kept as pleasant, positive, and reassuring as possible. These publications should not be filled with the unnecessarily realistic details of surgical procedures but should emphasize the positive benefits to be achieved by regular periodic visits to the dentist. Many such attractive brochures are available—primarily through the American Dental Association. However, Sandell adds a word of caution:

> Many dentists feel that, by placing an assortment of pamphlets in the reception room, they have met their responsibility for patient education. Making pamphlets available to patients in the reception room may have some incidental or accidental value. But, pamphlets are most effectively used when they are given to a patient by the dentist (or his auxiliary personnel) to amplify or reinforce what he has already told the patient about his particular problem.[25]

If the dental assistant or receptionist is alert and has noted previously exactly what procedures will be performed for this particular patient, she can be of value in helping to select and suggest appropriate dental health educational materials for the patient who is waiting. If the patient is coming for a first appointment—for examination, diagnosis, and treatment planning—a simple brochure (preferably developed by the dentist or a member of the dental health team) explaining the particular routine in that dental office can be given to the patient or mailed in advance. Ideally, the dental hygienist and dental assistant would be called in at the time of treatment planning or case presentation, so that they can be briefed and a more effective educational program can be planned for the individual patient. Explanations can be given, for example, about the necessity for dental radiographs as a diagnostic aid, the safety of modern dental radiographic procedures, and the office's particular practices regarding routine recall of patients. Or if the patient is a candidate for dentures, the receptionist or assistant can select the proper materials relating to the positive benefits of modern prosthetic appliances. Then, too, if the assistant is alert, she can volunteer to answer any questions the patient might have and explain the procedures which will be followed during the appointment. Many patients are apprehensive about dental procedures even though they appear calm outwardly. It is helpful if the patient can talk out these fears with the dental assistant and be reassured. By adroit questioning, the assistant sometimes can elicit some of these apprehensions and alert the dentist.

Usually, the patient is called directly from the reception room into the operatory. Perhaps the patient first should be called into a private office where the dentist, the patient, and as appropriate, the entire dental health team sit down together around a conference table to discuss the patient's problems, his needs, and the procedures to be employed for him. This initial conference should give the members of the dental health team some insight into how to communicate with the individual patient. One wonders how any member of the dental health team can expect to be a good educator if no time is spent with the patient in an attempt to understand his vocabulary, his perceptions, and what he already knows. One wonders, also, if dentists realize just how threatening they appear in their white operating gowns — sometimes with head lamps and face masks — peering down from on high on the helpless patient seemingly trapped in the dental chair. Even if patients are given the opportunity to talk, it is difficult for many to express themselves freely under these circumstances which dramatically emphasize the dentist's role as an "authority figure."

It seems so obvious, that perhaps it is overlooked, that most dental patients have little opportunity to ventilate their feelings. Ventilation — freely talking out fears, apprehensions, and anxieties — is one of the tools of the medical profession but rarely is made available to the dental patient. All too often the patient is seated in the chair, his mouth (so it seems to the patient) stuffed with cotton rolls and a variety of gadgets and props. If the dentist or hygienist would take but a few minutes to query the patient, allowing him to ventilate and express his fears, and if the treatment procedure to be followed could be explained, time might be saved in the long run and many misunderstandings might be eliminated.

When the dentist talks with a patient, he must remember to do so in a language that can be understood. Dental jargon, such as "buccal," "MOD," and "prophy," is incomprehensible to many patients. A professional person does not create respect for his knowledge by using scientific language when it is not appropriate. In general, the smaller the words and the simpler the terms, the more likely that they will be effective in communication. If technical language must be used, it should be explained carefully. Most patients will appreciate the dentist's courtesy if, before launching into a discussion of periodontal disease, he takes a moment to explain the disease and possibly note that it has sometimes been referred to as "pyorrhea." The health professional can satisfy his own need to appear to be "scientific" by using both the scientific term and the common term — actually "translating" for the patient as he goes. He can avoid "talking down" to the patient by indicating that he assumes the patient already knows both terms. For instance, he might say, "Mrs. Kirkpatrick, as you know, periodontal diseases, commonly called pyorrhea, are diseases of the gums and bones supporting the teeth."

Ordinarily, patient education is directed toward a particular problem in a patient's mouth. If the patient exhibits extensive carious lesions or periodontal disturbances, the cause, measures necessary to correct the problem, and the possible sequelae if these measures are not taken should be discussed, in a general way, with the patient. The average dentist can do much better in this regard if he has a knowledge of the educational tools available and knows how to use them. The American Dental Association has a wide variety of educational material, such as *Teeth, Health and Appearance* and *The Chairside Instructor*, which cover many dental topics and are useful in the reception room as well as in the operatory. In addition, the Association produces a variety of pamphlets for specific purposes such as *X-Rays and Your Teeth*, which explains why radiographs are essential in a complete dental examination and diagnosis, and *They're Your Teeth*, which gives the essential information about periodontal diseases. Obviously, educational materials must be kept in a place convenient to the dentist when he is providing care to a patient or counseling him about his dental problems.

Although the nature of dental treatment procedures usually makes it difficult for patients to "ventilate," it does provide the dentist with an opportunity to talk about dental health with the patient all the while he is operating. Many dentists provide patients with a large hand mirror so they can watch the procedures being performed, and they explain to the patient exactly what is going on step-by-step. For other patients, however, such a procedure is not indicated. Instead, the dentist should use positive suggestion and discuss more pleasant activities, such as hobbies or fishing.

Arnim of the University of Texas has described a program of oral hygiene for the arrestment of dental caries and the control of periodontal diseases which apparently works well in his hands.[2] It is suggested that the serious reader may wish to review this program for ideas which he can adapt to his own practice.

The Role of the Dental Hygienist

Practically everything that has been said about the dentist refers also to the dental hygienist, except that the hygienist has even greater opportunities to provide patient education. In the first place, she rarely is performing a procedure which is uncomfortable to the patient. Second, her professional education should have stressed the technics of patient education. After a thorough discussion with the dentist, and perhaps participating as an observer in treatment-planning sessions and the case presentations for the individual patients, the dental hygienist soon will know the dentist's ways of operating and types of procedures he recommends or performs. The dental hygienist can then develop a planned educational program for each patient. Such a planned educational program should be tailored to the individual needs and interests of the patient and should not only stress toothbrushing, fluoride, restriction of carbohydrates, and regular visits to the dentist, but should also provide for the patient an exposure to the total realm of dentistry and dental procedures. It would seem wise for the dental hygienist to spend a few minutes at the beginning of the day or before each appointment studying the history and treatment plan of her patients. With this information, she should be able to raise pertinent questions regarding previous treatment or conditions and personalize her dental health instruction for the patient. She also would convey to the patient her interest in his particular oral condition.

With her special skills in dental health education, the dental hygienist can help develop individualized teaching materials for the dental practice in which she is employed. Flip charts and other visual aids can be designed by the dental hygienist for use both in her operatory and in the dentist's. She also can help to develop leaflets and other printed materials for the dental office.

The dentist has the ultimate responsibility for the conduct of the practice and must create an atmosphere in his office which is conducive to dental health education, and he must set the example. If the dental hygienist is expected by the dentist to perform a certain number of prophylaxes per day and if she is reimbursed on a percentage basis rather than by salary, it may make it more difficult for her to utilize the patient educational experience which has been an important part of her dental hygiene education.

Evaluation of Dental Health Education in the Private Office

Evaluation of the educational efforts in the private office can be a difficult problem because of the multiple socioeconomic variables that influence patients' behavior. The members of the dental health team can never be sure that their actions have directly caused a patient's change in behavior. For instance, the patient's sudden interest in toothbrushing may not be the result of the educational program in the dental office. Even though it is difficult to ascertain just exactly who or what is responsible for or contributed to a change in behavior, the members of the dental health team still have an important role in evaluation.

The dental behavior of patients can be identified as a continuum — starting with the patient's initial or present behavior at one end and placing optimum dental behavior at the other. The necessity of planning the educational approach becomes apparent, because in order to evaluate it one must determine (1) what is the optimum dental behavior for each individual patient; (2) where the logical starting point for the patient's dental behavior should be; (3) the logical sequence for the respective behaviors leading up to the optimum dental behavior; and, finally, (4) the means that will be used to determine if the behavior has been accomplished. For example, disclosing solution may be an objective indicator of toothbrushing behavior. The purpose of evaluation in dental health education is not to identify who or what caused the changes, but whether the various changes in behavior have occurred which have led to optimum dental behavior.

Patient education is particularly important for the parents of young children, since many will seek for their children advantages that they have not had themselves. Mothers, and fathers too, are concerned about having a better life for their children. Many thoughtful parents include, in that definition of a better life, better dental health for their children. Therefore, it would seem wise to capitalize upon all opportunities to educate parents.

Patient education in the dental office can reach directly only those patients (or their parents) who come into a dental office. Although only about 40 percent of the population visits the dental office at all during a given year, the opportunities to educate this group should not be lost. Those people who visit the dentist are usually the better educated, have a better income, and are frequently the opinion leaders in the community. If dentists and their office personnel use every chance to educate those who do get into the dental office, there is hope that these people will spread the information through their families, through their neighborhoods, through child study groups, and through parent-teacher associations.

DENTAL HEALTH EDUCATION IN THE COMMUNITY

Other Professional Personnel

After establishing an effective program of education in the dental office, including regular in-service education of the entire dental staff, the dentist and dental hygienist should give first priority to reaching the nondental professional people in the community, such as physicians, pharmacists, nurses, teachers, school administrators, social workers, and hospital administrators. Informal contacts with these people present excellent opportunities for dental health education and should not be overlooked.

Formal opportunities to provide dental health education, such as invitations to speak to a group of physicians or nurses, do occur, although less frequently. Dentists and dental hygienists often make one of two mistakes in responding to such requests. They may plunge in and do the job, completely forgetting that the dental or dental hygiene society has a responsibility and therefore should be consulted. On the other hand, they may back off, feeling that participation would be considered "advertising" by their colleagues. The *Principles of Ethics* of the American Dental Association (and usually of local societies) may appear conflicting and confusing in this area but it is actually quite clear. What it says, in effect, is that: (1) dentists have an obligation to share their knowledge with others in those areas where they have special competence; and (2) before making public appearances they should consult with the officers or appropriate committees of their professional society. Dental hygienists might follow the same pattern within their own association and clear any technical subject matters with an advisory committee from the local dental society.

In any event, the dental health education of dentistry's professional colleagues is of high priority. If the opportunities are not available, consideration should be given to judicious ways of creating them. The best chance to increase knowledge about oral health among professional personnel is to reach them while they are still in school — in medical schools, pharmacy schools, schools of nursing, teachers' colleges, and practical nurses' courses. When this task has been accomplished, it is time to attempt to reach other groups.

School Programs

Long-range educational efforts may be more successful in modifying public attitudes than short-term efforts. Today, and probably for many years to come, most dental health problems can be prevented or controlled only by daily, continuous effort by the individual. Prevention of periodontal diseases, for example, depends on a modification of patterns of daily living. This objective, of course, entails a more profound change in attitudes than is needed to benefit from single, infrequently repeated actions such as immunization. Short-term educational approaches which urge people "to do a specific thing now" are useful in attacking some problems, but are inadequate to change dietary patterns, toothbrushing habits, and patterns of visiting the dentist.

In general, patterns of living cannot be taught — at least not in the sense that skills such as arithmetic or reading are taught. Instead they must develop out of the life experience of the individual. But how are they to be developed? One suggestion is to focus long-term educational goals not on the adults of today, but on the adults of subsequent generations — to try to develop in children patterns of life in accord with sound health practices. This approach includes improved dietary practices, periodic visits to the dentist, and learning effective personal hygiene habits. It includes also learning about dental diseases, the impact they have on the person and on the family, and the kind of preventive and remedial actions that are available.

Haefner has stated that, if one is willing to settle for long-range gains rather than a short-term approach, the school setting offers a great potential for effective dental health education.[8] It provides an excellent opportunity for communication with virtually all persons within the entire school-age group and in an explicitly educational context where learning is emphasized and rewarded. Having an entire population as a captive audience in this type of setting is a rare and wonderful occurrence that deserves to be capitalized upon fully. Furthermore, continuing educational influence can be exerted on the target audience over a considerable time period. The process can begin at an early age, when habit patterns are still in the process of being formed rather than having been firmly established and resistant to change, as is true of adults. The school setting also offers the advantage that the dental health educator can use both mass communication and face-to-face communication approaches on the same audience and derive maximum benefit from each. The mass communication approach can be used to present health information efficiently to groups via lectures, motion pictures, books, pamphlets, and in other ways. This approach in turn can be supplemented by face-to-face communication between teacher and students. The face-to-face aspects can provide an opportunity for individualizing instruction to meet the needs and problems of individuals, and can also serve as a powerful motivating force. The school classroom setting also offers the possibility of making use of the powerful forces of group dynamics in inducing students to take appropriate dental health actions.

Rosenstock contends that health teaching cannot be merely didactic.[21] It must be embedded into the socialization process so that rewards for successful learning occur at all levels of society. This objective, of course, means that parents of children must cooperate; it also means that school systems must participate actively instead of relegating dental health efforts to intermittent dental inspections or occasional and sporadic lectures. Modifying health educational programs in the schools poses no theoretical problems, but the practical problems are great.

Working With School Personnel. One needs only to spend a few hours in the office of a busy school superintendent to begin to realize the extent of the practical problems. In today's school system there are all sorts of problems and pressures. Many groups want the school program to include a particular item or to place special emphasis on a certain aspect of the curriculum. Dentistry is only one of the groups with "special interests." Some dental societies have even gone so far as to appoint a delegation to demand that the superintendent arrange to have a certain number of hours of "dental health" taught each week. Educators and school systems are faced also with a tremendous increase in knowledge which must be included in the curriculum, an increase easily demonstrated by comparing a textbook on chemistry or physics of a few years ago with one of today. Then there are the pressures on the superintendent and his curriculum specialist to "get back to teaching the three R's" or the pressures on the school system which have been brought about by developments in the "cold war."

How, then, should a dental society approach a busy school superintendent in an effort to improve dental health education in the schools? Following an axiom of public health that one should start where the people are and with their problems, an effort should be made to ascertain what is going on currently in the school system and to determine the problems faced by the school staff. The dental society should first attempt to meet the most pressing dental problem as seen by the school personnel. Frequently this problem is voiced by a harassed school nurse who sees rampant dental disease in the mouths of the school children with whom she comes in contact, and who wants help in meeting the dental emergencies which occur every day. She wants to know if she can work out some way of getting children in pain cared for or fractured teeth restored. If the dental society can work out a mutually satisfactory solution to these pressing problems of the school staff, then it has moved one step closer to gaining a sympathetic hearing from the school superintendent in regard to demands for more dental health education in the curriculum. A current problem such as the regulation that mouth guards be provided to all athletes engaged in contact sports is an excellent starting place for the dental society to achieve good relations with the school people. If the dental society cooperates in this program, as indeed it should, then another step has been taken toward forwarding its school dental health educational aims.

A similar approach has been suggested by Yoho:

> One fault common to professional groups and their individual members is that of limiting their interest and concern to those activities that have a direct relationship to, and bearing upon, their professional concerns. The educator or the school administrator reacts much as other individuals react and cannot be expected to be really enthusiastic about dental health unless the dentist demonstrates some sincere interest in education. In the school situation, the administrator is concerned about a number of things among which is general health, including dental health. Therefore, it is important that dentistry be actively represented in those situations where school and community health programs are determined. The attitude of the dentist who serves on the school board, the city council, in the state legislature, or is active in other community affairs will influence materially the kind of relationships that are developed between the dental and educational professions.[30]

If the dental profession hopes to utilize educational approaches to accomplish some of the objectives of dental health, those within the profession who are assigned this responsibility are obligated to become fairly sophisticated in educational methods, procedures, policies, and organizations. Dentists should: (1) become acquainted with the methods by which health education is incorporated in the school curriculum, the person or persons responsible for curriculum decisions, general policies, and the legal and moral responsibilities of the school that help determine these policies; (2) develop an understanding of the preparation of teachers in the field of health and how this preparation can be improved through cooperation with teachers' colleges and school systems; and (3) above all, find out what is being done already by the school in dental health education before initiating a new program or suggesting new approaches to the problem.

All too often dentists and dental hygienists may assume that, just because they don't happen to know about it, there is nothing going on in the schools in the way of dental health. Before suggesting a dental program, dentists and dental hygienists should review the courses of studies and teacher guides and should become familiar with the textbooks being used, find out what supplementary dental health instructional material already is being provided schools, and determine what assistance the school needs in order to improve its health educational program. This review should be approached not as if dental professionals were authorities "policing" or "checking" on what is or is not being done, but rather in a friendly, helpful manner of cooperative assistance in attaining a mutual goal—the health of the children. Several standard texts on various aspects of health education in the schools are listed at the end of the chapter under additional readings. They should be helpful to the dentist or dental hygienist acquainting himself with school health education. The approaches suggested here should be appreciated by educators and should be more effective. They probably will be less costly in time, effort, and money.

Direct Classroom Instruction. Dentists and dental hygienists sometimes are invited (or invite themselves) into classrooms to "give a talk on teeth." Health professionals should be cautious in answering requests to participate directly in classroom instruction. Teachers possess skills as unique to their profession as are the skills of the dentist, and they ordinarily are far better equipped to instruct than are dentists and dental hygienists. Teachers have the skills and years of preparation to do the job of direct classroom instruction; they know their children and their vocabulary levels; they know at what point in the school curriculum a project on dental health would be most appropriate. There are only a few occasions when health professionals should participate directly in classroom instruction. These situations would include: (1) when the class has been working on a project on dental health; (2) when the students have questions which the teacher cannot answer; and (3) when the teacher feels that they would benefit from having a guest expert come into the classroom. In such situations, the teacher and the guest expert should work closely together in planning the session. All too frequently, dentists and dental hygienists who go into classrooms do one of two things—they either speak in technical language above the heads of the audience or they underestimate the level of their audience, in some instances even talking "baby talk."

It would seem much better for health professionals to spend their time working with those who in turn will do the teaching. A well-prepared session with an elementary school faculty during a teachers' meeting would be of much more benefit than an isolated "talk" by a health expert to a classroom of elementary children.

There is much that dentists and dental hygienists can do in working with the faculties of the various schools in their communities. They can help prepare educational materials and serve as resource people to the teachers—providing them with information or guiding them to suitable teaching materials. They also can review the content of textbooks for accuracy and for appropriateness to the local situation. In cooperation with the teachers they can offer to make their dental offices available for field trips by a class of children or by a committee of the class who then in turn will report to the class on the experience. Health professionals can participate in science fair activities serving as resource people to the youngsters working on science projects. They can participate in career days and numerous other appropriate activities. But, unless they are adequately prepared teachers themselves, they have no business, except under the conditions mentioned, participating in direct classroom instruction.

Other Community Opportunities

Dentistry has been so concerned with the attempt just to get school-age children into the dental office—let alone reaching younger children—that the important area of educating the parents of the newborn child frequently has been overlooked. One wonders how often a dentist or a dental hygienist has been associated with courses of instruction for expectant parents. Dentists or dental hygienists also could participate in the child health conferences sponsored by health departments. Dentists and dental societies could work closely with the pediatricians and obstetricians or with the public health nurses and nutritionists who participate in well-child conferences. Recommendations concerning fluoridation and topical applications of fluoride could be included in recommended immunization procedures.

At the other extreme are the health problems and developing community programs for the ever increasing number of persons in the older age groups. Dental health education is important for these individuals also. This group, for example, should know about the signs and symptoms of oral cancer and what to do about them.

Between the extremes of youth and old age is the vast group of neglected breadwinners and homemakers. In addition to attempting to reach them as parents through their concern for their children, there remain many unexplored pathways—industrial health programs, farm extension groups, service clubs, and other community activities in which this group already participates. Much remains to be done in the field of dental health education. The opportunities are numerous; they only need to be used to their full potential.

Community Organization

In Chapter Nine, special attention was given to some of the facets of community organization as they related to fluoridation campaigns. The concepts of identifying potential leaders and gaining community support should be of special interest to dentists and dental hygienists, and should not be limited to fluoridation campaigns. As indicated in the foregoing paragraphs, the members of the dental health team may find many programs that have dental implications which would benefit by professional support. Although the members of the dental health team will seldom be solely responsible for organizing a community dental health effort, their active support and assistance in planning and implementing such a program can be invaluable. A key principle to be remembered, regardless of the type of program, is to attempt to develop participation by a broad range of members of the community. If this principle were applied zealously instead of often being ignored, more community programs would have broad community support instead of indifference or a negative reaction on the part of the community. Some basic references on community organization and leadership have been included in the additional readings at the end of this chapter.

Resources Available

Local Resources. Fortunately there are many competent sources to which a dentist or dental society can turn for help in problems of dental health education. Frequently the local dental society itself has a committee on dental health education which has had experience working with the schools and the community. The members of the committee often are quite knowledgeable about the ongoing programs of the school and community in dental health education and the teaching materials that have been developed by the local school system or provided by the dental society. They can often suggest materials that are available to help the individual dentist if he is called upon by a school or community group. Therefore, it would seem wise for the dentist or dental hygienist to turn first to the local dental society's committee on dental health education. If there is no such committee, the practitioner will have to work with officers of his local society and, perhaps, together they may wish to organize one. Most school systems of any size today have available a curriculum director or consultant, usually a person with an advanced degree in education. Such individuals are specialists and know the overall curriculum plan and organization for a total school system. The committee can work with the curriculum director to find out what already is going on in the schools.

The local health department or voluntary agencies may employ health educators who can be of help. Sometimes there is a qualified public health dentist or dental hygienist working for the local health department or school system who may be called upon for consultation.

State Resources. Almost all state dental societies have active committees on dental health education. Some state dental societies have developed informational materials and guides which they will make available to local school systems and other community groups, either for their adoption in toto or to be modified and tailored to suit the local situation. Official state agencies should not be overlooked, either. Often the state health department, even if it does not have an individual trained in dental health education on its staff, has a division of general health education with competent health educators who can provide assistance. The director of the health department's dental division, too, usually is able to provide suggestions from which the local dental society and local school system can select those that are appropriate. The state department of education frequently has a specialist in health education on its staff who works closely with the state health department, its dental division, and its health educators in general programs of health education. This person usually has many years of teaching background and experience and advanced education in health education. He frequently has a well-established liaison with almost every school system in the state. The assistance that such an individual can offer should not be overlooked.

National Resources. If local and state resources are not sufficient, the dentist can turn to the American Dental Association. Several units of the Association can be of help in dental health education. Foremost of these is the Bureau of Dental Health Education which has a staff of health education specialists ready, as their time and budget permit, to assist state and local dental societies with their problems of dental health education. The Bureau of Public Information makes materials available, primarily for the mass media. The Bureau of Audiovisual Service can provide films, film strips, slides, recordings, and other audiovisual aids which, when used judiciously, can be of considerable help. All of the dental health educational materials which are available from the American Dental Association are listed in a catalog of materials which is published annually. Every dentist should know what is available from the Association so that he can apply those he thinks will be valuable immediately to his own practice and stand ready to suggest various materials to community groups and the schools.

The regional dental consultant of the Public Health Service often can provide state and local dental directors with suggested approaches that have worked in other states and regions and can be tailored to fit the local situation. He frequently knows of specialists who may be called upon to help solve particular problems.

Evaluation of Dental Health Education in the Community

Evaluation of educational efforts in the community is similar to the evaluation approach suggested for the private office setting. The emphasis should be placed on planning a logical educational sequence and determining whether the desired behavior—for example, fluoridation—was accomplished. The difficult job of evaluating just who is responsible and which methods were the most successful for achieving the desired behavioral outcome for the community should be left to the controlled investigations of social scientists.

SELECTIVITY IN THE USE OF EDUCATIONAL MATERIALS AND METHODS

Materials available from state and national agencies, as well as those provided by the American Dental Association, must of necessity be of a general nature since they are used in many areas. Therefore, before they are recommended for a particular group in a local community, they should be reviewed to be sure that they are appropriate. Even though they may not be completely appropriate for the particular problem or a particular locality, they still can be used if doubtful points are explained to the group which will be using them and special exception taken. If audiovisual aids (films, especially) are used in teaching, they should be previewed, their showing planned carefully, their appropriateness for the audience checked, their limitations and errors clarified, and the important points of their message emphasized beforehand. Once films have been shown, they should be followed with a planned discussion—perhaps reemphasizing the message or reexplaining their shortcomings.

Warner has pointed to the dangers inherent in the showing of some dental films.[29] The palatable coating which surrounds a dental health fact should not so absorb the child's interest that his mind is distracted from the real issue. Attracting children's interest is sometimes confused with entertaining them. This danger is illustrated by the reaction of a first grader to a dental health film in which the cast consisted of dogs dressed as people. The first grader's awestruck comment after seeing this apparently far more interesting than educational film was, "Did you know that dogs could walk around on their hind legs all the time if they want?"

Some would contend that this misinterpretation could have been avoided if the teacher had prepared the class for the dental health film; that is, if she had used the film as an enrichment to, rather than as a substitute for, her own teaching. This contention may be true, but too liberal mixing of fantasy with fact still is likely to create confusion in the imaginative minds of young children. In contrast, consider the meaningful discussions which can take place in lower-grade classrooms following the showing of a dental health film which effectively combines interest with fact rather than using "walking, talking dogs." This type of film tells its dental health message through pleasant everyday experiences of an average family. Almost any child can relate to the situations depicted without being so carried away by bizarre phenomena that the dental health message is lost.

For use in his own office, each dentist should review the materials available from the American Dental Association and other sources in the light of his own dental practice. If he finds materials acceptable to him, he should go ahead and use them. However, if there are one or two items in these publications with which he does not agree, he still may wish to use the publications but should explain to his patients (and his office personnel) just exactly where he differs with the publications and why. If he finds that the publications for the most part are not suitable for him, it might be better for him not to use them at all. Instead, it would be preferable to develop materials which are tailored individually for his own practice. In this regard, his dental hygienist can be of considerable help. If he has no dental hygienist, it might be wise for him to turn to one of the educational specialists in his local school system or health department to help him in preparing his own materials.

Some dentists have found that "before and after" intraoral photographs (or 2 × 2 slides) of his patients can be used effectively to show other patients what can be done for similar conditions in their mouths. Several commercial companies have developed a series of expensive slide or movie projectors with an accompanying recorded narrative to be placed in reception rooms for patient self-instruction. Some of these impersonal devices appear to be little better than the "canned spiel" of the medicine-show hawker aimed at "selling dentistry" rather than education of the patient.

Unfortunately, many of the dental health educational materials which have been available in the past, and even some available today, contain inaccuracies and misinformation. For this reason, educational materials need to be reviewed carefully for accuracy as well as for appropriateness for the particular audience. Although the dentist is able to check the accuracy of materials for his own use, there are many dental health educational materials of dubious quality available to teachers, health departments, nurses, and others who also are educating the public about dental health. Hence, the importance of working with fellow professionals and offering consultation to them is reemphasized.

All too frequently, dentistry's efforts and expenditures for mass education of the public may have been relatively fruitless. Many competent educators would question the wisdom of some of the projects used during observances of National Children's Dental Health Week—the "smile contest," the poster contest, the essay contest. In spite of conscientious efforts in health education, there are incidents in which well-meaning intentions have produced unexpected and even detrimental outcomes. Warner cites the example of a pretty little girl made unhappy because she was not even considered in the competition for the "best smile contest."[29] She was undergoing orthodontic treatment and the unsightly braces on her teeth ruled her out at first glance. In dental health as in most other aspects of health, all children cannot meet a single, ideal standard. Too many factors which the child, the parents, or even the dentist cannot control determine the dental health status. Esthetics, heredity, the socioeconomic level of the family, and the availability of dental care can be either assets or handicaps to a child's dental health status. Rather than setting a standard goal for children, dental health education should aim toward helping each child achieve his own highest potential for dental health, whatever that may be. It was inconsistent to exclude the little girl from competition in the "best smile contest" because she was wearing orthodontic appliances, since the appliances represented a major effort to reach a higher level of dental health. Educators have recognized the contradictions of health contests for many years. Dental health competition of various types which still are staged are seldom initiated by educators. However, health specialists probably are remiss in not being ready with alternate plans when community groups (and dental societies) propose "best smile contests." In one instance, a local dental society was persuaded to provide mouth guards for all children engaged in contact sports with the funds which originally had been designated for a "king and queen of smiles contest."

The emphasis in current dental health educational materials on the structure and function of the teeth can be questioned, too. This emphasis parallels the outmoded "hygiene" lectures of several generations ago wherein the student was expected to memorize the names of the bones in the body. It would seem that patients, and school children in particular, could be motivated to better dental health habits without having to know technical information about the dentition such as the relation of the dentin to the pulp, or the functions of the incisors or molars. Since there appears to be so little time available for dental health in the presently crowded curriculum, it would appear wiser to be more selective in the dental health teaching that is done.

The responsibility for dental health education—of patients, auxiliary dental personnel, nondental professional health workers, school people, community leaders, parents, and the public—placed upon dentists and dental hygienists is formidable indeed. Dentistry has no voluntary agencies such as the March of Dimes, heart, cancer, or tuberculosis societies, or national health foundations working for it. Yet dentistry has come far in its relatively short professional history. Each dentist and dental hygienist who gives that little extra effort to dental health education will further the dental health of the public and, in so doing, elevate the status of dentistry.

Bibliography

1. American Dental Association, Bureau of Economic Research and Statistics. Family dental survey. I. Dental health concepts. Am. Dent. A. J., 47:575-80, Nov. 1953.
2. Arnim, S. S. An effective program of oral hygiene for the arrestment of dental caries and the control of periodontal disease. South. Calif. S. Dent. A. J., 35:264-80, July 1967.
3. Aronoff, Joel. Contemporary directions in motivational theory. p. 85-111. (In Hutchins, D. W., ed. Motivation in preventive dentistry. Columbia, Mo., University Missouri, c1968. XII + 287 p.)
4. Cartwright, D. P. Some principles of mass persuasion. Human Relations, 2:253-67, July 1949.
5. Festinger, Leon, et al. Theory and experiment in social communications. Ann Arbor, Institute Social Research University Michigan, 1950. 123 p.
6. Freidson, Eliot, and Feldman, J. J. The public looks at dental care. Am. Dent. A. J., 57:325-35, Sept. 1958.
7. Griffith, William, and Knutson, A. L. The role of the mass media in public health. Am. J. Pub. Health, 50:515-23, Apr. 1960.
8. Haefner, D. P. Dental health education. p. 80-94. (In Striffler, D. F., ed. The scope of dental public health; report of a training course in dental public health administration. New York, American Public Health Association, 1964. 193 p.)
9. Haefner, D. P., et al. Preventive actions in dental disease, tuberculosis, and cancer. Pub. Health Rep., 82:451-9, May 1967.
10. Hochbaum, G. M. Public participation in medical screening programs: a sociopsychological study. Washington, Government Printing Office, 1958. 23 p.
11. ———. Some principles of health behavior. p. 7-19. (In Proceedings; 1959 Biennial Conference of the State and Territorial Dental Directors with the Public Health Service and the Children's Bureau. Washington, Government Printing Office, 1959. VII + 62 p.)
12. Katz, Elihu, and Lazarsfeld, P. F. Personal influence; the part played by people in the flow of mass communications. Glencoe, Ill., Free Press, [1955]. XX + 400 p.
13. Kesel, R. G. Dental practice. p. 95-238. (In Hollinshead, B. S., dir. The survey of dentistry; the final report. Washington, American Council Education, c1961. XXXIV + 603 p.)
14. Koos, E. L. The health of Regionville; what the people thought and did about it. New York, Columbia University Press, 1954. XIV + 177 p. (p. 69-71)
15. Lewin, Kurt. Group decision and social change. p. 330-44. (In Newcomb, T. M., and Hartley, E. L., eds. Readings in social psychology. New York, Holt, 1947. 688 p.)
16. Metzner, C. A. Attractions and blocks; the A and B of the utilization of dental service. Am. Dent. A.J., 60:3-8, Jan. 1960.
17. National Opinion Research Center, University of Chicago. Marginal results and basic cross-tabulations; public attitudes and practices in the field of dental care. [Chicago], National Opinion Research Center, 1960. n. p. mimeog.
18. ———. Factors associated with preventive dental practice. Report No. 69. [Chicago], National Opinion Research Center, 1959. IV + 161 p. mimeog. (p. 27-31)
19. Robbins, P. R. Some explorations into the nature of anxieties related to illness. Genetic Psychol. Monogr., 66:91-141, 1st Half, Aug. 1962.
20. Rosenstock, I. M. What research in motivation suggests for public health. Am. J. Pub. Health, 50:295-302, Mar. 1960.
21. ———. Presenting a public health program. Ann Arbor, University Michigan School Public Health, 1962. 34 p. mimeog.
22. ———. Why people use health services. Milbank Mem. Fund Quar., 44:94-124, (part 2) July 1966.
23. Rosenstock, I. M., Derryberry, C. M., and Carriger, B. K. Why people fail to seek poliomyelitis vaccination. Pub. Health Rep., 74:98-103, Feb. 1959.

24. Rosenstock, I. M., et al. The impact of Asian influenza on community life; a study in five cities. Washington, Government Printing Office, 1960. V + 98 p.
25. Sandell, P. J. Technics of dental health education. Mich. S. Dent. A. J., 44:312-4, 317, Nov. 1962.
26. ―――. Effective methods in dental health education. Dent. Clin. No. Am., n. v.: 205-14, Mar. 1961.
27. Striffler, D. F. Dental health education; some essentials for a state dental association's programs. Mich. S. Dent. A.J., 43:323-30, Dec. 1961.
28. Traeger, C. H. Action potentials in health research and practice. p. 3-6. (In National Health Council. 1961 National Health Forum on better communication for better health. New York, National Health Council, 1961. 30 p.)
29. Warner, Elizabeth M. Guidelines to dental health education programs for children. J. School Health, 31:193-8, June 1961.
30. Yoho, Robert. Some views on dental health education. Mich. S. Dent. A. J., 44: 291-4, Oct. 1962.
31. Young, W. O. Dental health. p. 5-94. (In Hollinshead, B. S., dir. The survey of dentistry; the final report. Washington, American Council Education, c1961. XXXIV + 603 p.)

Additional Readings

Adult Education Association. Taking action in the community. Chicago, Adult Education Association, c1955. 48 p.
Birch, David, and Veroff, Joseph. Motivation: a study of action. Belmont, Calif., Brooks/Cole, c1966. IX + 98 p.
Feldman, J. J. The dissemination of health information; a case study in adult learning. Chicago, Aldine, 1966. 274 p.
Fodor, J. T., and Dalis, G. T. Health instruction: theory and application. Philadelphia, Lea and Febiger, 1966. 178 p.
Grout, Ruth E. Health teaching in schools; for teachers in elementary and secondary schools. 5th ed. Philadelphia, Saunders, 1968. XII + 390 p.
Kirscht, J. P., et al. A national study of health beliefs. J. Health and Human Behav., 7:248-54, Winter 1966.
Luft, Joseph. Group processes; an introduction to group dynamics. Palo Alto, National Press, c1963. V + 57 p.
Mayshark, Cyrus, and Shaw, D. D. Administration of school health programs; its theory and practice. St. Louis, Mosby, 1967. XIV + 483 p.
Miller, H. L. Teaching and learning in adult education. New York, MacMillan, c1964. XI + 340 p.
Moss, Bernice R., Southworth, W. H., and Reichert, J. L., eds. Health education; a guide for teachers and a text for teacher education. 5th ed. Washington, National Education Association, 1961. XI + 429 p.
Oberteuffer, Delbert, and Beyer, Mary K. School health education. 4th ed. New York, Harper and Row, c1966. X + 534 p.
Rosnow, R. L., and Robinson, E. J., eds. Experiments in persuasion. New York, Academic Press, 1967. XIX + 519 p.
Ross, M. G., and Lappin, B. W. Community organization; theory, principles, and practice. 2nd ed. New York, Harper and Row, 1967. 290 p.
Schramm, Wilbur, ed. The science of human communication. New York, Basic Books, c1963. VIII + 158 p.
Young, Marjorie A. C. Review of research and studies related to health education practice (1961-1966): what people know, believe, and do about health. Health Education Monographs, No. 23. New York, Society Public Health Educators, 1967. 76 p.
―――. Review of research and studies related to health education communication: methods and materials. Health Education Monographs, No. 25. New York, Society Public Health Educators, 1967. 70 p.
Young, Marjorie A. C., and Simmons, Jeanette J. Review of research and studies related to health education practice (1961-1966); psychosocial and cultural factors related to health education practice. New York, Society Public Health Educators, 1967. 64 p.

Section Six

THE DENTIST, HIS PRACTICE, AND HIS COMMUNITY

CHAPTER 15

The Role of the Dentist and Dental Hygienist in Maintaining the Health of the Community

Graduation is only a month away. In what now seems a surprisingly short time, Mr. Larry Jackson will become Dr. Jackson — dentist — licensed to provide oral health care for the public.

Some six years ago, Larry chose to study dentistry, one of the most important decisions of his life. This decision will affect profoundly the course of the rest of his life.

Once he is licensed to practice dentistry, Larry will be faced with a different but equally important decision: What kind of dentist will he be? Instructors will no longer determine the type of professional standards that must be maintained. In fact, the chances are that there will be few outside checks on his practice.

Actually, the development of a professional career is determined by many decisions, not just one. Each day the dentist will be called upon to decide whether every restoration and procedure will be completed as expertly as possible or just well enough to get by; whether to continue to study and develop or to stagnate; whether to discharge the obligations of a professional man to his community or to abdicate his responsibilities and let others carry the load.

CHAPTER 15

THE ROLE OF THE DENTIST AND DENTAL HYGIENIST IN MAINTAINING THE HEALTH OF THE COMMUNITY

The professional skills of the dentist and the dental hygienist should be of value not only in the clinical practice of dentistry for individual patients, but also in working with groups of individuals toward improving the health of the community. The dental public health skills and technics which are of particular value in community health promotion have been outlined. This chapter will consider the application of this knowledge and these skills in the community in which the dentist will establish his practice.

Although the basic methods for improving dental health are the same in any area, the approach will differ according to local circumstances. In a large metropolitan area the dentist and the dental hygienist will work primarily within the framework of their local professional societies in relations with other organized community agencies. A variety of resources should be available including a well-staffed local health department, active voluntary agencies (such as councils on social welfare and heart and cancer associations), health specialists in the schools, and possibly a dental school. In the smaller community, on the other hand, extensive resources may not be available, but there is an opportunity to work more directly to influence health services rather than having to channel efforts through a variety of organizations. As Hill has pointed out:

> The problem which should confront each young graduate is not whether he has an obligation to the public, but how he can best meet his community responsibility.... A new member of the profession who has been permitted to add certain letters after his name is recognized as belonging to a learned group. He should accept a certain amount of responsibility and leadership in solving civic problems of his community. He should have particular interests in all civic matters related to health and health facilities.... In these and related matters, the public needs guidance and rightfully expects those trained in these fields to provide it.[9]

IN DENTAL PRACTICE

The first obligation of the dentist and the dental hygienist is to conduct a practice that will provide the best service of which they are capable to the public.

Location

In general, the primary consideration for the dental hygienist, once she has decided in which geographic area she wishes to practice, is to find a dental practice in which her skills can be utilized most effectively. For the dentist, however, the location chosen will determine to a large extent the personal satisfaction he derives from practice, the income he will enjoy, and the degree to which he can meet public demand for dental care. Establishing a practice in a metropolitan area already overcrowded with dentists ordinarily is not in the best interests of either the dentist or the public. Similarly, the wisdom of locating in a community too small to utilize the full-time service of a dentist is questionable. There is no arbitrary formula which can be used in selecting a location, but intelligent study of available guides is recommended. The dentist and his family should first determine those aspects of community life which are of greatest personal importance, such as the availability of educational and cultural opportunities or ready access to hunting and fishing. With these priorities established, available sites can be evaluated in terms of the need for dentists and the ability of the community to support additional personnel. Important guides are trends in population growth, income and educational levels, economic stability, and the number and age of dentists presently practicing. This type of information is published by the American Dental Association and frequently also can be obtained from state dental societies, local and state chambers of commerce, and the dental divisions of state health departments.

When a number of possible locations have been selected, the dentist should visit the area to interview representatives of dental supply companies, public health dentists, dental society officials, and business and civic leaders. (The desire of civic officials to have an additional dentist locate in the community may color their analysis of the ability of the community to support an additional dentist.) Frequently the dentist must determine the portion of the population which may be expected to seek dental care in its own community, and the number who probably will go to a larger adjacent trading center. A rough measure of the ability of a community to support a dentist is that an area that can support three active medical practices has sufficient demand for service to support a dentist.

In a community of any size the location within the city may have a significant influence on the rapidity with which a practice will become established. A location near a rapidly expanding suburban area that is not supplied with dentists, for example, is usually more desirable than a downtown location. A number of publications are available to assist in the selection of a location, some of which are listed in the recommended readings.

Auxiliary Personnel

The proper use of auxiliary personnel is an important factor in ensuring an adequate income for the dentist and maximum productivity to serve the public. The key to the effective use of auxiliary personnel is careful planning. The dentist must determine the kind of practice that he wishes to have and the ways in which he can use auxiliary personnel to build and maintain such a practice. Auxiliaries should be employed to compensate for the dentist's weaknesses and complement his strengths. If the dentist tends to be somewhat forgetful, for example, it would be foolish to employ an auxiliary with the same characteristic. The dentist who finds it difficult to meet the public should seek to employ an auxiliary with a warm outgoing personality.

Dental Assistants. If at all possible, the dentist should employ a full-time assistant immediately. As soon as demand is sufficient, a second assistant should be added so that one assistant may serve full time at the chair as the dentist's "second pair of hands."

The functions of dental assistants are not well standardized. Because of the general lack of formal training programs, the proper selection, training, and utilization of dental assistants require careful planning and effort by the dentist. An important tool in the employment of dental assistants is the preparation of a written "job description." It spells out clearly the duties that are to be performed by an assistant, and it suggests the type of training that may be needed following employment. The job description makes it possible for both the dentist and the prospective employee to determine if the individual is the type of person for the job. Recruitment of potential employees should be continued until there are sufficient candidates to make a selection based on the needs of the office. Interviewing potential employees should be done at a time when the dentist will not be interrupted or rushed.

If possible, dental assistants with formal training should be employed. Otherwise, the dentist must provide systematic training following employment of an assistant. This task can be eased by utilizing correspondence courses in dental assisting, a basic text, or evening classes offered through the dental assistants' association or local vocational training agency. Assistants should have a clear understanding of the duties they are to perform, and the dentist should standardize his operating procedures so that his assistants can anticipate his every move.

Dental Hygienists. When the practice has grown to the point that the dentist is booked one month in advance, it has been suggested that he is busy enough to utilize a dental hygienist.[16] (Later, a full- or part-time dental laboratory technician may be utilized if the practice is large and includes a high proportion of prosthetic service.)

By performing the professional duties for which she has been educated and licensed, the hygienist usually can be expected directly to increase the gross income of the practice sufficiently to cover the cost of her employment. She can relieve the dentist of part of the time-consuming but essential duties to allow him to concentrate on more complicated aspects of his practice — all for the mutual benefit of the patient and the practice.

The dentist may find it necessary to conform to local custom regarding the recruitment of a dental hygienist. Although a straight salary is the most common method of payment, many dental hygienists are paid a minimum salary plus a percentage of the receipts from certain procedures (such as oral prophylaxes), and some receive commissions only. In some areas, it is common for dental hygienists to be employed by several dentists, spending only one or two days a week in each office. The custom of remuneration based on a percentage of receipts and employment by more than one dentist appears to discourage the proper utilization of hygienists in dental practice. Under ideal circumstances, a hygienist should devote all of her efforts to one practice, providing a balanced service of patient recall, chairside health education, appropriate preventive measures, and oral prophylaxes. It is the responsibility of the dentist to organize his practice so that the hygienist may work effectively and make her maximum contribution. For example, the hygienist should have an operatory of her own, and duties such as "housekeeping" should be held to a minimum (although all of the office personnel, including the dentist, should be willing to help each other as necessary).

Financing Care

Obviously, the dentist has a personal interest in collecting for the services that he performs. He also has a responsibility to his patients to make payment for dental care as easy as possible. The most common method for the payment of dental care has been, and probably will continue to be, a cash transaction—either immediate payment or a billing at the end of the month. The dentist also may utilize a personal note form to finance care for patients considered good credit risks who do not have sufficient funds to meet the cost of a large bill at the time of treatment. For this type of patient, the dentist may feel fortunate if he can utilize a budget-payment plan sponsored by his dental society. To obtain maximum benefit, however, he must learn how to use the plan properly. Whenever possible a budget-payment plan should be made available for routine conservative care for entire families and not limited to financing major prosthetic reconstruction. In areas in which the group purchase of care is administered by dental service corporations or similar agencies, problems of collections will be eased for that part of the practice covered by the plan.

The dentist and his staff can do much to simplify the payment for care by organizing the office so that patients receive a careful explanation of the care to be provided, are given a clear idea of the cost, and are presented with alternative methods of payment, and perhaps alternative methods of treatment, for example, by phasing the treatment over a period of time. The dentist is a figure of authority in his own office. The dentist has the responsibility, therefore, to initiate the discussion of finances in a helpful, sympathetic manner that recognizes the possible unvoiced fears and misgivings of the patient.

The responsibility to provide treatment for indigent families is primarily that of the community, not the dentist. The obligation of the dentist is to provide the leadership to ensure that community facilities for the indigent are available. Also, it would seem that a member of a health profession is obligated to provide relief of pain and infection in an emergency regardless of the possibility of payment, although neither the *Principles of Ethics* nor rulings by the Judicial Council of the American Dental Association clearly spell out the responsibility of the dentist in this field.[15] Over the years, many dentists, as a public service, have given freely of their time to provide treatment to the less fortunate members of the community. Commendable as such efforts by individual dentists may be, they do not fulfill the full responsibility of the profession. In this regard, Hill has said, "This does not mean that the profession should provide free dental service to the indigent, but, inasmuch as the oral health care of the community can be provided only by those so licensed, they should provide leadership in finding ways for such service."[9]

Continuing Education

"Every dentist has the obligation of keeping his knowledge and skills freshened by continuing education through all of his professional life."[15] Graduation from professional school is but the first step in professional dental education, not its termination. The bare minimum accomplishment for all dentists and dental hygienists should be regular attendance at the scientific session of their local and state professional associations and the systematic reading of dental periodicals. The "study club" mechanism is one of the most valuable methods of maintaining professional skills and well might be utilized more widely. In addition, every dentist and hygienist should plan to enroll periodically in postgraduate refresher classes sponsored by dental schools or professional societies. Both the dentist's practice and his personal finances should be arranged to encourage regular attendance by himself and his dental hygienist at such courses.

Preventive Services

If the dentist is to render the highest caliber of professional service to his patients, his practice must be organized to utilize all available preventive procedures. These include the operation of a recall system, provisions for adequate patient education, the use of topical applications of fluoride, recommendations for dietary fluoride supplementation routinely where indicated, routine oral prophylaxes, treatment of incipient periodontal disturbances, judicious use of radiographic procedures, and proper sterilization technics. Emphasis on patient education helps to ensure that patients will accept these services. The dentist also should attempt to establish fees which include reasonable remuneration for preventive services.

A dentist should explore the resources that are available to strengthen the preventive and educational aspects of his practice. The state or local health department or the dental school in his area can inform him where to obtain caries activity tests, determinations of the fluoride content of home water supplies, and biopsy services. He also will wish to obtain listings of audiovisual aids and printed material which may be rented or purchased from the American Dental Association or obtained from state and local health departments.

WORKING WITH OTHERS

The American Dental Association* and the American Dental Hygienists' Association

The new dentist and dental hygienist are indebted to past members of their professional societies for standards of modern dental education, prestige enjoyed by dentistry, and development of knowl-

---

*It should be noted that there is another national dental group—the National Dental Association. The National Dental Association was founded in 1913 to provide an organization through which Negro dentists could improve themselves and better serve their patients, because for most of these men it was not possible to join the local and state societies of the American Dental Association. Through the growing cooperation between the American Dental Association and the National Dental Association over the years, particularly through the formation of the liaison committee between the two

edge and skill on which modern dental practice is based. The organizational structure of the dental and dental hygiene professions is essentially the same — the major differences relate to the much smaller number of dental hygienists.

The basic membership unit of organized dentistry is the local or component dental society which usually covers a city or district. A dentist, locating in a community, can contact the secretary of the local dental society about membership. Membership in the component dental society automatically makes a dentist a member of his state constituent dental society and the American Dental Association. (Members of the uniformed services and dental students may join the American Dental Association directly.)

The local dental society provides an opportunity for close professional association with fellow dentists. The scientific programs of the component society are the most convenient method of keeping abreast of new developments in the profession. The work of the committees and business meetings is concerned primarily with problems of immediate local importance, such as how to improve the teaching of dental health in the local school, how to promote a fluoridation program, or the best ways of working cooperatively with the Office of Economic Opportunity's local Community Action Program relating to dental care for Headstart children. Any question of local, state, or national significance may be raised for discussion at the local level. If it be of state or national significance, the expression of opinion of the local society can be transmitted to the state dental society and, if appropriate, to the American Dental Association.

A variety of other important functions may be handled either on the local or state level, depending on the relative size of dental societies. A number of societies, for example, maintain active committees to work with law enforcement agencies and the state board of dental examiners to help ensure that the dental practice act is administered properly. These activities protect the public against illegal and unethical practitioners and, by so doing, protect the privileges of those who conduct conscientious, ethical practices. An additional service of many local and some state dental societies is the operation of budget-payment plans. Some societies also have insurance plans for their members. Among the group insurance plans offered for the dentist are health and accident, life, group hospitalization, professional liability, and fire and theft insurance.

Associations, real progress in the elimination of restrictive racial clauses in the various constitutions of the American Dental Association's constituent and component societies has been made.[17] Indeed, one of the leaders of the National Dental Association has stated, "The fight for equality of opportunity to participate in and join the American Dental Association is largely won, and the mechanism for dealing with discrimination by local or state dental societies is now available. . . . Surely, we must remain vigilant, and organized, and be ever careful that no Negro is denied equal opportunity in the profession and its organized activities. But this must be done within the mainstream and not from the outside looking in, as essentially we are doing now."[8]

State dental associations are governed by their members, either directly through an annual meeting or through a representative governing body named by the local dental societies. The primary function of state dental societies is to deal with problems that can be served best at the state level. As local dental societies deal with local organizations such as health departments, boards of education, and county welfare agencies, so do state dental associations play an important function in dealing with state agencies. Since the legal basis for dental practice is established by legislation at the state level, one of the important responsibilities of a state dental association is to represent the dentists of the state in relations with the state legislature. With a few exceptions, the annual scientific sessions are larger and more comprehensive than those sponsored by local dental societies. State societies also frequently sponsor other types of continuing education such as postgraduate courses, touring seminars, and workshops. Most state groups publish journals, bulletins, or newsletters.

In many ways, the functions of the American Dental Association at the national level parallel the services carried out by component and constituent dental societies. The *Journal of the American Dental Association*, one of several scientific journals published by the Association, is the basic scientific publication serving the entire profession. A wide variety of services is made available by the Bureaus of Audiovisual Service, Data Processing Services, Dental Health Education, Economic Research and Statistics, Library and Indexing Service, and Public Information. The 17 councils of the Association study problems within their frame of reference and make recommendations to the Board of Trustees and the House of Delegates. Besides participating in the development of standards and policies, the councils provide national leadership for the profession. The Council on Dental Education, for example, studies ways of ensuring that the professional education of dentists, dental hygienists, and auxiliary personnel is of the highest possible caliber and recommends policies for adoption by the Association. In addition, this council has the responsibility for accrediting professional schools and internship and residency programs; maintains a program of aptitude testing to aid in the selection of dental and dental hygiene students; and directs a recruitment program to acquaint young people with the advantages of a career in dentistry.

The other councils are Dental Care Programs, Dental Health, Dental Materials and Devices, Dental Research, Dental Therapeutics, Dental Laboratory Relations, Federal Dental Services, Hospital Dental Service, Insurance, International Relations, Journalism, Judicial, Legislation, National Board of Dental Examiners, Relief, and Scientific Session.

The governing body of the American Dental Association is a House of Delegates composed of more than 400 elected representatives of the 52 constituent state and territorial dental societies. The

House of Delegates establishes the overall policy of organized dentistry and elects the Board of Trustees and the officers of the Association. The Board of Trustees is the instrument of the House of Delegates which supervises the administration of Association activities and serves as the governing body between the annual meetings of the House of Delegates. The constituent state associations are organized into 14 trustee districts of roughly comparable membership size, and a member of the Board of Trustees is selected from each district.

The Association has over 100,000 members. In an organization of this size, representative procedures for government are necessary. The affairs of the Association are conducted in such a manner, however, that any member may be heard on an issue through appropriate channels. A resolution calling for the establishment of a new policy or a change in an existing policy ordinarily should follow the following procedure: discussion and adoption by the local dental society and transmittal to the state dental association; discussion and adoption by the state dental association and transmittal to the American Dental Association; review by the Board of Trustees for study, recommendation, and transmittal to the House of Delegates; assignment of the resolution to a reference committee; open hearings by the reference committee at which any member of the Association can express his views; transmittal to the House of Delegates with the recommendations of the reference committee; and last, final action by the House of Delegates, which may be acceptance, rejection, or modification of the original resolution and the reference committee recommendations.

Whereas dental service corporations have been established only at the state level to date, there is a National Association of Dental Service Plans which was established in 1965 under the directive of the House of Delegates of the American Dental Association and became operative in January 1966.[13] It is the national coordinating agency for the nation's voluntary, nonprofit, state-dental-society-sponsored dental service plans. Its purpose is to increase the availability of dental services to the public by encouraging the expansion of dental prepayment programs administered through dental-society-approved service plans and to assist in the development of multistate and national group coverage. In 1968 the first multistate dental service program was coordinated by the National Association of Dental Service Plans for the Northwest International Association of Machinists' Benefit Trust of Seattle, Washington.[4] In 1969, the NADSP adopted the name "Delta Dental Plans" and a triangular symbol to represent professionally sponsored dental prepayment programs.

Health Departments

Most dentists and dental hygienists will practice in communities served by some type of local health department. The range of services provided, however, will vary from comprehensive programs in large metropolitan areas to minimum services in small district, county, or city offices containing no more than perhaps a sanitarian, a public health nurse, and a clerk. In those areas in which there is no local health department, minimum health protective services are provided by state health department personnel.

Regardless of its size, the local health department is the community agency primarily concerned with the protection and promotion of the health of the population. One of the first services of health departments, and still one of the most fundamental, was the protection of the public against hazards of the environment by ensuring a pure water supply, safe supplies of food and milk, and adequate disposal of excreta and other wastes. In recent years, the traditional problems of environmental sanitation have become more complex because of the development of new hazards such as air pollution and dislocations caused by suburban development.

Public health laboratory personnel provide the diagnostic services necessary to aid in maintaining a safe environment and in controlling and preventing disease outbreaks. Epidemics of serious communicable diseases are rare today because physicians, nurses, and epidemiologists exercise constant epidemiological surveillance. The registration of births, deaths, birth defects, and causes of illness and death provide guidelines vital in the planning of programs. The health of mothers and children traditionally has been a prime concern to public health agencies. The health department works with the medical and dental professions, hospitals, schools, and other community agencies to ensure adequate prenatal care of mothers, medical care at the time of delivery, optimum health supervision of the infant and preschool child, and school health services designed to protect the health of children and to teach habits of healthful living. The public health nurse plays a vital role in all public health activities — serving as a liaison between home, school, and community. The most important role of the public health nurse is that of a teacher and counselor, whether she is working with the classroom teacher in the school, participating in immunization clinics, conducting classes in child care, or visiting a home to demonstrate proper methods of child care or of managing the sick.

The dentist and hygienist also will find that the local health department is an invaluable resource in dental health activities. Even if the department does not have dental health personnel on its staff, it has much to offer. The public health nurse, for example, has many opportunities to influence community attitudes toward dental health in her work with mothers and children, with parent groups, and with school personnel. The engineer and sanitarian are invaluable allies in any effort to fluoridate a community water supply. The health officer can provide liaison with the local medical society to encourage support for dental projects. He, also, should take an active part in any program for community water fluoridation.

Larger health departments should attempt to employ dental personnel and operate regular dental health programs. In some communities, a dental hygienist may be employed to serve as a consultant in dental health within the department and to schools and interested community agencies. Other health departments may be able to employ both a public health dentist and a supporting staff of dental hygienists.

The health department must have sufficient financial support to be able to maintain basic health services if it is to be expected to initiate a dental program. If the dentists in a community can help in obtaining a budget sufficient to employ both an adequate nursing staff and a dental hygienist, for example, the establishment of a dental program will be easier. The members of the dental profession, also, have an obligation to participate in the planning of dental programs, in the establishment of policies, and in working to ensure that salaries are adequate to employ competent dental personnel. This type of counsel usually is provided through an advisory committee selected from members of the local dental society.

The resources of the local health department are reinforced by the staff and programs of the state health department, including divisions of dental health in all states except Alaska.

Other Agencies

Schools not only have a responsibility for the health education of school-age children, but they also provide a mechanism through which a major share of children can be reached easily and economically. Health programs for school-age children include three essential elements: (1) maintenance of a school environment which will protect the health of children, facilitate their emotional adjustment, and be conducive to learning; (2) instruction in health which will provide both essential information and motivate children to follow proper health practices; and (3) provision of health services such as medical and dental supervision to ensure the early detection and correction of illness and disability. Many administrators feel that the function of a school should be limited to the protection of the environment and health instruction. In some school systems, however, health appraisal and treatment programs are carried out directly. In order to work effectively in the community the dentist must determine local philosophy and tradition regarding the scope of services provided by the school system.

Departments of public welfare usually attempt at least to ensure a minimum level of economic support for that segment of the population which has an income inadequate for the necessities of life. The types of aid granted and the administrative mechanisms utilized vary widely throughout the United States. In some areas the state department of public assistance will provide casework services, financial determinations, and direct aid on the local level for all needy families. In other areas, the state agencies deal only with certain categories of the needy, and general assistance is the responsibility of city or county welfare departments. The degree of responsibility that will be assumed by welfare agencies for the provision of dental care to the indigent will depend upon Medicaid. A few state departments of public welfare have programs to finance care for indigent children. In other areas, care of indigent children is handled by health departments or other community agencies, including voluntary organizations. In each community will be found a variety of clubs and associations with an interest in dental health. Parent-teacher groups often play a key role in the organization and promotion of community health programs. They also provide one of the best opportunities to reach parents.

Other professional workers in the health field, particularly physicians and nurses, influence public attitudes toward dental care. Close liaison, therefore, should be maintained with the professional associations in related health fields.

Hospitals

Hospitals, important health resources in any community, provide significant opportunities for the dentist. Unfortunately, the dental profession has not capitalized on the opportunities in this area. An editorial in *Hospitals* summarized the problem:

> ... the most striking example of professional insularity today [is] the practice of dentistry. Some holes have been made in the traditional fabric of the solo practice of dentistry but, by and large, the dentist practices as an individual in the four walls of his office ... he is not integrated into the hospital, the institution which represents centricity in our society in the delivery of health care.
>
> Fault lies on both sides. The dentist too often looks at the mouth as if there were no man. In the hospital, too often is the man looked at as if there were no mouth.[12]

The nature of hospital dental services varies widely. On one extreme will be found complete hospital dental departments offering a broad range of surgical, restorative, and diagnostic services for both inpatients and outpatients. Other hospitals maintain only inpatient oral surgical services. In small hospitals, dental services often are nonexistent or limited to some types of staff membership for dentists and the occasional admittance of a patient requiring general anesthesia or hospital management for dental service.

Regardless of the type of the hospital service, dentists should recognize both the opportunity and obligation to participate fully in hospital affairs by applying for staff privileges. The dentist should attend staff meetings regularly and expect to function as an equal member of the health team. Such participation can improve relations between physicians and dentists. Also, many dentists' wives will find volunteer service in the hospital auxiliaries a rewarding activity. The dentist should interest himself in the total concerns of the hospital, including such seemingly mundane problems as balancing the budget and raising funds for expansion. Hospital privileges should be earned by the dental profession through the acceptance of responsibility for hospital services in the community. The dentist should acquaint himself with hospital regulations and procedures and with recommended hospital operative technics. If this type of training has not been received in dental school, it is incumbent upon the local dental society to organize courses for this purpose.

The Federal Services

Other available resources are the programs of the federal services: the U.S. Air Force, Army, Navy, Public Health Service, and the Veterans' Administration. Dental, dental hygienists', and dental assistants' societies often can turn to a nearby federal installation for assistance in the development of community dental health programs. Most federal services—whether military bases, V.A. hospitals, or area offices of the Division of Indian Health of the Public Health Service, for example—emphasize the importance of good community relations and stand ready to help worthy programs in their area with manpower, material, and facilities, and most place a high priority on preventive dentistry activities.

For the dentist about to go into federal service, an acquaintance with the preventive dentistry programs of the various services is important. Frequently the recent dental graduate entering the service is named "preventive dentistry officer" at his station or post. All too often he does not know quite what this assignment entails—in fact, he finds it hard to verbalize a concept of "preventive dentistry." It is suggested that he read some of the recent articles[1-3, 5, 7, 10, 14] published on preventive dentistry in the federal services, search out the latest preventive dentistry manuals and directives for his branch of the service, and reread Chapter Nine and 14 in this book. He should consider the assignment an opportunity to learn about various approaches to preventive dentistry and to improve his clinical skills and efficiency. Also, most of the services provide opportunities for their officers to enroll in various formal and informal courses of study offered either by the service itself or by outside educational institutions. Hopefully, he should be able to carry over the appropriate technics and philosophy to his own practice when he leaves the service—if he decides not to make a career in the service.

PRIORITIES FOR COMMUNITY EFFORT

The dentist who conducts a modern dental practice and who is active in community affairs will participate in many different kinds of activities to enhance the health of his community. In order of relative priority, these efforts will be directed toward: (1) maximum use of preventive procedures; (2) provision of the highest quality of dental service to the most people; (3) the promotion of the total health of the community in which the dentist lives; and (4) the organization and support of specific efforts to improve *oral* health. From time to time during his years of practice the dentist should expect to be involved, to varying degrees, in these activities.

As the dentist and dental hygienist participate in the life of their community, they may serve on planning committees and participate in community surveys. It is within this context that they work to identify the major *dental* health problems of the community, investigate the resources available to solve these problems, and participate with others in developing a community attack on the dental health problem.

The first step in studying dental health problems is to review the activities of official and voluntary agencies to determine the dental health activities now being carried out. It is unwise to assume that there are none. A dental public health program should be adequately staffed, financed, and tailored to fit the needs and resources of its locale. It should be planned to (1) apply community methods for the prevention of dental diseases; (2) carry out effective education in dental health through the schools and the community organizations; and (3) attempt to ensure that all members of the community receive dental care.

Prevention

The first priority of any community dental health program should be to ensure that the community water supply contains an optimum amount of fluorides. The second objective should be to provide topical applications of fluoride (or fluorides through other means) for all children who cannot use a fluoridated water supply. Experience to date indicates that relatively few children will receive benefits of topically applied fluorides unless organized community programs provide these on a mass basis.[6]

Dental Health Education

Schools. The first priority in any school health education program should be assigned to enhancing the knowledge of the teacher and providing aids which will improve her effectiveness in the classroom. A great deal of health teaching, including dental health, is taking place in the schools. The effectiveness of this teaching, however, may be improved through the guidance and counsel of the practicing dentist, the dental society, and the public health worker. The teacher is a professional in the field of instruction just as the dentist is a professional in the provision of health care. The average dentist is no better qualified to attempt classroom instruction in a grade school than is the teacher qualified to restore teeth. The dentist can perform a valuable function by participating in workshops and in-service training for teachers to give them the technical dental information needed for effective teaching. The teacher should have available the tools and materials needed for effective teaching—perhaps provided by the dental health education committee of the local dental society. Textbooks, curriculum guides, and audiovisual aids should be reviewed to be sure that their dental content is accurate. The materials available in the school frequently need to be supplemented by teachers' guides, audiovisual aids, and other materials.

Other important aspects of school health activities are the policies and practices of the school system itself. For example, permitting the sale of soft drinks and confections in the school building largely negates any teaching directed against indulgence in between-meal snacks. Dentists should cooperate with school systems in the observance of special events in accordance with the overall philosophy and objectives of the school. A school system that has an active year-round dental health education program, for example, may prefer not to participate in special events for National Children's Dental Health Week on the valid grounds that to do so would interfere with, not strengthen, the regular dental health activities. If so, the dental society should direct its efforts to areas of the community not receiving any regular dental health education. Career days, student guidance programs, and science fairs provide valuable opportunities to recruit students for dentistry, dental hygiene, and dental assisting.

Community. Regardless of their field of specialization, professional health workers tend to be seen by the public as experts in all fields, and their advice frequently is sought and followed. Furthermore, individuals such as physicians, nurses, dental hygienists, dental assistants, laboratory technicians, and physical and occupational therapists have many opportunities to teach about dental health in the course of their regular activities. For this reason, every opportunity should be utilized to communicate to fellow health workers accurate and current information about dentistry—and one of the best opportunities is preservice education of health professionals.

The staff of the health department has many opportunities to improve peoples' attitudes toward dental health in the course of routine activities such as well-child conferences, prenatal clinics, and future parents' classes. A primary difficulty in conducting general dental health educational programs is that of reaching any large segment of people. Voluntary health agencies and civic groups provide an opportunity to reach a certain segment of the population with relatively effective person-to-person teaching. Groups which should not be overlooked are labor unions, granges, home demonstration clubs, service clubs, Future Farmers and 4-H groups, and fraternal organizations. Although there are great limitations in the effectiveness of mass media (such as radio and television), they should be utilized whenever possible, but not relied upon entirely. The strength of these media lies in their ability to impart information or to sensitize individuals to accept more intensive education. They are weak in their ability to motivate action.

Treatment

The ultimate objective of the dental profession, and of any dental health program, is to ensure that every individual receives complete treatment and that the natural teeth are maintained throughout life in a healthy mouth. A more realistic immediate objective, although still somewhat visionary, is to see that every child in the community receives treatment regularly from the time the primary teeth have come into the mouth until the child is old enough to assume the responsibility for his own care.

The most valuable device for promoting regular dental care among school children probably is the use of a referral card system operated as part of the school health program. The distribution of the referral card can be utilized as an opportunity for concurrent educational activities in the classroom, as a mechanism for distributing health educational materials, as a means of encouraging parents to seek care from their own family dentist, and as a rough screening device to identify children whose families cannot afford to purchase dental care. Good results for the expenditure of effort can be expected from those families who can obtain dental care for their children if sufficiently motivated. But such a program is not feasible unless there are facilities for treatment, including facilities for treatment of children from indigent families and children with special health problems, and should not be recommended unless someone is responsible for follow-up, such as the school nurse, public health nurse, or the school dental hygienist. If necessary, programs to motivate or to provide dental care for the school-age population can be instituted on an incremental basis, thus limiting the initial drain on the manpower resources.

THE PROFESSIONAL OBLIGATIONS OF THE DENTIST AND DENTAL HYGIENIST

Lyons, noting the unique status of health professionals in the community, points out that they are sometimes referred to as "professional gentlemen [or gentlewomen]":

> How may one define or describe a professional gentleman? He may be described as a gentle man who professes certain things. He professes that he is educated beyond the general level of his community. He professes that he has special knowledge and skills. He professes his dedication to the public's welfare over his own. He professes that he gives more than he receives, willingly and by design. He professes his indebtedness to his predecessors from whom he inherited the knowledge, the skills, and the tradition of his

profession. He professes that he, in turn, will enrich and further endow the profession in which he enjoys membership.

The professional gentleman professes these attributes and the public accepts his professions in full faith. This faith of the public compounds the responsibilities of the professional gentleman. He holds a public trust within himself.

The obligations of the young dentist just entering the profession are deeply rooted in these attributes of a professional gentleman, in the definition of a profession, and in the American tradition of dentistry as a healing art. They involve not only fulfillment of duty and responsibility to the public but also preservation of professional status and self.[11]

Bibliography

1. Bernier, J. L. The preventive dentistry program of the Army Dental Corps. J. Dent. Educ., 28:31-6, Mar. 1964.
2. Bernier, J. L., and Sumnicht, R. W. The emergence of preventive dental practice in the U.S. Army. Military Med., 131:520-4, June 1966.
3. Bishop, E. M. A report on the Veterans Administration Office of Dentistry. Am. Dent. A. J., 70:977-84, Apr. 1965.
4. Dental service plans sign first multistate program. Am. Dent. A. J., 76:249, Feb. 1968.
5. Elwell, K. R. USAF preventive dentistry program—its first decade. Am. Dent. A. J., 66:711-7, May 1963.
6. Galagan, D. J. A public health dentist looks at topical fluorides today. J. Dent. Child., 26:164-72, 3rd Quar. 1959.
7. Grossman, F. D. Practical approaches to large-scale stannous fluoride applications. Am. Col. Dent. J., 35:58-64, Jan. 1968.
8. Henry, J. L. Where do we go from here? Nat. Dent. A. Bul., 26:5-9, Oct. 1967.
9. Hill, T. J. The obligation of the dentist to his community. Am. Dent. A. J., 60:327-9, Mar. 1960.
10. Howard, R. L. Army motivation study. Am. Col. Dent. J., 35:65-73, Jan. 1968.
11. Lyons, Harry. Obligations of the new dentist to society, to his profession, and to his fellow dentists. Am. Dent. A. J., 64:46-9, Jan. 1962.
12. Man and mouth. Edit. Hospitals, 34:37, Jan. 16, 1960.
13. National Association of Dental Service Plans. What is the National Association of Dental Service Plans? Chicago, National Association Dental Service Plans, n.d. n.p.
14. Preventive dentistry at United States Naval Academy. Am. J. Orthodont., 53:458-61, June 1967.
15. Principles of ethics with official advisory opinions as revised June, 1967. Am. Dent. A. J., 76:678-84, Sept. 1967.
16. Stearns, Patricia A. Incorporating a dental hygienist in a private dental office. N. Mex. Dent. J., 7:9-12, Aug. 1956.
17. Wallace, J. C., Jr. The National Dental Association and its contribution to American dentistry. Nat. Dent. A. Bul., 24:43-8, Jan. 1966.

Additional Readings

Bureau of Economic Research and Statistics, American Dental Association. Distribution of dentists in the United States by state, region, district and county. Chicago, American Dental Association. (Published annually.)

Campbell, R. H. The dental hygienist in private practice. Dubuque, Iowa, Brown, c1964. XIV + 130 p. (p. 55-65)

Facts about states for the dentist seeking a location. Chicago, American Dental Association. (Published annually.)

Hollander, L. N. Modern dental practice: concepts and procedures. Philadelphia, Saunders, 1967. XVII + 197 p.

Stinaff, R. K. Dental practice administration. 3rd ed. St. Louis, Mosby, 1968. XVI + 214 p.

INDEX

Adenocarcinoma, 136
Adults, chronically ill, dental care for, 251
  institutionalized, dental care for, 252
Advertising, in health education, 301-302
American Dental Association
  dental health education and, 316
  dentist and, 330-333
  health program of, for children, 261-263
  policies on dental prepayment plans, 218-219
  services of, 332
American Dental Hygienists' Association, 330
Assistant, dental, 148, 149, 281-282, 327
Auxiliary personnel
  experimental studies with, 284-286
  future role of, 283-289
  use of, 279-289, 327-328

Buccal cancer, 135

Cancer, oral, 134-138
Carbohydrates, fermentable, restriction of, and dental caries, 177-178
Caries, dental, 89-119. See also *Dental caries.*
Chi square, 66
Classroom instruction, in dental health, 313-314
Cleft lip, 139, 249
Cleft palate, 139, 249
Clinical trial, 57-60
Community
  dental health education and, 315

Community (*Continued*)
  dental health in, 309-317
  dental programs in, 337-340
    dental hygienist and, 325-341
    dentist and, 325-341
  fluoridation in, 338
  preventive dental programs in, 151-178

Dean, H. Trendley, dental fluorosis studies by, 39
def index, 49
Defects, enamel, 138-139
Delta Dental plans, 225, 333
Dental assistant, 148, 149
  use of, 281-282, 327
Dental care programs, public, 236-263
  1700 to 1935, 239-242
  1935 to 1965, 242-253
  1965 and future, 253-255
  federal, 243-244
  future of, 259-261
  history of, 237-239
  state and local, 244-253
Dental caries
  antibiotics and, 113
  dextrans and, 112-113
  dietary control of, 116-117
  dietary supplements and, 112
  epidemiology of, 73-78
  fermentable carbohydrates restriction and, 177-178
  fluoride and, 78
  indices of, 46-50
  nutrition and, 114-117
  nutritional deficiencies and, 77
  prevention and control of, 89-119
  sugar and, 75, 115-116
  vaccine for inhibition of, 113
Dental epidemiology, 35-60

343

344 INDEX

Dental health education, 149-150, 295-320
 definition of, 296-297
 dental hygienist and, 307-308
 in community, 309-317, 338-340
  evaluation of, 317
  professional personnel and, 309-310
 in dental office, 302-309
  evaluation of, 308-309
 in schools, 310-314, 338
 materials and methods for, 317-320
 opportunities for, 304-307
Dental hygienist, 149, 328
 and community health, 325-341
 in dental health education, 307-308
 in public health, 17-31
 professional obligations of, 340-341
 use of, 279-280
Dental insurance, 211-216
 commercial, 227-228
 cost-control and, 216
 demand for, 211-212
 fee schedules and, 215
 indemnity and service plans, 214
 independent nonprofit, 227
 leadership and, 212-213
 selection of risks in, 213-214
Dental laboratory technicians, use of, 282-283
Dental payment plans
 American Dental Association policies on, 218-219
 budget, 210-211
 delta, 225, 333
 history of, 217-221
 merits of, 228-231
 organization of, 221-228
 postpayment, 210-211
 prepayment, 211-233
 utilization of, 232-233
Dental practice
 closed-panel group, 223-224
 location of, 326-327
 management of, 149
 open-panel group, 222
 preventive, 143-150, 330
  characteristics of, 143-145
  development of, 145-150
Dental profession, society and, 5-6
Dental programs, community, 337-340
Dental public health, 18-25
Dental service corporation, 224-225
Dental specialists, 272-274
Dental surveys, in preventive programs, 152-154
Dental treatment
 attitudes toward, 198-202
 availability of, 202-203
 demand for, 193-205
  future levels of, 203-205
  increase in, 275-276

Dental treatment *(Continued)*
  demand for, increasing productivity and, 278-279
  increasing supply of dentists and, 277
  knowledge and, 197-198
  past experience and, 202
  reducing dental needs and, 276-277
 financing of, 208-233, 328-329. See also *Dental payment plans.*
 for children, 186-188
  handicapped, 248-251
 for school children, cost of, 188-189
 in community, 340
 in public health, evaluation of, 15
  financing of, 14
 incremental, 192-193
 initial, need for, 185
 maintenance, need for, 185-186
 need for, 183-193
  among adults, 190-192
 utilization of, 194-197
Dentifrices, fluorides in, 109-112
Dentist(s)
 American Dental Association and, 330-333
 and hospitals, 336-337
 and public health, 8-9, 17-31
 community health and, 325-341
 distribution of, 268-272
 federal services and, 337
 further education of, 329-330
 future need for, 274-276
 in fluoridation campaign, 163-168
 in specialties, 272-274
 interpersonal relations and, 303-304
 professional obligations of, 340-341
 supply of, 266-274
  trends in, 266-268
Diagnosis, of dental disorders, 11-12
DMF index, 46

Education, in dental health, 295-320. See also *Dental health education.*
Enamel defects, 138-139
Epidemiology
 dental, 35-60
  indices in, 44-57
 of dental caries, 73-78
 of periodontal diseases, 78-84
 research in, limitations of, 68-69
 statistics in, 63-68
Examination, dental, 10-11

F ratio, 65
Federal dental programs, public health dentist in, 24-25

INDEX

Federal services, dentist and, 337
Fees, for dental services, 147
Fluoridation, 78, 90-105, 154-169
  campaign for, 157-158
  dentist and, 163-168
  efficacy of, 98-105
  in community, 338
  of salt, 106-107
  opponents of, 158-161
  referendum on, 165-168
Fluoride(s)
  and dental caries, 105-112
  as dietary supplement, 171
  in dentifrices, 109-112
  physiology and metabolism of, 91-98
  topical application of, 107-109, 169-171
Fluoride tablets, 106
Fluorosis, 138

GB, 55
GI, 51
Gingival Bone Count, 55
Gingival Index, 51
Gingival-Periodontal Index, 53
Gingivitis, 126-127
GPI, 53
Group practice, closed-panel, 223-224
  open-panel, 222

Handicapped children, dental care for, 248-251
Health, public, 8-16. See also *Public health.*
Health agencies, 335-336
Health centers, neighborhood, 257, 259
Health departments, 255-259
  local, funding of, 256
Health education, basic principles of, 297-302
  dental, 149-150, 295-320. See also *Dental health education.*
Health service corporation, 228
Health workers, in community, 339
  in fluoridation campaign, 157-158
HLD index, 56
Hospitals, dentist and, 336-337
Hygienist, dental, 149, 328. See also *Dental hygienist.*

Indigents, dental care for, 248
Insurance, dental, 211-216. See also *Dental insurance.*
Interdepartmental Committee on Nutrition for National Defense (ICNND), 75

Jaws, malignant tumors of, 136

Kerr-Mills bill, 254

Labor unions, health programs of, 216-217
Laboratory technicians, use of, 282-283
Leukoplakia, 135
Lip, carcinoma of, predisposing factors in, 138
Literature, scientific, evaluation of, 69-71
Local dental programs, public health dentist in, 24

Malalignment Index, 56
Mass media, in health education, 300-302
McKay, Frederick S., dental fluorosis studies by, 37-39
Mean, arithmetic, 64
Medicaid, 254
Medicare, 253
Mouth protectors, 176-177

National Association of Dental Service Plans, 225, 333
Newburgh-Kingston study, of fluoridation, 96-97
Nutrition, and dental caries, 114-117

Office of Economic Opportunity (O.E.O.), 257
OFI, 56
OHI-S, 53
Oral cancer, 134-138

Payment plans, for dental care, 210-233
PDI, 52
PDR, 55
Periodontal disease
  age and, 79-82
  chronic destructive, 127-134
  control of, 129-134
  diet and, 82-84
  epidemiology of, 78-84
  indices of, 50
  social factors and, 82
Periodontal Disease Rate, 55
Periodontal Index (PI), 51

INDEX

PMA index, 51
"Poor Laws," 239
Population growth, and need for dentists, 274-275
Probability (P), 65
Public dental care programs, 236-263. See also *Dental care programs, public.*
Public health, 8-16
  analysis and, 11-12
  definition of, 8
  dental, as specialty, 18-25. See also *Public health dentist.*
  history of, 18-20
  dental hygienist and, 17-31
  dentist and, 8-9, 17-31
  survey in, 11
  treatment and, 13-15
Public health dental hygienist
  background of, 25-26
  education of, 26-27
  functions of, 27-28
  qualifications of, 28-31
Public health dentist
  background of, 20-21
  functions of, 22-24
  in federal dental programs, 24-25
  in local dental programs, 24
  in state dental programs, 24
  qualifications of, 28-31
Public welfare, 254-255
  health and, 335

Ramfjord Periodontal Disease Index, 52
Recall system, 148
Referendum, on fluoridation, 165-168
Referral programs, for control of dental diseases, 172-176

Schools, dental health education in, 310-314, 338
  health programs of, 335
School children, dental inspection of, 172-174
Screening, for detection of dental disease, 172-174
Simplified Oral Hygiene Index, 53
Specialists, dental, 272-274
Squamous cell carcinoma, 135, 136
Standard deviation, 64
State, and dental health education, 316
State dental programs, public health dentist in, 24
Surveys, dental, in preventive programs, 152-154

t test, 65
Teeth, DMF, 46
Trial, clinical, 57-60

Welfare, public, 254-255, 335